Handbook for
PRINCIPLES AND PRACTICE OF GYNECOLOGIC ONCOLOGY

SECOND EDITION

Handbook for
PRINCIPLES AND PRACTICE OF GYNECOLOGIC ONCOLOGY

EDITION 2

EDITORS

■ Douglas A. Levine, MD
Associate Attending Surgeon
Gynecology Service, Department of Surgery
Memorial Sloan Kettering Cancer Center
New York, New York

■ Don S. Dizon, MD, FACP
Clinical Co-Director, Gynecologic Oncology
Director, Oncology Sexual Health Clinic
Massachusetts General Hospital Cancer Center
Harvard Medical School
Boston, Massachusetts

■ Catheryn M. Yashar, MD
Professor, Department of Radiation Medicine and Applied Sciences
University of California—San Diego
Moores Cancer Center
La Jolla, California

■ Richard R. Barakat, MD, FACOG, FACS
Deputy Physician-in-Chief
Regional Care Network and MSK Cancer Alliance
Ronald O. Perelman Chair in Gynecologic Surgery
Memorial Sloan Kettering Cancer Center
New York, New York

■ Andrew Berchuck, MD
Director, Division of Gynecologic Oncology
Department of Obstetrics and Gynecology
Director, Gynecologic Cancer Program
Duke Cancer Institute
Duke University Medical Center
Durham, North Carolina

■ Maurie Markman, MD
Senior Vice President for Clinical Affairs
National Director of Medical Oncology
Cancer Treatment Centers of America
Philadelphia, Pennsylvania

■ Marcus E. Randall, MD, FACR, FASTRO
Professor and Chair, Department of Radiation Medicine
Markey Foundation Endowed Chair
University of Kentucky
Chief, Ambulatory Services
UK HealthCare
Lexington, Kentucky

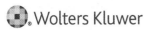
. Wolters Kluwer

Philadelphia · Baltimore · New York · London
Buenos Aires · Hong Kong · Sydney · Tokyo

Acquisitions Editor: Julie Goolsby
Senior Product Development Editor: Emilie Moyer
Editorial Assistant: Brian Convery
Marketing Manager: Stephanie Kindlick
Production Project Manager: David Saltzberg
Design Coordinator: Stephen Druding
Manufacturing Coordinator: Beth Welsh
Prepress Vendor: SPi Global

2nd Edition

Library of Congress Cataloging-in-Publication Data
Handbook for principles and practice of gynecologic oncology / editors, Douglas A. Levine [and 6 others]. — 2nd edition.
    p. ; cm.
    Abridgement of: Principles and practice of gynecologic oncology. 6th ed. / edited by Richard R. Barakat ... [et al.]. c2013.
    Includes bibliographical references and index.
    ISBN 978-1-4963-0642-5 (alk. paper)
    I. Levine, Douglas A., editor. II. Principles and practice of gynecologic oncology. Abridgement of (work):
    [DNLM: 1. Genital Neoplasms, Female.   WP 145]
    RC280.G5
    616.99'465—dc23
                                                                            2014044272

This book is dedicated to all those who care for our patients on the wards and in the operating rooms, and to our families who support us.

CONTRIBUTORS

Jose Alejandro Rauh-Hain, MD
Clinical Fellow, Gynecologic
  Oncology
Massachusetts General Hospital
Harvard Medical School
Boston, Massachusetts

Joyce N. Barlin, MD
Assistant Professor
Department of Obstetrics and
  Gynecology
Albany Medical College, Albany
  Medical Center
Attending Physician
Women's Cancer Care Associates
Albany, New York

Rachel M. Clark Sisodia, MD
Instructor
Department of Obstetrics,
  Gynecology, and Reproductive
  Biology
Harvard Medical School
Attending Physician
Division of Gynecologic Oncology
Department of Obstetrics and
  Gynecology
Massachusetts General Hospital
Boston, Massachusetts

Don S. Dizon, MD, FACP
Clinical Co-Director, Gynecologic
  Oncology
Director, Oncology Sexual Health
  Clinic
Massachusetts General Hospital
  Cancer Center
Harvard Medical School
Boston, Massachusetts

Tracilyn R. Hall, MD
Clinical Fellow in Obstetrics and
  Gynecology
Division of Gynecologic Oncology
Massachusetts General Hospital,
  Harvard School of Medicine
Boston, Massachusetts

Douglas A. Levine, MD
Associate Attending Surgeon
Gynecology Service, Department of
  Surgery
Memorial Sloan Kettering Cancer
  Center
New York, New York

Sharon M. Lu, MD
Resident Physician
Department of Radiation
  Oncology
Kaiser Permanente Southern
  California
Los Angeles, California

Samith Sandadi, MD, MSc
Gynecologic Oncologist
Florida Gynecologic Oncology
Fort Myers, Florida

Catheryn M. Yashar, MD
Professor, Department of Radiation
Medicine and Applied Sciences
University of California—
  San Diego
Moores Cancer Center
La Jolla, California

PREFACE

Medicine is a field in continual evolution, and gynecologic oncology is no exception. Indeed, the field is constantly changing as new data are published that further our understanding and treatment approaches to these cancers. As a result, we have created the PPGO Handbook as a complement to its parent textbook, *Principles and Practice of Gynecologic Oncology*, sixth edition. We have designed this handbook with an eye toward students, residents, nurses, and anyone new to gynecologic oncology who needs to rapidly acquire basic familiarity with the field, a summary of newer developments that have taken place since publication of the textbook, and who desire such critical information all in one place.

The PPGO Handbook has been shortened from the key chapters in the parent textbook, with an emphasis on introductory and summary information. It is organized by chapter, with each of the major cancer sites covered. In addition, we cover the basics of oncology practice to get the reader oriented not only to the field of gynecologic oncology but to the practice of cancer medicine. To help our readers, we have highlighted key points from each chapter to ensure that the most important information stands out, and incorporate treatment algorithms where appropriate. Finally, a few suggested articles for reading are listed with each chapter, and more extensive references can be found in the parent textbook. When desired, trainees can move easily from chapters in this handbook to the comprehensive chapters in the larger textbook for greater detail.

Several of the chapters in this new edition were coauthored by gynecologic oncology and radiation oncology fellows, and we extend our thanks to them for their contributions. As trainees, they lend an invaluable perspective on the information that fellows want to see in a clinical handbook.

We hope this handbook will meet its goals as a convenient introduction to a field that is exciting and changing rapidly—and one which we hope they will find as rewarding as we have.

ACKNOWLEDGMENTS

First and foremost, we thank the authors of *Principles and Practice of Gynecologic Oncology*, sixth edition, from whose excellent chapters the current handbook chapters in large part are derived. We also thank the gynecologic oncology and radiation oncology fellows who helped create new content and ensure that we are addressing those areas of most importance and interest. We are also grateful to Emilie Moyer, Senior Product Development Editor, and Julie Goolsby, Acquisitions Editor, of Wolters Kluwer, for their expert oversight and guidance throughout the development of this edition. We thank the staff of the Gynecology Surgery Academic Office at Memorial Sloan Kettering Cancer Center who were extensively involved with this project—Jennifer Grady, Alexandra MacDonald, and George Monemvasitis. Finally, we would like to acknowledge the work of the late Jonathan W. Pine, Jr. In his time as Senior Executive Editor at Wolters Kluwer, Jonathan was a driving force behind the PPGO Handbook project and several editions of the PPGO parent textbook. We are forever grateful for his enthusiasm and guidance.

Douglas A. Levine, MD
Don S. Dizon, MD
Catheryn M. Yashar, MD
Richard R. Barakat, MD
Andrew Berchuck, MD
Maurie Markman, MD
Marcus E. Randall, MD

CONTENTS

CHAPTER 1

Principles of Chemotherapy in Gynecologic Cancer

INTRODUCTION

> **KEY POINTS**
> ■ The principles of modern chemotherapy require a working knowledge of growth characteristics of normal and tumor tissues.

Tumor Biology

The rationale to explain the impact of chemotherapy rests on our ability to exploit differences in the growth kinetics of normal versus malignant cells. In addition, differences in the kinetics of these tissues also explain many of the toxicities associated with treatment. Three normal cell populations can be distinguished based on growth patterns. *Static cells* are well differentiated and rarely undergo cellular division. *Expanding cells* retain the capacity to grow but are normally quiescent in their adult state. *Renewing cells* exist in a continuous proliferative state with cell division balanced by terminal differentiation. Of these, renewing cells are the most susceptible to treatment-related toxicities, including alopecia, mucositis, and bone marrow suppression.

Among mechanisms governing cellular regulation, apoptosis has emerged as a major mechanism for regulating growth and development of tissues and the susceptibility of tumors to treatment. For example, overexpression of functional *bcl-2* and nonfunctional *p53* genes is associated with chemotherapy resistance.

Gompertzian Growth of Tumors

The exponential enlargement of tumors has been characterized in a pattern termed gompertzian growth. This describes a pattern of exponential growth during initial cell divisions that slows as the tumor grows. The importance of this pattern is to recognize that exponential growth is not strictly maintained throughout a tumor's history. Other potentially important implications of gompertzian growth include the following: (i) metastatic spread may occur even before detection of the primary lesion and (ii) at later stages, a small number of doublings may be required to produce a marked change in tumor size.

Host–Tumor Interactions

Tumor growth is dependent on the manipulation of host factors, including angiogenic pathways that represent their access points to nutrients and oxygen. Growth generally does not rely upon the induction of host lymphatics, but rather through the induction of a disordered capillary network composed of leaky vessels. The net result is regional hypoxia and necrosis, which, practically speaking, may limit the effective delivery of chemotherapy.

The Cell Cycle

Another important aspect to understand is the cell cycle. Cells can remain in a postmitotic compartment (G_0) for an extended period of time; at this point, the cell is not cycling, though it is capable of reentering the cell cycle when triggered by growth factors.

Cell cycling begins at the G_1 checkpoint, which is associated with diverse cellular processes including protein and RNA synthesis and DNA repair. After passing G_1, cells enter the synthetic phase (S). This phase is marked by replication, when a complete copy of cellular DNA is created. Cells then enter the G_2 checkpoint, allowing another control point prior to entering active mitosis (M) consisting of prophase, metaphase, anaphase, and telophase. After separation into two daughter cells, the postmitotic checkpoint (G_3) is reached, at which point cells can further differentiate, stop cycling, or divide once more.

Most chemotherapeutic agents disrupt this process by inhibiting or interfering with DNA, RNA, or protein synthesis. In addition, rapidly proliferating cells are characterized by a short G_1 checkpoint and are also the more sensitive cells to chemotherapy's effects. Cell cycle–specific agents commonly used in gynecologic cancers include antifolates (G_1, S), doxorubicin (S), platinum compounds (G_1, G_2, S), taxanes (M), and bevacizumab (G_0, G_1, S, G_2).

PHARMACOLOGIC PRINCIPLES OF CHEMOTHERAPY

KEY POINTS

- The route of administration depends on many factors that are drug specific (solubility, requirements for activation) and patient specific (feasibility, tolerability).
- The maximal effectiveness of an agent depends on optimizing the area under the time concentration curve (AUC) at critical tumor sites.
- The inactivation and excretion of chemotherapeutic agents occur primarily by the liver, kidneys, and body tissues, with lesser elimination through the stool.
- It is critical that the concomitant administration of other drugs be understood due to the potential of drug–drug interactions that may increase the risk of more serious toxicities or less effective therapy.

Absorption, Distribution, and Transport

Drugs may be given orally, intravenously, intramuscularly, intra-arterially, or intraperitoneally. The selection of the most appropriate route is dependent on drug solubility, the requirements for drug activation, tolerance levels of local tissue, individual patient feasibility (usually based on values and preferences), and the optimal tumor drug exposure. Ultimately, maximal effectiveness depends on optimizing the area under the concentration time curve (AUC) at critical tumor sites.

The increasing utilization of oral chemotherapy and the development of oral molecular-targeted agents have renewed interest in bioavailability in the setting of meals and other factors that can modulate local intestinal transport. For example, the bioavailability of one tyrosine kinase inhibitor was increased over threefold in the setting of a high-fat meal. Another interesting association concerns grapefruit juice, which can alter absorption through the intestinal mucosa by inhibiting the cytochrome P450 isozyme, cytochrome P450 (CYP)-3A4, and possibly the drug efflux pump, P-glycoprotein. Drugs that are substrates for either of these compounds can be more efficiently absorbed after the ingestion of grapefruit juice due to reduced local metabolism, leading to increased serum levels.

The extent of drug binding to serum proteins may have an impact on tumor drug exposure. Many chemotherapeutic agents are lipophilic and highly protein bound in plasma, particularly to albumin. It is generally the unbound "free" drug that mediates toxicity, and any condition associated with variability in protein binding can have an impact on cumulative drug exposure. For example, the toxicity of chemotherapy is frequently accentuated in patients with poor nutritional status, which is associated with reduced protein levels.

Intraperitoneal Chemotherapy

Intracavitary chemotherapy has been used for tumors confined to the peritoneum, pleura, or pericardium. The rationale for this approach is based on the fact that clearance from a body cavity is delayed compared to clearance from the systemic circulation, resulting in a more prolonged exposure to higher regional concentrations of active agents. However, penetration of peritoneal tumor nodules by passive diffusion is limited by fibrotic adhesions, tumor encapsulations, and high interstitial pressures as a consequence of intratumoral capillary leak without functional lymphatic drainage. Therefore, it has been postulated that the major role for intracavitary chemotherapy administration would be in patients with minimal residual disease.

Cisplatin is well absorbed from the peritoneum into the bloodstream and has received the greatest attention for intraperitoneal delivery in ovarian cancer, achieving a laparotomy-confirmed response rate of greater than 32%. In view of the risk of systemic toxicity from cisplatin, there has been renewed interest in the use of intraperitoneal carboplatin, which differs in terms of protein binding and overall time required for activation.

In contrast to cisplatin, paclitaxel is poorly absorbed from the peritoneal compartment, suggesting that patients might benefit from combined intravenous and intraperitoneal administration to optimize tumor drug exposure. As a single agent, intraperitoneal paclitaxel demonstrated a 61% pathology-confirmed complete response rate among 28 assessable patients with initial microscopic disease. However, only 1 of 31 patients (3%) with greater than microscopic disease achieved a complete response.

Some agents, such as cyclophosphamide and ifosfamide, are prodrugs and must undergo irreversible metabolism to the active form, most commonly in the liver. For these agents, intraperitoneal administration would be ineffective, as it would achieve high local concentrations of the native compound, but without an opportunity for bioconversion.

Renal Excretion

The inactivation and excretion of chemotherapeutic agents occur primarily by the liver, kidneys, and body tissues, with lesser elimination through the stool. Table 1.1 lists drugs that require modification in the setting of renal or hepatic dysfunction.

Acute or chronic renal insufficiency is common in gynecologic cancer patients due to tumor-mediated obstruction, drug-induced toxicity, or advanced age. The incidence of moderate renal insufficiency dramatically increases with advanced age. For example, in the 60- to 69-year age group, over one third of women have an estimated glomerular filtration rate (GFR) of less than 60 mL/min/1.73 m^2 (Fig. 1.1). In addition, serum creatinine levels can be inappropriately low as a consequence of reduced muscle mass, malnutrition, or alterations in fluid balance, and any of the standard formulae will overestimate GFR. This has potential clinical consequences for drugs such as carboplatin, where dosing is based on renal clearance.

Several methods are available to estimate GFR (Table 1.2). All of these formulae are based on stable normalized biologic parameters and are less useful in the setting of dynamic changes following acute renal injury or nonrenal fluctuations in serum creatinine and fluid status, such as those that might occur in the postoperative setting or in the presence of large-volume ascites or in patients with abnormal muscle mass. While urine collection for the measurement of creatinine clearance might be thought to provide a better estimate of GFR, it is also subject to great variability in clinical practice. The use of ^{51}Cr-ethylenediamine tetraacetic acid clearance remains the standard for the measurement of GFR, but it is rarely used in clinical practice due to the cost and complexity associated with radioisotopes.

Metabolism and Pharmacogenomics

With the expanded knowledge of metabolic pathways and awareness of polymorphisms in key enzymes, it is sometimes possible to identify individuals with a dramatic increased risk of toxicity. For example, dihydropyrimidine dehydrogenase (DPD) controls the rate-limiting step in fluoropyrimidine metabolism, and approximately 10 variant DPD alleles can occur with sufficient frequency to merit consideration of screening, as patients with less active DPD can be at risk for life-threatening mucosal injury and bone marrow suppression after receiving a single standard dose of 5-fluorouracil. While methods are available for screening, current assays can be expensive, and the potential reduction in risk needs to be balanced against the costs of a widespread screening program.

Uridine diphosphoglucuronosyl transferase 1A1 (UGT1A1) is responsible for the glucuronidation of bilirubin and a number of drug metabolites, most notably SN-38, the major active metabolite of irinotecan. Patients with a deficiency in UGT1A1 are at increased risk for life-threatening diarrhea and bone marrow suppression after receiving irinotecan. While the UGT1A1*28 promoter mutation has been studied most extensively, mutations in the coding region can also occur, particularly in Asian populations,

Table 1.1 Modifications in the Setting of Renal and Hepatic Dysfunction

Agents That Should Be Considered for Modification in the Presence of Moderate to Severe Renal Dysfunction	Agents That Generally Do Not Require Modification in the Presence of Moderate Renal Dysfunction	Agents That Should Be Considered for Modification in the Presence of Hepatic Dysfunction
Actinomycin D	Anastrozole	Docetaxel
Bleomycin	Bevacizumab	Doxorubicin
Capecitabine	Cetuximab	Epirubicin
Carboplatin	Docetaxel	Mitoxantrone
Cisplatin[a]	Doxorubicin	NAB-paclitaxel
Cyclophosphamide	Epirubicin	Paclitaxel
Etoposide	Erlotinib	PEG-liposomal doxorubicin
Ifosfamide	Fluorouracil	Vinblastine
Irinotecan	Gefitinib	Vincristine
Methotrexate	Gemcitabine	Vinorelbine
Topotecan	Letrozole	
	Leucovorin	
	Leuprorelin	
	Megestrol	
	NAB-paclitaxel	
	Paclitaxel	
	Oxaliplatin	
	PEG-liposomal doxorubicin	
	Tamoxifen	
	Trastuzumab	
	Vinblastine	
	Vincristine	
	Vinorelbine	

[a]Can be administered at full doses in anephric patients receiving hemodialysis.

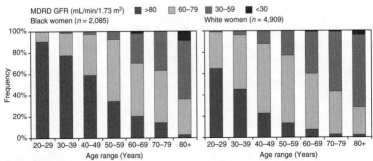

FIGURE 1.1   Distribution of renal function in nondiabetic adults. Weighted distribution of predicted GFR (mL/min/1.73 m²) based on the MDRD formula from the Third National Health and Nutrition Examination Survey (NHANES III). *Source:* Adapted from Clase CM, Garg AX, Kiberd BA. Prevalence of low glomerular filtration rate in nondiabetic Americans: Third National Health and Nutrition Examination Survey (NHANES III). *J Am Soc Nephrol.* 2002;13:1338–1339, with permission.

Table 1.2	Commonly Utilized Formulae to Estimate Creatinine Clearance (CRCL, mL/min)	
Formula Name	Formula
Cockcroft–Gault	$(140 - \text{age}) \times \text{weight (kg)} \times (0.85$ if female$)$/serum Cr (mg/dL) $\times 72$
Jelliffe	$\{98 - [0.8 \times (\text{age} - 20)]\} \times (0.9$ if female$)$/serum Cr (mg/dL)
MDRD for GFR [mL/min/1.73 m²]	$170 \times [\text{serum Cr (mg/dL)}]^{-0.999} \times (\text{age})^{-0.176} \times (0.762$ if female$) \times (1.180$ if African American$) \times [\text{SUN (mg/dL)}]^{-0.170} \times [\text{Alb (g/dL)}]^{+0.318}$

Alb, serum albumin concentration; BSA, body surface area; Cr, creatinine; GFR, glomerular filtration rate; MDRD formula, the Modification of Diet in Renal Disease study equation; SUN, serum urea nitrogen concentration.

and may predict for efficacy in addition to toxicity. Gilbert syndrome is associated with a mild unconjugated hyperbilirubinemia and reduced activity of UGT1A1 that is also associated with an increased risk of toxicity in both homozygous and heterozygous patients.

Drug Interactions

During routine care, patients may receive a variety of drugs, including antiemetics, antihistamines (H1 and H2), steroids, nonsteroidal anti-inflammatory agents, anticoagulants, narcotics, and anti-infective agents. Particular attention should be placed on drugs that could alter renal function, such as aminoglycoside antibiotics, nonsteroidal anti-inflammatory agents, and diuretics in patients with reduced fluid intake.

Increased attention has been focused on drug metabolism and potential interactions at the level of CYP isozymes, particularly CYP-3A4, which is potentially linked to the metabolism of nearly half of all pharmaceutical agents. Drugs that are *substrates* for the same isozyme may competitively inhibit metabolism, but these interactions are usually not of clinical consequence. Drugs that *directly inhibit* CYP isozymes without being a substrate for that isozyme are more likely to have clinical consequences. These include itraconazole, ketoconazole, fluconazole, and erythromycin. Other drugs act as *inducers* of CYP isozymes by increasing gene expression or protein levels, such as glucocorticoids, barbiturates, and rifampin, which can increase the net activity of CYP-3A4, resulting in decreased concentrations of susceptible compounds. Among the anticancer agents that are substrates for CYP-3A4 are cyclophosphamide, ifosfamide, docetaxel, etoposide, paclitaxel (also CYP-2C8), vincristine, vinblastine, tamoxifen, and gefitinib.

Owing to the diversity and rapid adoption of new chemotherapy and nonchemotherapy compounds, information regarding drug interactions is best obtained from online databases (e.g., http://www.medicalletter.com, http://www.micromedex.com, or http://www.druginteractioninfo.org/Home.aspx) or from the drug manufacturer.

DRUG RESISTANCE AND TUMOR CELL HETEROGENEITY

KEY POINTS

- The emergence of drug resistance limits the curative potential of chemotherapy.
- Dosing of chemotherapy must consider the setting and objective of treatment. More intense regimens are best utilized in the adjuvant or neoadjuvant setting.
- Treatment monitoring often encompasses repeat measurements of tumor sites identified on imaging. The common standard to interpret tumor measurements on clinical trial utilizes RECIST criteria.
- Chemotherapy can result in significant toxicities. Patient education and provider knowledge are key to managing the complications of treatment.

The curative potential of chemotherapy is limited by the emergence of drug resistance, which can be either intrinsic or acquired, and may involve one drug or multiple agents (pleiotropic resistance). Of note, tumors with intrinsic drug resistance to natural products tend to arise from duct or other cells lining excretory organs.

Intrinsic drug resistance is likely due to the clonal selection of tumor subpopulations that have survived previous chemotherapy exposure. In contrast, acquired drug resistance develops through somatic mutations, regulation of gene expression, or other phenotypic alterations. Of these, acquired resistance mechanisms may have a reversible component that could influence the timing and selection of subsequent chemotherapy.

There are two major patterns of drug resistance in gynecologic oncology: (i) pleiotropic drug resistance associated with the overexpression of membrane-associated transport proteins, such as MDR1 (P170 glycoprotein), which has maximal impact on natural products, including the anthracyclines, vinca alkaloids, and taxanes and (ii) resistance due to reduced cellular uptake as a result of the loss of membrane transport proteins, increased detoxification of intermediates by glutathione production, increased damage tolerance due to defective detection, and/or apoptotic signaling, and expanded capacity of DNA repair. These second mechanisms are predominantly responsible for resistance to alkylating agents, including the platinum compounds (Table 1.3).

Platinum Resistance and DNA Repair

Multiple mechanisms are associated with platinum resistance and point to potentially important clues to increase the cytotoxicity of these agents.

As a highly polar compound, cisplatin enters cells relatively slowly. Thus, the uptake of platinum can be influenced by several factors, including cation concentrations, pH, and the presence of reducing agents. Membrane transporter proteins, particularly the copper transporter-1 (CTR1), have been shown to play a substantial role in platinum influx. In addition, down-regulation of CTR1 has been shown to be a mechanism of platinum resistance.

Another mechanism of platinum resistance is associated with elevated levels of cellular glutathione (GSH), which also is associated with resistance

Table 1.3	Specific Mechanisms of Tumor Drug Resistance	
Resistance Mechanism	Examples	Specific Cellular Target or Effects
Impaired activation	5-Fluorouracil	Reduced levels of thymidylate synthase, thymidylate phosphorylase, or DPD
	Methotrexate	Reduced intracellular polyglutamation
	Doxorubicin	Low P450 enzymes
	Cyclophosphamide, ifosfamide	Decreased microsomal transformation
	Gemcitabine	Decreased deoxycytidine kinase
Increased drug efflux	Natural products	Increased MDR 1 (P170)
	Topotecan, mitoxantrone	Increased BCRP (ABCG2)
Increased drug inactivation	Alkylating agents, platinum	Elevated glutathione and other cellular thiols
Accelerated DNA repair	Alkylating agents, platinum, radiation	Induction of DNA repair enzymes
Increased damage tolerance	Alkylating agents, platinum, radiation	Loss of DNA mismatch repair
Transport defects	Melphalan	Reduced carrier-mediated uptake
	Gemcitabine	Decreased nucleoside transporter
	Platinum	Decreased copper transporter-1
Target alterations	Methotrexate	*DHFR* gene amplification
	Paclitaxel, docetaxel	Increased tubulin-$\beta3$ isoforms or mutations
	Hydroxyurea and gemcitabine	Decreased ribonucleotide reductase
	Glucocorticoids	Decreased receptor binding
	Camptothecins	Decreased topoisomerase-I
	Anthracyclines, etoposide	Decreased topoisomerase-II

to other alkylating agents and radiation therapy (RT). However, the exact mechanism by which GSH and other thiol compounds modulate cytotoxicity is unknown.

Enhanced capacity for DNA damage tolerance and repair can play a role in drug resistance to alkylating agents and cisplatin. Loss of DNA mismatch repair system genes such as *MLH1* is not uncommon in ovarian cancer, and this appears to increase after exposure to platinum compounds. In addition, functional loss of *MLH1* activity in patients with ovarian cancer can occur through hypermethylation-mediated silencing of the *MLH1* gene following platinum exposure.

Nucleotide excision repair (NER) is the primary mechanism to remove platinum–DNA adducts from genomic DNA. Excision repair cross-complementing 1 (*ERCC1*) is a critical gene in the NER pathway, and increased mRNA levels of *ERCC1* have been associated with platinum resistance. In addition, *ERCC1* may also be prognostic, independent of chemotherapy. In one study of patients with lung cancer, patients assigned to observation who had *ERCC1*-positive tumors had better survival compared to those whose tumors were *ERCC1*-negative.

The association between ovarian cancer risk and mutations in *BRCA1* and *BRCA2* sparked interest in DNA repair after it was recognized that patients with *BRCA1/2*-associated tumors had improved outcomes compared with those without such mutations. One explanation of this was the association of *BRCA1/2* mutations and increased response to agents that target DNA, such as the platinum compounds. How to incorporate drugs that inhibit DNA repair in tumors with loss of *BRCA1/2* remains an area of active investigation.

Taxane Resistance

The subject of taxane resistance continues to be an area of active investigation. Overexpression of the drug efflux protein MDR-1 has consistently been associated with resistance to paclitaxel in cells and in retrospective analyses. However, prospective trials that combined an MDR-1 inhibitor with taxanes failed to improve clinical outcomes.

Mutations in the β-tubulin subunit have been associated with paclitaxel resistance in some preclinical models, but this does not appear to be a common mechanism. Still, expression of the tubulin-β3 isoform has been linked to cell survival pathways with a potential impact on clinical outcome.

Still, these molecular mechanisms do not adequately explain the clinical behavior associated with paclitaxel therapy in women with ovarian cancer. For example, patients who progress or recur following exposure to paclitaxel delivered every 3 weeks may still respond to paclitaxel on a weekly schedule.

Dose Intensity and Density

Dose intensity is a standardized measure of the amount of drug administered over time, most commonly expressed as $mg/m^2/week$. Preclinical studies demonstrate a sigmoidal relationship between dose and tumor response. The hypothesis that greater dose intensity would produce greater benefit has been extensively evaluated in the setting of advanced ovarian cancer, beginning with a series of retrospective studies suggesting a correlation between actual delivered dose intensity and clinical outcomes. However, within practical dose ranges that can be achieved in the clinical setting, prospective randomized trials have not demonstrated significant improvements in either disease-free or overall survival. These frontline studies focused on platinum dose intensity. The question of paclitaxel dose intensity was also addressed in the setting of recurrent disease, again without any evidence of improved outcomes.

By contrast, there is a renewed interest in "dose-dense" therapy, in which agents are sequentially administered at maximal tolerated doses using short cycle intervals. This approach has been favorably evaluated in the adjuvant therapy of breast cancer, although it has not been clearly established if the clinical benefit is secondary to dose density or weekly scheduling of specific components.

Chemotherapy Settings

Adjuvant chemotherapy refers to the initial use of systemic chemotherapy after surgery and/or RT has been performed with curative intent, and there is no evidence of residual disease. Adjuvant chemotherapy is considered if the subsequent risk for recurrence after initial definitive therapy is relatively high (generally >20%), but it is not routinely recommended when the risk of recurrence is less than 10%.

Concurrent chemotherapy with radiation (chemoradiation) refers to the use of chemotherapy to sensitize tumors to the effects of radiation generally delivered with curative intent. This has been most extensively studied in the primary management of locally advanced cervical cancer, where platinum-based chemoradiation has been proven to be superior to radiation alone.

Neoadjuvant chemotherapy generally refers to the use of chemotherapy in the management of locally advanced disease in situations where it would be difficult or impractical to perform immediate surgery or radiation. Following a response to initial chemotherapy, there is an expectation that morbidity associated with the overall treatment program can be minimized in conjunction with a reduction in the radiation treatment volume or the extent of surgery. This approach has been considered in advanced cervical cancer, where high initial response rates to neoadjuvant therapy have been observed. However, the long-term benefit of this approach has not been established. Neoadjuvant therapy is also a consideration in advanced ovarian cancer, particularly in patients with large-volume ascites, pleural effusion, diffuse small-volume disease, or comorbidities that might increase surgical risk.

Monitoring of Tumor Response

Generally accepted criteria for the evaluation of response are necessary to facilitate treatment decisions and comparisons among different regimens. The Response Evaluation Criteria In Solid Tumors (RECIST) are the most commonly used criteria in current clinical trials. RECIST is based on the prospective designation of at least one "target lesion" that measures at least 2 cm in one dimension, as well as "nontarget lesions" that are used to corroborate response (Table 1.4).

The summary response designation within RECIST integrates the findings from target and nontarget lesions, as well as serum tumor markers (if applicable). Serum tumor markers are not sufficient to declare response but, if initially elevated, must normalize to designate a complete response. In the case of ovarian cancer, international criteria to declare disease progression on the basis of a serial elevation in CA-125 have been widely adopted, but there is incomplete agreement on criteria to define a partial response during treatment.

Table 1.4	Overall Disease Response Categories (RECIST)
Complete response (CR)[a]	Disappearance of all *target*[b] and *nontarget* lesions and normalization of tumor marker levels (if appropriate).
Partial response (PR)	At least a 30% decrease in the sum longest diameter (LD) of *target* lesions (taking as reference the baseline sum LD) without the progression of *nontarget* lesions or the appearance of new lesions. *Note*: In the case where the only *target* lesion is a solitary pelvic mass measured by a physical examination (not radiographically measurable), a 50% decrease in the LD is required.
Progressive disease (PD)	At least a 20% increase in the sum LD of *target* lesions, taking as reference the smallest sum LD recorded since the start of the treatment, or the appearance of one or more new lesions, or the progression of any *nontarget* lesion. *Note*: In the case where the only *target* lesion is a solitary pelvic mass measured by a physical examination (not radiographically measurable), a 50% increase in the LD is required.
Stable disease (SD)[c]	Neither sufficient shrinkage of *target* lesions to qualify for PR nor sufficient increase to qualify for PD, taking as reference the smallest sum LD since the start of the treatment. No appearance of new lesions (*target* or *nontarget*).

[a]To be assigned PR or CR, changes in tumor measurements must be confirmed by repeat assessments not <4 weeks after the criteria for response are first met. The duration of overall response is measured from the time that criteria are met for CR or PR (whichever status is recorded first) until the first date that recurrence or PD is objectively documented, taking as reference for PD the smallest measurements recorded since the treatment started.

[b]All measurable lesions up to a maximum of five lesions per organ and ten lesions in total, representative of all involved organs, should be identified as *target* lesions and recorded and measured at baseline. *Target* lesions should be selected on the basis of their size (lesions with the LD) and their suitability for accurate repeated measurements (either by imaging techniques or clinically). All other lesions (or sites of disease) should be identified as *nontarget* lesions and should also be recorded at baseline. Measurements of these lesions are not required, but the presence or absence of each lesion should be noted throughout follow-up.

[c]In the case of SD, follow-up measurements must have met the SD criteria at least once after study entry at a minimum interval (in general, not <6 to 8 weeks) that is defined in the study protocol. SD is measured from the start of the treatment until the criteria for disease progression are met, taking as reference the smallest measurements recorded since the treatment started.

Measurable lesions—lesions that can be accurately measured in at least one dimension with LD $\geq$ 20 mm using conventional techniques or $\geq$10 mm with spiral CT scan.

Nonmeasurable lesions—all other lesions, including small lesions (LD < 20 mm with conventional techniques or <10 mm with spiral CT scan), that is, bone lesions, leptomeningeal disease, ascites, pleural/pericardial effusion, inflammatory breast disease, lymphangitis cutis/pulmonis, cystic lesions, and also abdominal masses that are not confirmed and followed by imaging techniques.

MANAGEMENT OF TOXICITY

KEY POINTS

- Bone marrow toxicity is the most common serious toxicity of chemotherapy.
- Erythropoiesis-stimulating agents (ESA), such as erythropoietin, have been associated with decreased survival in randomized trials.
- Effective antinausea therapy is critical and should be tailored to the emetogenic potential of the regimen.
- Carboplatin hypersensitivity reactions typically occur with the second dose of the second course of therapy and may be severe.

Toxicity Assessment, Dose Modification, and Supportive Care

Chemotherapeutic regimens are universally toxic, with a narrow margin of safety. Initial chemotherapy dosing is based on body surface area, weight, renal function, and hepatic function, using guidelines from clinical trials. However, patient tolerance of treatment varies widely, and it is necessary to monitor toxicity with ongoing modifications to avoid serious acute and cumulative side effects.

The Cancer Therapy Evaluation Program (CTEP) of the National Cancer Institute has developed a detailed and comprehensive set of guidelines for the description and grading of acute and chronic organ-specific toxicities. The current version of the Common Terminology Criteria for Adverse Events (CTCAE) is available in electronic format from CTEP (http://ctep. info.nih.gov). Basic hematologic parameters are summarized in Table 1.5.

Bone Marrow Toxicity

Bone marrow toxicity is the most common dose-limiting side effect associated with cytotoxic drugs, and neutropenia is the most common manifestation of bone marrow toxicity, occurring 7 to 14 days after the initial drug treatment and persisting for 3 to 10 days. For purposes of dose modification, the absolute neutrophil count is preferred to total white blood count. Dose-limiting thrombocytopenia is less common than neutropenia, but it may be problematic with carboplatin.

Radiation, alkylating agents (e.g., melphalan and carboplatin), and other DNA-damaging agents (e.g., nitrosoureas and mitomycin C) can have cumulative long-term effects on the bone marrow. Most other agents, including the taxanes and topotecan, show no evidence of cumulative toxicity and can be administered for multiple cycles without any dose modification.

In view of the frequent occurrence of neutropenia and the risk of infectious complications, utilization of granulocyte colony–stimulating factors (G-CSF), including filgrastim or the longer-acting polyethylene glycol (PEG)-filgrastim, has increased. Although these agents promote more rapid granulocyte recovery, avoiding potential complications and facilitating the maintenance of dose intensity, their use has not been shown to improve long-term survival for patients with gynecologic cancer, compared to conservative management

Table 1.5	**CTCAE Grading of Myelosuppression**			
	Grade			
Element	1	2	3	4
Leukocytes (per mm³)	LLN to 3,000	<3,000 to 2,000	<2,000 to 1,000	<1,000
Neutrophils (per mm³)	LLN to 1,500	<1,500 to 1,000	<1,000 to 500	<500
Hemoglobin (g/dL)	LLN to 10.0	<10.0 to 8.0	<8.0; transfusion indicated	Life-threatening consequences; urgent intervention indicated
Platelets (per mm³)	LLN to 75,000	<75,000 to 50,000	<50,000 to 25,000	<25,000

LLN, lower limit normal (institutional).
Source: CTCAE, Common Terminology Criteria for Adverse Events, version 4.03, June 2010, National Institutes of Health, National Cancer Institute. Available at: http://evs.nci.nih.gov/ftp1/CTCAE/CTCAE_4.03_2010-06-14_QuickReference_5x7.pdf

with dose reduction and cycle delay. In addition, G-CSF is not effective in the management of thrombocytopenia and may actually increase the degree of thrombocytopenia by the diversion of immature marrow elements.

Moderate degrees of anemia are quite common in cancer patients receiving chemotherapy, which may contribute to chronic fatigue. ESA, including erythropoietin (epoetin alfa) and darbepoetin, can ameliorate the anemia associated with chemotherapy, but there has been concern about data with regard to the potential risks associated with ESA, including cardiovascular events, thrombosis, and reduced tumor-related survival in placebo-controlled randomized trials. A Medicare decision memo limits reimbursement to patients with confirmed hemoglobin of less than 10 g/dL. In addition, these agents should not be used in patients being treated with curative intent.

Gastrointestinal Toxicity

There are three major categories of nausea and vomiting: *anticipatory*, occurring prior to the actual administration of chemotherapy; *acute onset*, beginning within 1 hour of chemotherapy administration and persisting for less than 24 hours; and *delayed*, beginning more than 1 day after chemotherapy administration and persisting for several days.

The antiemetic regimen is tailored to the emetogenic potential of the treatment, which reflects the incorporation of specific drugs, as well as the dose and schedule of drug administration. Table 1.6 categorizes chemotherapy agents according to their emetic potential. Mild nausea and vomiting can often be managed effectively with H-1 antihistamines (diphenhydramine), phenothiazines (prochlorperazine or thiethylperazine), steroids (dexamethasone or methylprednisolone), benzamides (metoclopramide), or

Table 1.6	Emetogenic Potential of Antineoplastic Agents (NCCN Practice Guidelines)
Level	Agent
High emetic risk (>90% frequency of emesis)[a]	▪ AC combination defined as either doxorubicin or epirubicin with cyclophosphamide ▪ Altretamine ▪ Carmustine > 250 mg/m^2 ▪ Cisplatin ≥ 50 mg/m^2 ▪ Cyclophosphamide > 1,500 mg/m^2 ▪ Dacarbazine ▪ Mechlorethamine ▪ Procarbazine (oral) ▪ Streptozocin
Moderate emetic risk (30%–90% frequency of emesis)[a]	▪ Aldesleukin > 12–15 million units/m^2 ▪ Amifostine > 300 mg/m^2 ▪ Arsenic trioxide ▪ Azacitidine ▪ Bendamustine ▪ Busulfan > 4 mg/d ▪ Carboplatin ▪ Carmustine ≤250 mg/m^2 ▪ Cisplatin < 50 mg/m^2 ▪ Cyclophosphamide ≤ 1,500 mg/m^2 ▪ Cyclophosphamide (oral) ▪ Cytarabine > 1 g/m^2 ▪ Dactinomycin ▪ Daunorubicin ▪ Doxorubicin ▪ Epirubicin ▪ Etoposide (oral) ▪ Idarubicin ▪ Ifosfamide ▪ Imatinib (oral)[b] ▪ Irinotecan ▪ Lomustine ▪ Melphalan > 50 mg/m^2 ▪ Methotrexate ≥ 250 mg/m^2 ▪ Oxaliplatin > 75 mg/m^2 ▪ Temozolomide (oral) ▪ Vinorelbine (oral)
Low emetic risk (10%–30% frequency of emesis)[a]	▪ Amifostine ≤ 300 mg ▪ Bexarotene ▪ Capecitabine ▪ Cytarabine (low dose) 100–200 mg/m^2 ▪ Docetaxel ▪ Doxorubicin (liposomal) ▪ Etoposide ▪ Fludarabine (oral) ▪ 5-Fluorouracil ▪ Gemcitabine ▪ Ixabepilone ▪ Methotrexate > 50 mg/m^2 < 250 mg/m^2 ▪ Mitomycin

Table 1.6	Emetogenic Potential of Antineoplastic Agents (NCCN Practice Guidelines) (continued)
Level	**Agent**
	▪ Mitoxantrone ▪ Nilotinib ▪ Paclitaxel ▪ Paclitaxel albumin ▪ Pemetrexed ▪ Topotecan ▪ Vorinostat
Minimal emetic risk (<10% frequency of emesis)[a]	▪ Alemtuzumab ▪ Alpha interferon ▪ Asparaginase ▪ Bevacizumab ▪ Bleomycin ▪ Bortezomib ▪ Busulfan ▪ Cetuximab ▪ Chlorambucil (oral) ▪ Cladribine (2-chlorodeoxyadenosine) ▪ Decitabine ▪ Denileukin diftitox ▪ Dasatinib ▪ Dexrazoxane ▪ Erlotinib ▪ Fludarabine ▪ Gefitinib ▪ Gemtuzumab ozogamicin ▪ Hydroxyurea (oral) ▪ Lapatinib ▪ Lenalidomide ▪ Melphalan (oral low dose) ▪ Methotrexate ≤ 50 mg/m^2 ▪ Nelarabine ▪ Panitumumab ▪ Pentostatin ▪ Rituximab ▪ Sorafenib ▪ Sunitinib ▪ Temsirolimus ▪ Thalidomide ▪ Thioguanine (oral) ▪ Trastuzumab ▪ Valrubicin ▪ Vinblastine ▪ Vincristine ▪ Vinorelbine

[a]Proportion of patients who experience emesis in the absence of effective antiemetic prophylaxis.
[b]Daily use of antiemetics is not recommended based on clinical experience.

benzodiazepines (lorazepam). For drugs with more severe emetogenic potential, a 5-hydroxytryptamine (5-HT3) receptor antagonist, such as ondansetron or granisetron, should be given prior to chemotherapy and repeated at 8- to 12-hour intervals. This may be combined with dexamethasone or the neurokinin-1 receptor antagonist, aprepitant. Longer-acting 5-HT3 antagonists have also become available, including palonosetron and dolasetron, which require only a single dose prior to chemotherapy. Anticipatory nausea and vomiting can become a significant problem during repeated cycles of chemotherapy and can sometimes be modulated by pretreatment with benzodiazepines, such as lorazepam. Unfortunately, this particular schedule produces significant sedation and can be used only in hospitalized patients or outpatients with independent transportation.

Diarrhea, oral stomatitis, esophagitis, and gastroenteritis are also potential problems. Patients with significant oral or esophagogastric symptoms may have their symptoms managed with oral viscous lidocaine (2%), other topical anesthetics, or parenteral narcotics in severe cases. Randomized controlled trials have demonstrated that multiple intravenous doses of recombinant keratinocyte growth factor (palifermin) before and after treatment can reduce the incidence and severity of chemotherapy-induced oral stomatitis associated with bolus 5-fluorouracil or high-dose chemotherapy. In general, dose-limiting mucosal injury is uncommon with platinum-based combinations, taxanes, and other single agents used in the treatment of gynecologic cancer.

Alopecia

Scalp alopecia is one of the most emotionally taxing side effects of chemotherapy. Aside from long-lasting alopecia that follows cranial irradiation, it is almost always reversible, but it can be a major deterrent to successful chemotherapy. A variety of physical techniques have been devised to minimize alopecia, including scalp tourniquets and ice caps designed to decrease scalp blood flow. Although partially effective, they are rarely successful with extended chemotherapy.

Skin Toxicity

Skin toxicities that occur during chemotherapy include allergic or hypersensitivity reactions (HSRs), skin hyperpigmentation, photosensitivity, radiation recall reactions, nail abnormalities, folliculitis, palmar-plantar erythrodysesthesia (PPE, hand-foot syndrome), and local extravasation necrosis.

PPE is a reversible but painful erythema, scaling, swelling, or ulceration involving the hands and feet. This occurs more often with chronic oral or intravenous medications, weekly treatment regimens, and formulations that increase drug circulation time, such as prolonged oral etoposide, weekly and continuous-infusion 5-fluorouracil, capecitabine, and PEG-liposomal doxorubicin, where it has emerged as a major dose-limiting toxicity.

Extravasation necrosis is a serious complication seen after tissue infiltration of vesicant drugs such as doxorubicin, dactinomycin, mitomycin C, and vincristine. Any suspected infiltration should prompt immediate removal of the intravenous line and application of ice packs to the infiltrated area every 6 hours for 3 days. Small series have reported a limited experience with local infiltration or topical application of steroids, N-acetylcysteine, dimethyl sulfoxide, and hyaluronidase with variable results, and recommendations are imprecise. However, single or multiple intravenous doses of dexrazoxane, a topoisomerase II catalytic inhibitor, appear to offer specific protection against injury from anthracyclines, including doxorubicin and daunorubicin. Skin necrosis from some extravasations may eventually require surgical debridement and skin grafting.

Neurotoxicity

Peripheral neuropathy is the most common neurotoxicity encountered in gynecologic oncology and is a particular risk with the administration of cisplatin and paclitaxel. Although less common with carboplatin than cisplatin, neuropathy can still occur, particularly in combination with paclitaxel. Peripheral neuropathy generally begins with symptoms of paresthesia (numbness and tingling) accompanied by a loss of vibratory and position sense in longer nerves associated with the feet and hands. It then progresses to functional impairment, with gait unsteadiness and loss of fine motor coordination, such as trouble buttoning clothes and writing. In moderate cases with paclitaxel and other nonplatinum agents, this is almost always reversible but may require several months posttherapy for substantial improvement. In more severe cases, symptoms may persist for the lifetime of the patient. If related to cisplatin, neuropathy can continue to progress after therapy has been discontinued, with long-term persistence of symptoms. Cisplatin has also been associated with permanent ototoxicity and, at higher doses, with a loss of color vision and autonomic neuropathy.

Patients with underlying neurologic problems, such as diabetes, alcoholism, or carpal tunnel syndrome, are particularly susceptible to neurotoxicity, and substitution of docetaxel for paclitaxel can be a useful strategy in some situations. All patients who receive potentially neurotoxic therapy should be routinely queried regarding symptoms so that severe damage can be avoided.

There has been an interest in agents that might prevent nerve damage, encourage recovery, or ameliorate symptoms. However, thus far, small studies with glutamine, vitamin E, and other agents have been inconclusive. Amifostine appears to be of borderline effectiveness, and there are no agents that can be recommended for the prevention of neuropathy in routine practice. Clinical management of painful paresthesias has been reported with amitriptyline and gabapentin.

Other neurotoxicities include acute and chronic encephalopathies, usually associated with intrathecal chemotherapy. Of particular relevance to the gynecologic cancer population, an acute reversible metabolic encephalopathy has been well described in association with ifosfamide and attributed to the toxic metabolite chloroacetaldehyde. This syndrome can potentially be prevented or treated by infusion of methylene blue, which may act through inhibition of monoamine oxidase activity with reduced chloroacetaldehyde formation in the liver.

Genitourinary Toxicity

Renal toxicity is a well-recognized side effect of cisplatin, even though only a small fraction of cisplatin is cleared by renal excretion. By contrast, carboplatin undergoes extensive renal clearance with little risk of toxicity. Careful attention to hydration status and saline-driven urinary output before, during, and immediately after cisplatin therapy is required to reduce the risk of renal failure.

Hemorrhagic cystitis can be seen with cyclophosphamide or ifosfamide, attributed to the metabolite acrolein. With moderate-dose cyclophosphamide, this complication can be prevented by maintaining a high urinary output, which reduces the overall urothelial exposure to the toxic metabolites. The risk of cystitis is essentially 100% with ifosfamide unless there is simultaneous administration of mesna, which binds and neutralizes acrolein in the urine.

Hypersensitivity Reactions

Paclitaxel is formulated in Cremophor-EL, a mixture of polyoxyethylated castor oil and dehydrated alcohol, which has been associated with mast cell degranulation and clinical HSR. Over 80% of reactions to paclitaxel occur within minutes during either the first or the second cycle of drug administration and can usually be managed with prophylactic medication (corticosteroids, histamine H1/H2 blockade, etc.) followed by rechallenge beginning at a lower rate of infusion. Similar reactions have been reported with docetaxel and PEG-liposomal doxorubicin, which are not formulated in Cremophor-EL, but their frequency is lower. Emerging data with NAB-paclitaxel indicate a marked reduction in the risk of HSR.

With improved survival and an increased utilization of second-line therapy, patients can also experience more traditional allergic reactions to selected chemotherapy agents. Carboplatin, an organoplatinum compound, has emerged as a major source of late allergic reactions. These occur most often during the second cycle of a second course of therapy, suggesting a process of antigen recall and priming of the immune response. Patients receiving the second course of carboplatin-based therapy should be closely monitored for early signs of hypersensitivity to avoid more serious reactions. Unlike the situation with paclitaxel, carboplatin reactions are not readily prevented or circumvented with prophylactic medication, although inpatient and outpatient strategies for desensitization have been reported and successfully utilized for patients who are responding to retreatment. However, the desensitization routine must generally be repeated with each cycle of treatment.

Other Significant Toxicities

These include cardiac toxicity from cumulative doxorubicin exposure, radiation recall vasculitis from doxorubicin, pulmonary fibrosis from bleomycin, gonadal dysfunction in premenopausal women from alkylating agents, and secondary acute leukemia from the chronic administration of alkylating agents, particularly melphalan in ovarian cancer.

SUGGESTED READINGS

Lee CW, Matulonis UA, Castells MC. Rapid inpatient/outpatient desensitization for chemo-therapy hypersensitivity: Standard protocol effective in 57 patients for 255 courses. *Gynecol Oncol.* 2005;99:393–399.

Li YF, Fu S, Hu W, et al. Systemic anticancer therapy in gynecological cancer patients with renal dysfunction. *Int J Gynecol Cancer.* 2007;17:739–763.

Markman M. Intraperitoneal antineoplastic drug delivery: Rationale and results. *Lancet Oncol.* 2003;4:277–283.

Mouridsen HT, Langer SW, Buter J, et al. Treatment of anthracycline extravasation with Savene (dexrazoxane): Results from two prospective clinical multicentre studies. *Ann Oncol.* 2007;18:546–550.

Pelgrims J, De Vos F, Van den Brande J, et al. Methylene blue in the treatment and prevention of ifosfamide-induced encephalopathy: Report of 12 cases and a review of the literature. *Br J Cancer.* 2000;82:291–294.

Therasse P, Arbuck SG, Eisenhauer EA, et al. New guidelines to evaluate the response to treatment in solid tumors. European Organization for Research and Treatment of Cancer, National Cancer Institute of the United States, National Cancer Institute of Canada. *J Natl Cancer Inst.* 2000;92:205–216.

2 Biologic and Physical Aspects of Radiation Oncology

INTRODUCTION TO RADIOBIOLOGY

KEY POINTS

- A typical course of radiation therapy is given in 10 to 40 fractions administered over 2 to 8 weeks, with each fraction killing a percentage of cells.
- Radiation exerts most of its deleterious effects by creating free radicals that cause breaks in two opposing strands of DNA, although hypofractionated regimens may exert additional biologic effects via endothelial cell damage and enhanced antitumor immunity.
- Oxygen chemically modifies radiation-induced DNA damage, making it irreparable.
- Hypoxia, conversely, shifts the cell survival curve to the right.
- Both the total dose of radiation and how fast it is delivered affect outcomes.
- Cell sensitivity to radiation varies in different phases of the cell cycle with late S phase being most radioresistant and M phase being most radiosensitive.

Radiobiology is the study of the action of ionizing radiations on living things. The size and histology of the tumor, as well as the relationship of the tumor to the normal organs within the radiation field, help determine the total dose and the dose per fraction.

Tumor Control Probability and Cell Survival Curves

Radiation effects exhibit a sigmoidal dose–response curve. The following is a theoretical dose–response curve for tumor control probability and normal tissue complications in the presence and absence of chemotherapy (Fig. 2.1). Ideally, there is a great deal of separation between the curve on the left, representing chances of tumor control, and the curve on the right, representing the chance for toxicity.

A typical course of radiation therapy is given in 10 to 40 fractions administered over 2 to 8 weeks. Each fraction kills a fixed percentage of cells. The log cell kill model describes cell kill in very simplistic terms such that a given radiation dose will kill a certain percentage of cells and that a tumor receiving a fractionated course of radiation gets progressively smaller with time. Additionally, tumor cells may have undergone clonogenic cell death wherein they are still present but unable to reproduce. Therefore, one does not necessarily have to kill all cancer cells in order to achieve cure if the remaining ones are unable to reproduce.

The shape of the cell survival curve is best described by the linear–quadratic model with DNA as the lethal target. Radiation exerts most of

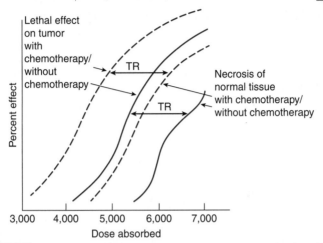

FIGURE 2.1 Theoretic curves for tumor control and complications as a function of radiation dose both with and without chemotherapy. TR, therapeutic range, or the difference between tumor control and complication frequency. *Source*: From Perez CA, Thomas PRM. Radiation therapy: Basic concepts and clinical implications. In: Sutow WW, Fernbach DJ, Vietti TJ, eds. *Clinical Pediatric Oncology*, 3rd ed. St. Louis, MO: Mosby; 1984:167, with permission from Elsevier.

its deleterious effects by causing breaks in two opposing single strands in the DNA backbone. Attempted repair of a double-stranded break may result in two possible outcomes: lethal outcomes and nonlethal outcomes. Nonlethal repair may result in a reciprocal translocation and preservation of the genetic information. In some instances, the reciprocal translocation results in the activation of an oncogene, which may manifest as a malignancy.

When a high dose of radiation (>10 Gy) is given in a single fraction, such as for stereotactic radiosurgery (SRS) or stereotactic body radiation therapy (SBRT), lethal DNA damage may not be the only resulting biologic effect. Other proposed effects include radiation-induced damage to tumor microvasculature and enhancement of antitumor immunity. These additional mechanisms of actions may explain the excellent clinical outcomes seen with SRS and SBRT.

DNA Damage Repair and the Shape of Cell Survival Curves

The concept that DNA damage repair drives the shapes of cell survival curves is well illustrated by experiments showing the effectiveness of oxygen as a sensitizer. Oxygen is known to chemically modify radiation-induced DNA damage, making it irreparable. This is known as the oxygen fixation hypothesis. Therefore, under anoxic conditions, DNA damage repair would be expected to increase considerably. Hypoxia causes the cell survival curve to shift to the right and change shape.

Biologically Equivalent Dose

Both the total dose of radiation and how fast it is delivered can produce very different outcomes. The same holds true for fractionated courses of radiation. The linear–quadratic equation can be used to derive an equation to be used as a guide to predict various biologic end points and is given by the following equation:

$$BED = D\left[1 + d/(\alpha/\beta)\right]$$

BED is the biologically equivalent dose, D is the total dose, d is the dose per fraction, and α/β is the dose where the alpha component of cell kill equals the beta component. These formulas are useful for conversion between different fractionation schemes: between standard and hypofractionation or between high-dose rate (HDR) and low-dose rate (LDR). This conversion is important so that doses can be compared between regimens.

The Cell Cycle

The cell cycle is an ordered set of events that results in cell growth and division into two daughter cells. The steps are G_1-S-G_2-M. G_1 stands for "GAP 1," and S phase stands for "synthesis" and is the point at which DNA replication occurs. Late S phase is the most radioresistant phase of the cell cycle since the DNA repair machinery for replication also can repair radiation damage. The G_2 stage stands for "GAP 2," and M phase stands for "mitosis" and is when nuclear division occurs. M phase is also the most radiosensitive phase of the cell cycle. Therefore, any DNA damage caused generally will be passed along to the daughter cells and may be fatal. This is one important reason why rapidly dividing cells such as cancers are radiosensitive. G_0 is a stable state of the cell and is typically observed with well-differentiated cells that have reached the end stage of development and are no longer dividing (e.g., neuron).

INTRODUCTION TO RADIATION PHYSICS

KEY POINTS

- The most common forms of radiation used in therapy are photons (x- and γ-rays) and electrons.
- There is an increased penetration as the energy of x- or γ-rays is increased.
- X- and γ-rays differ in their source of production: x-rays are artificially produced, whereas γ-rays arise through the natural process of radioactive decay within the nucleus of an atom.
- Exposure is the amount of ionization produced in air by photons, and its unit is roentgen (R).
- Radiation deposits energy in tissue by transferring energy from photons to ionized particles, which in turn transfer energy to the medium (usually tissue).
- The SI unit for absorbed dose is also joule per kilogram or gray, which has replaced the previously used term "rad." I gray = 100 cGy = 100 rads.

Radiation physics is the study of the interaction of radiation with matter. In the treatment of patients with radiation, this matter is either tumor tissue or normal tissues.

Units Used in Radiation and Radiation Therapy

Radiation is an abbreviation for electromagnetic radiation. It can occur in numerous forms. The most common forms used in radiation therapy are x-rays, γ-rays, and electrons. X- and γ-rays are also known as photons. Electrons are a form of particle beam radiation. Other particles or forms of radiation include protons, neutrons, and heavier alpha particles.

X- and γ-rays are forms of electromagnetic radiation, similar to visible light, but with a much smaller wavelength, that is, greater energy. The difference between x- and γ-rays is only their respective origins. Modern radiotherapy treatment machines termed linear accelerators or linacs create x-rays artificially by bombarding an atom or tungsten target with high-speed electrons. Linacs can produce both photon and electron beams of different energies depending on their construction. There is an increased penetration as the energy of x- or γ-rays is increased. The x-rays produced by linacs are much more penetrating than cobalt (^{60}Co) γ-rays.

While x-rays are artificially produced, γ-rays arise through the natural process of radioactive decay within the nucleus of an atom. These radioactive isotopes can occur naturally or be created artificially. Examples include the brachytherapy sources cesium (^{137}Cs) and iridium (^{192}Ir) as well as cobalt (^{60}Co) teletherapy treatment machines. Table 2.1 lists many of the more common radioactive isotopes and their physical properties. Use of radium 226 (^{226}Ra) sources is now historic.

Electrons are negatively charged particles and will usually only penetrate a few millimeters to centimeters in tissue. Similar to photons, the higher the energy of the electron, the farther it will penetrate into the tissue, but as opposed to photons, the skin dose increases rather than decreases. Electrons are used to treat tumors or tissues close to the skin surface such as superficial inguinal nodes and tumors of the skin, including vulvar cancers.

Regarding photon interactions with tissue, the dominant process at megavoltage (MV) energies used in radiation therapy is termed the Compton effect.

Table 2.2 lists some basic units of radiation and radiation therapy, both in historic context and in terms of modern SI units. Exposure is the amount of ionization produced in air by photons, and its unit is the roentgen (R). The SI unit for exposure is coulomb per kilogram (C/kg) with 1 R = 2.58 × 10^{-4} C/kg air. Kerma (kinetic energy release per unit mass) defines the transfer of energy from photons to directly ionized particles. These directly ionized particles, in turn, transfer some of their energy to the medium (usually tissue). This transfer of energy is defined as the absorbed dose to the medium from the radiation beam. The SI unit for kerma is joule per kilogram (J/kg) or gray (Gy). The SI unit for absorbed dose is also joule per kilogram or gray, which has replaced the previously used term "rad." Often the term centigray (cGy) is used. The cGy is equivalent to the rad, and 1 gray equals 100 cGy.

Table 2.1	Physical Properties and Uses of Brachytherapy Radionuclides					
Element	Isotope	Energy (MeV)	Half-Life	HVL-Lead (mm)	Source Form	Clinical Application
Obsolete Sealed Sources of Historic Significance						
Radium	^{226}Ra	0.83 (avg)	1,626 y	16	Radium salt encapsulated in tubes and needles	LDR intracavitary and interstitial
Radon	^{222}Rn	0.83 (avg)	3.83 d	16	Radon	Permanent interstitial Temporary molds
Currently Used Sealed Sources						
Cesium	^{137}Cs	0.662	30 y	6.5	Cesium salt encapsulated in tubes and needles	LDR intracavitary and interstitial
Iridium	^{192}Ir	0.397 (avg)	74 d	6	Seeds in nylon ribbon encapsulated source on steel cable	LDR temporary interstitial HDR interstitial and intracavitary
Cobalt	^{60}Co	1.25	5.26 y	11	Encapsulated spheres	HDR intracavitary
Iodine	^{125}I	0.028	59.6 d	0.025	Seeds	Permanent interstitial
Palladium	^{103}Pd	0.020	17 d	0.013	Seeds	Permanent interstitial
Gold	^{198}Au	0.412	2.7 d	6	Seeds	Permanent interstitial
Strontium	^{90}Sr–^{90}Y	2.24 MeV β_{max}	28.9 y		Plaque	Superficial ocular lesions

Developmental Sealed Sources

Americium	^{241}Am	0.060	432 y	0.12	Tubes	LDR intracavitary
Ytterbium	^{169}Yb	0.093	32 d	0.48	Seeds	LDR temporary interstitial
Californium	^{252}Cf	2.4 (avg) neutrons	2.65 y			LDR temporary interstitial
Samarium	^{145}Sm	0.043	340 d	0.060	Seeds	LDR temporary interstitial

Unsealed Radioisotopes Used for Radiopharmaceutical Therapy

Strontium	^{89}Sr	1.4 MeV β_{max}	51 d	SrCl$_2$ IV solution	Diffuse bone metastases
Iodine	^{131}I	0.61 MeV β_{max} 0.364 MeV γ	8.06 d	Capsule NaI oral solution	Thyroid cancer
Phosphorus	^{32}P	1.71 MeV β_{max}	14.3 d	Chromic phosphate colloid instillation Na$_2$PO$_3$ solution	Ovarian cancer seeding: peritoneal surface polycythemia vera, chronic leukemia

Table 2.2	SI Units for Radiation Therapy		
Quantity	SI Unit (Special Name)	Non-SI Unit	Conversion Factor
Exposure	C kg^{-1}	roentgen (R)	1 C kg^{-1} ≈ 3,876 R
Absorbed dose, kerma	J kg^{-1} (gray [Gy])	rad	1 Gy = 100 rad
Dose equivalent	J kg^{-1} (sievert [Sv])	rem	1 Sv = 100 rem
Activity	s^{-1} (becquerel [Bq])	curie	1 Bq = 2.7 × 10^{-11} Ci

RADIATION PRODUCTION

KEY POINTS

■ Intensity-modulated radiation therapy (IMRT) is accomplished by using small computer-controlled leaves in the head of the machine (multileaf collimators or MLCs) to block the beam in different patterns, modulating beam intensity and creating multiple complex treatment fields. The result is improved target coverage and increased sparing of normal tissues.

■ Image-guided radiation therapy (IGRT) refers to the imaging of treatment fields prior to treatment delivery in order to precisely align patient and improve treatment accuracy.

Radioactive Isotopes

As mentioned before, γ-rays are typically derived from radioactive isotopes, for example, ^{60}Co. Electrons or beta particles also come from radioactive isotopes. Radioactivity is the result of an atom changing its "energy" state, usually to a lower "energy" state, by the emission/absorption/internal conversion of photons or electrons in the atom.

Radioactivity, or activity, is denoted by the symbol A and is defined as the number of disintegrations per unit of time. The equation describing radioactive decay is $A = A_o e^{-\lambda t}$, where A_o is the initial activity, λ is the decay constant, and t is some unit of time later. Other important units for radioactivity and radioactive decay are the half-life ($T_{1/2}$) and the average life (T_a). The half-life is the amount of time necessary to reduce the original amount of material by half. $T_{1/2}$ is related to the decay constant by $T_{1/2} = 0.693/\lambda$. T_a is related to the decay constant and the half-life by $T_a = 1/\lambda = 1.44 \, T_{1/2}$.

Cesium 137 (^{137}Cs) has replaced radium as a safer, equally effective radioisotope. It is typically used for LDR gynecologic brachytherapy in tandem and ovoid and cylinder applicators. Iridium 192 (^{192}Ir) comes in various activities and can be used for interstitial and intracavitary gynecologic implants. It is the primary isotope for HDR applications.

Linear Accelerators

Linacs produce radiation by accelerating an initial beam of electrons across a variable electric field. This electron beam can be adjusted to control its shape and intensity before delivery to the patient. Alternatively, the electron beam can be directed to a tungsten target. The electron–target interaction creates a forward scattered photon beam or x-ray. The resulting photon beam can then be modified by the machine using filters and collimators to produce the desired radiation field shape.

Photon beams of different energies have a different absorbed dose pattern within tissues. This pattern is normally characterized as a percent depth dose or variation of dose as a function of depth within tissue. The higher-energy photons deposit dose at greater depths, and less dose is deposited at shallow depths. This is called "skin sparing" and is a characteristic of high-energy photons.

Modern linacs come equipped with MLCs and asymmetric jaws to control the shape of the radiation beam directed before it reaches the patient. MLCs are small (projected size at the patient approximately 1 cm) adjustable collimators built into the linac gantry that work together to create a shaped opening mimicking the effects of a poured block. With the advent of computer-controlled motion of the MLCs, the radiation field can be controlled to produce an IMRT treatment. In IMRT treatments, the MLCs are used to create many small fields of radiation within a larger treatment field. This adaptability allows the radiation treatment planner to create and deliver very complex treatment fields that improve target coverage while attempting to spare normal tissues.

IMRT for gynecologic cancers is currently an active subject of investigation. Published benefits of IMRT treatment plans compared to conventional three-dimensional conformal include improved dose sparing to normal tissue while simultaneously delivering higher tumor dose. One major challenge to the implementation of IMRT for gynecologic cancers has been the variation among radiation oncologists in target and normal organ delineation. To address this concern, the Radiation Therapy Oncology Group (RTOG) has defined parameters for contouring of targets and normal organs, margin size, and dose volume constraints in the postoperative setting in early cervical or endometrial cancers. An accompanying online atlas is available to improve consistency between multiple contouring physicians. The RTOG (Lim et al.) has also developed an MRI atlas for contouring the intact cervix for IMRT.

Currently, the RTOG has completed two phase II studies of postoperative IMRT to the pelvis for gynecologic cancers. RTOG 0418, which investigated postoperative pelvic IMRT alone in endometrial patients and with weekly cisplatin in cervical cancer patients, found low rates of hematologic toxicity, allowing for high rates of weekly cisplatin use. Similarly, RTOG 0921 examined postoperative IMRT with concurrent cisplatin and bevacizumab followed by carboplatin and paclitaxel for endometrial cancer; 1-year results from this phase II study show that this regimen is both feasible and well tolerated. The RTOG is currently conducting a randomized phase III study of standard versus IMRT pelvic radiation for postoperative treatment of endometrial and cervical cancer (RTOG 1203). Figure 2.2 shows a side-by-side comparison of IMRT and conventional four-field pelvic irradiation plans.

Due to the highly precise and conformal nature of IMRT delivery, organ and tissue motion is a significant concern and potential obstacle to the widespread implementation of IMRT for gynecologic cancers. A relatively new and increasingly relevant technology in radiation therapy is IGRT. Modern linacs have added on board imaging that allows the treatment fields to be recorded electronically at every treatment setup using an electronic portal imaging device. By comparing computer-generated radiographs (DRRs or digitally reconstructed radiographs) with the actual patient images, discrepancies in field shape and patient setup can be corrected before the delivered treatment. This type of corrective behavior before treatment is the foundation of IGRT. The latest variations on IGRT are the addition of computed tomography (CT) scanners or magnetic resonance imagers within the linac to verify more completely the correct alignment of the patient on the treatment table prior to treatment.

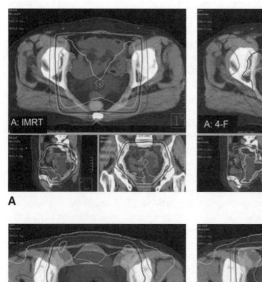

A

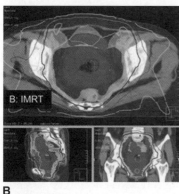 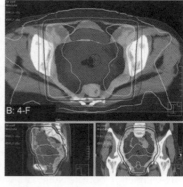

B

FIGURE 2.2 Intensity-modulated radiotherapy (IMRT) and four-field plans for (**A**) a large involved uterus and (**B**) a small uninvolved uterus. *Source*: From Forrest J, Presutti J, Davidson M, et al. A dosimetric planning study comparing intensity-modulated radiotherapy with four-field conformal pelvic radiotherapy for the definitive treatment of cervical carcinoma. *Clin Oncol.* 2012:24:e63–e70, with permission from Elsevier.

Simulation

The conventional simulator uses a diagnostic (kV) photon beam to reproduce all the gantry, collimator, and table rotations used in a linac treatment and therefore "simulates" the actual treatment. CT-based simulators ("CTSims") have largely replaced conventional simulators and combine a diagnostic CT scanner with a software package that allows for the simulation of the necessary gantry angles and table angles modeled in the computer. Following the scan, the treatment isocenter and the full CT images are transferred to the computer planning system for further treatment planning. DRRs of the treatment field are created for later comparison to actual treatment images.

Computerized Dosimetry

In a modern radiotherapy department, computers are necessary to accurately calculate the absorbed doses to tissues. These absorbed doses within tissues are termed isodoses or lines of the same dose. To initiate this process, CT images are acquired of the area of interest at a pretreatment planning session or simulation. These scans are typically obtained on the CT simulator. Treatment targets such as pelvic lymph nodes, the uterus, or the vagina are identified through contouring on these images, as are normal tissues such as the rectosigmoid, bladder, and small bowel. Dose goals are identified for the targets and normal tissues. A dosimetrist uses this information to design the radiation treatment plan, which is reviewed by the treating physician and a physicist and is altered as needed to best address the tumor and avoid the normal organs and tissues.

The goal for most treatment plans is to treat the target to a specified dose while minimizing dose to adjacent normal tissues. Figure 2.3 illustrates the

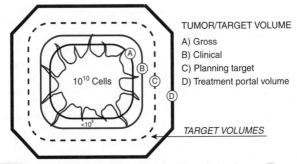

**DEFINITION OF "VOLUMES"
IN RADIATION THERAPY**

TUMOR/TARGET VOLUME

A) Gross
B) Clinical
C) Planning target
D) Treatment portal volume

10^{10} Cells

$<10^8$

TARGET VOLUMES

FIGURE 2.3 Schematic representation of "volumes" in radiation therapy. The treatment portal volume includes the GTV, potential areas of local and regional microscopic disease around the tumor (clinical), and a margin of surrounding normal tissue (planning). *Source*: From Perez CA, Purdy JA. Rationale for treatment planning in radiation therapy. In: Levitt SH, Khan FM, Potish RA, eds. *Levitt and Tapley's Technological Basis of Radiation Therapy: Practical and Clinical Applications*, 2nd ed. Philadelphia, PA: Lea & Febiger; 1992. Modified in Perez CA, Brady LW, Roti JL. Overview. In: Perez CA, Brady LW, eds. *Principles and Practice of Radiation Oncology*, 3rd ed. Philadelphia, PA: Lippincott-Raven Publishers; 1998:1, with permission.

gross target volume (GTV), the clinical target volume (CTV), the planning target volume (PTV), and the treated volume. The CTV includes all of the GTV plus possible microscopic extensions. The PTV includes all of the CTV plus a margin to account for possible geometric uncertainties of the patient or treatment margin. The irradiated volume includes all of the PTV plus any margins that might be included in the treatment plan to provide minimum dose coverage to the PTV.

BRACHYTHERAPY PRINCIPLES

KEY POINTS
- Brachytherapy delivers a concentrated dose of radiation to immediately adjacent tissues by implanting radioactive sources within a patient.
- Implants can be temporary or permanent.
- In gynecologic malignancies, temporary implants are used most frequently and are categorized as interstitial (sources are directly inserted into tumor-bearing tissues) or intracavitary (sources are placed into naturally occurring body cavities or orifices such as the vagina or uterus).
- Dose rate is the amount of dose delivered over an interval of time. LDR is defined as 40 to 100 cGy per hour. HDR is defined as 20 to 250 cGy per minute.

Brachytherapy is a term with Greek roots where "brachy" means "short distance." With brachytherapy, a highly concentrated dose of radiation is delivered to immediately surrounding tissues within millimeters to several centimeters of the applicators that carry the radioactive sources. This allows for a high dose of radiation to be delivered to closely approximated tumor and to relatively spare surrounding normal tissues such as the rectosigmoid, bladder, and small bowel.

There are different types of brachytherapy or radioactive implants. For gynecologic carcinomas temporary implants are used most frequently and are categorized as interstitial or intracavitary. With interstitial brachytherapy, the radioactive sources are transiently inserted into tumor-bearing tissues directly through placement in hollow needles or tubes. With intracavitary brachytherapy, radioactive sources are placed into naturally occurring body cavities or orifices such as the vagina or uterus using commercially available hollow applicators such as a vaginal cylinder or tandem and ovoids. Permanent interstitial implants entail the insertion of radioactive seeds (iodine 125 [^{125}I], gold 198 [^{198}Au], and palladium 103 [^{103}Pd]) directly into tumor-bearing tissues to emit radiation continuously as they decay to a nonradioactive form.

Dose rate is also an important variable in brachytherapy. Traditional LDR irradiation has been used for decades in gynecologic cancers using ^{226}Ra and ^{137}Cs sources for intracavitary insertions and low-activity ^{192}Ir sources for interstitial insertions. HDR brachytherapy has gradually been introduced over the last several decades and entails the use of a highly radioactive (^{10}Ci) ^{192}Ir source. Standard ranges for LDR are 40 to 100 cGy per hour and for HDR, 20 to 250 cGy per minute (1,200 to 15,000 cGy per hour). Pulsed dose rate uses a medium strength ^{192}Ir source of 0.5 to 1.0 Ci with dose rates of up to 3 Gy per hour and delivers the treatment in a "pulsed" method over only 10 to 30 minutes of each hour as opposed to LDR techniques, which deliver 30 to 100 cGy per hour continuously over several days. PDR delivers the same total dose over the same total time at the same hourly rate as LDR, but with an instantaneous dose rate higher than LDR, and was developed to combine the isodose optimization of HDR brachytherapy with the biologic advantages of LDR.

The term "afterloading" refers to an unloaded applicator that has radioactive sources introduced after insertion. Nearly all modern brachytherapy exploits afterloading. Remote afterloading, which eliminates all personnel exposure, entails the use of a computer-driven machine to insert and retract the source(s), which are attached to a cable.

CLINICAL APPLICATIONS

KEY POINTS

- The Manchester system approach for prescribing brachytherapy dose relied on predetermined doses and dose rates directed to fixed points in the pelvis.
- "Point A" was defined as 2 cm lateral to the central canal of the uterus and 2 cm from the mucous membrane of the lateral fornix in the axis of the uterus.
- Standard definitive total doses to points A and B when combined with external beam therapy at a dose rate of 50 to 60 cGy per hour are 85 and 60 Gy, respectively.
- Upper limit of total doses to normal tissue from combined external beam and brachytherapy are as follows: bladder more than 75 to 80 Gy, rectum less than 70 to 75 Gy, and vaginal surface 120 to 140 Gy.
- Patterns of Care Studies (PCS) have revealed that brachytherapy is the single most important treatment factor in multivariate analysis for stage III-B cervix cancer with respect to survival and pelvic control.
- Although prescription to point A has been used historically, a shift is occurring to transition to image-guided brachytherapy with dose prescribed to the high-risk volume.

Brachytherapy Systems for the Treatment of Cervical Cancer

Intracavitary brachytherapy for cervical carcinoma was profoundly impacted by the development of various "systems" that attempted to combine empiricism with a more scientific and systematic approach. Three systems developed in Europe, including the Paris System, the Stockholm system, and the Manchester System. The Manchester system principles are an integral part of modern brachytherapy.

The Manchester System

The Manchester system standardized treatment with predetermined doses and dose rates directed to fixed points in the pelvis. The fixed points A and B were selected on the theory that the dose in the paracervical triangle impacted normal tissue tolerance rather than the actual doses to the bladder, rectum, and vagina. "Point A" was defined as 2 cm lateral to the central canal of the uterus and 2 cm from the mucous membrane of the lateral fornix in the axis of the uterus (Fig. 2.4). It often correlates anatomically with the point of crossage of the ureter and uterine artery and was taken as an average point from which to assess dose in the paracervical region. "Point B" was located 5 cm from midline at the level of point A and was thought to correspond to the location of the obturator lymph nodes.

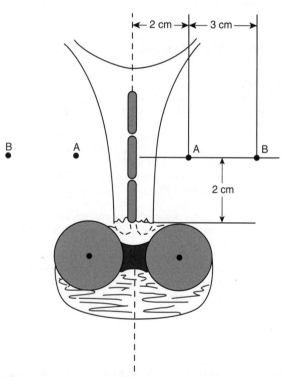

FIGURE 2.4 The Manchester system. Definitions of points A and B in the classical Manchester system are found in the text. In a typical application, the loading of intrauterine applicators varied between 20 and 35 mg of radium and between 15 and 25 mg of radium for each vaginal ovoid. The resultant treatment time to get 8,000 R at point A was 140 hours. *Source*: From Meredith WJ. *Radium Dosage: The Manchester System.* Edinburgh, UK: Livingstone; 1967, with permission.

To achieve consistent dose rates, a set of strict rules dictating the relationship, position, and activity of radium sources in the uterine and vaginal applicators was devised. With current LDR applications using cesium rather than radium, it is considered standard to have a point A dose rate of 50 to 60 cGy per hour and to deliver a total dose of 85 Gy to point A and 60 Gy to point B when combined with external beam therapy.

The Fletcher (M.D. Anderson) System

The Fletcher system was established at M.D. Anderson Hospital in the 1940s. The Fletcher applicator was subsequently developed and remains an integral part of gynecologic brachytherapy. The primary prescription parameter in the Fletcher system was tumor volume and prescription rules were based on maximum mg-hours and maximum time, taking into account the total external beam dose and the calculated sigmoid dose. Standardized source arrangements and limits on the vaginal surface dose and mg-hours were all used to help specify treatment. Individualization to fit the anatomical situation was an essential aspect of this system.

The Fletcher colpostats were further evolution of the Manchester ovoids. They were made with the same diameters of 2, 2.5, and 3 cm but were more cylindrical than Manchester "ovoids" and were attached to handles, with shielding in the direction of the bladder and rectum. Initially, these were preloaded with radium, but later an afterloading model was developed and loaded instead with ^{137}Cs. Recommended loadings were 15, 20, and 25 mg of radium for the 2-, 2.5-, and 3-cm colpostats, respectively, and 5 to 10 mg for the mini-ovoids. Recommended tandem loadings were usually 15–10–10 mg of radium with the amount of radium in the tandem usually greater than that in the ovoids.

More modern adaptations include CT and MRI compatible devices that are designed similarly but lack the shielding seen in the non-CT/MRI compatible devices. With these devices, avoidance of normal tissues is accomplished using image guidance.

The M.D. Anderson approach to treatment specification reflects a policy of treating advanced cervical carcinoma to normal tissue tolerance. This includes integrating standard loadings and mg-hours with calculated doses to the bladder, rectum, sigmoid, and vaginal surface. The activity in the ovoids is limited by the vaginal surface dose, which is kept below 140 Gy. Calculated bladder and rectal doses are noted and are sometimes used to limit the duration of the intracavitary system, with the combined external beam and implant doses for the bladder kept at less than 75 to 80 Gy and for the rectum at less than 70 to 75 Gy. Mg-Ra-eq hours are usually limited to 6,000 to 6,500 after 40- to 45-Gy external beam. In a retrospective review of cervical cancer patients treated definitively at M.D. Anderson, the median total dose to point A from external beam and intracavitary irradiation was 87 Gy, and the median doses to the bladder and rectum were 68 and 70 Gy. The total dose delivered to the vaginal surface was limited to 120 to 140 Gy or 1.4 to 2.0 times the point A dose. These total doses to point A and the vagina, bladder, and rectum are used as contemporary guidelines for determining implant duration and therefore dose.

The latest development in image-guided adaptive brachytherapy is the integration of MRI into the treatment planning process. Advances in MRI such as diffusion-weighted imaging can help to increase diagnostic accuracy by differentiating malignant from benign tissue. Potter et al. from the University of Vienna recently published their data on clinical outcomes in 156 patients with locally advanced cervical cancer patients treated with MRI-guided brachytherapy combined with 3D conformal radiotherapy with or without chemotherapy. Local control rates at 3 years reached 95% to 100% in stage IB/IIB patients and 85% to 90% in stage III/IV patients and stage IIB patients with poor treatment response. Compared to historical data, results from this study demonstrated improved pelvic control with a relative risk reduction of 65% to 70%, as well as a reduction in major treatment-related morbidity.

Dose Specification Points for Cervical Cancer

Most institutions use a derivation of the Manchester (point A) or Fletcher systems (mg-hours combined with qualitative assessment of implant geometry) to specify dose and implant duration, and though variations exist, most will attempt to quantify doses in the paracervical region (point A), and at either point B or the pelvic wall (C or E), and the rectum and bladder.

Importance of Brachytherapy in Cervical Cancer

When curative treatment is planned, patients with cervical carcinoma treated with definitive irradiation should receive a combination of external beam irradiation and brachytherapy. As revealed in the patterns of care studies (PACS) and the retrospective series of Perez et al., recurrences and complications are decreased when brachytherapy is used in addition to external beam. Use of an intracavitary implant was the single most important treatment factor in multivariate analysis for stage III-B cervix cancer with respect to survival and pelvic control in the 1973 and 1978 PCS. Retrospective series with external beam alone have proven marginal outcomes with this approach.

INTRACAVITARY APPLICATORS: CERVICAL CANCER

Low-Dose Rate

The best-known LDR applicators are the Fletcher-Suit and Henschke tandem and ovoid (colpostat) applicators. In the 1970s, the Delclos mini-ovoid was developed for use in narrow vaginal vaults. The mini-ovoids do not have shielding added inside the colpostat, and this together with their smaller diameter produces a higher surface dose than regular ovoids with resultant higher doses to the rectum and bladder.

The Fletcher-Suit-Delclos tandem and cylinder applicator was designed to accommodate narrow vaginas where ovoids may be contraindicated and to treat varying lengths of the vagina when mandated by vaginal spread of disease. The cylinders vary in size from 2 to 5 cm to accommodate varying vaginal sizes. Vaginal cylinders increase the length of the vagina and rectum treated with an associated increase in complications including vaginal fistulae, rectal ulcers, and strictures. Interstitial implantation should also be a consideration for patients with a narrow vagina or with distal vaginal disease.

Interstitial Applicators: Cervical and Vaginal Cancers—LDR and HDR

Interstitial implantation is appropriate in select patients with bulky tumors, anatomical distortion such as an obliterated endocervical canal or narrow vagina, or recurrent disease. The development of prefabricated perineal templates, through which stainless steel needles were inserted and after-loaded with ^{192}Ir or ^{125}I, was pivotal in advancing interstitial techniques for the treatment of cervical and vaginal cancers. The Syed-Neblett (Best Industries, Springfield, VA) is one well-known commercially available template system. Typically, total LDR doses to the tumor volume or reference isodose from the implant range from 23 to 40 Gy over 2 to 4 days. The total HDR dose will be approximately 60% of the total LDR dose and will be given in divided fractions.

External whole pelvic irradiation (39.6 to 45.0 Gy) generally precedes implantation. The total LDR dose to the reference volume from the combined implant and external beam approximates 70 to 85 Gy over 8 weeks.

HDR Brachytherapy for Cervical Cancer

Though LDR techniques have been the traditional standard for decades for gynecologic brachytherapy, HDR techniques have gained increased acceptance and are being used more recently due to some inherent advantages.

The advantages of HDR techniques include the following:

1. Outpatient therapy: because treatment time is very short, treatment is performed on an outpatient basis.
2. Reproducibility: the shortened treatment time provides a greater degree of certainty that applicator displacement as a function of time will be decreased.
3. Dosimetric advantages: the newer systems, which allow a single source to "dwell" at a site for a calculated period of time, combined with dose optimization software programs, provide a significant further improvement in the ability to shape the dose distribution.
4. Improved dose distributions may allow for a reduction in normal tissue doses.
5. Potential reduction in treatment duration: integration of HDR one to two times per week with external beam irradiation two to four times per week can lead to a shorter overall treatment duration, which may be pivotal in maximizing cure.
6. Health care providers receive decreased exposure due to the use of remote afterloading systems.
7. Potential radiobiologic advantages: reoxygenation of hypoxic cells can take place between fractions, and this may in fact be a radiobiologic advantage of HDR.

HDR disadvantages are the following:

1. Lower therapeutic ratio: HDR lowers the therapeutic ratio compared to LDR, and there is a potential increase in late tissue effects with large fraction sizes.
2. Labor intensity: there is an increase in the number of implants per patient from 1 to 3 to 3 to 6 (range, 2 to 16).
3. The need for sedation may still exclude high-risk patients even though bed rest is not required.

Conversion from LDR to HDR

A basic concept is that the total dose with HDR must be less than with LDR and the number of fractions must increase (70 to 74). This concept comes from early radiobiologic studies, and calculations have shown that one must give approximately 60% of the LDR dose with HDR.

HDR Applicators

The tandems and ovoids used with HDR are variations of the traditional Fletcher and Henschke LDR applicators but are lighter, narrower, and smaller. The ovoids are 2.0, 2.5, and 3.0 cm in diameter with and without shielding.

The ring applicator, which is an adaptation of the Stockholm technique, has become a popular applicator. The ring applicator is ideal for patients without lateral vaginal fornices. Its ease of insertion and predictable geometry make it a popular alternative to tandem and ovoids.

Tandem and cylinder applicators are used in the setting of a narrow vagina or vaginal extension of disease and are available in diameters of 2.0 to 4.0 cm. As with LDR tandem and cylinder applicators, the bladder and rectal doses may increase with this applicator, and the dose distribution will be more cylindrical than pear shaped, which can underdose bulky tumors.

Dose-Fractionation Schemes

Different fractionation schedules have been reported for HDR brachytherapy, with the dose per fraction at point A varying from 3 to 10.5 Gy, the number of fractions from 2 to 13, and the number of fractions per week from 1 to 3. Currently, the most common approach in the United States is to use 5 fractions of 5 to 6 Gy in combination with whole pelvis irradiation of 45 to 50 Gy.

Sequencing with External Beam

In nonbulky disease presentations, HDR insertions are often integrated early in the treatment course after approximately 20 Gy of external beam RT. Alternatively, some institutions choose to take the whole pelvis to 40 to 45 Gy initially, preceding the five HDR insertions, unless the patient has very early disease or evidence of early vaginal stenosis. Compressing the duration of treatment to less than 60 days may be desirable. HDR and external beam fractions should not be given on the same day.

Brachytherapy for Endometrial Cancer

Hysterectomy is the cornerstone of treatment for endometrial carcinoma. Selective use of vaginal brachytherapy, external beam irradiation, or both in the postoperative setting is based on the histopathologic risk factors identified in the tissues removed at the time of surgical staging. Vaginal brachytherapy is typically performed using Fletcher colpostats or a variety of vaginal cylinders (Delclos, Burnette). Both LDR and HDR techniques are used. Vaginal ovoids are available in diameters of 2 to 3 cm with associated caps and shielding and treat approximately the upper third of the vagina. Vaginal cylinders are available in diameters of 2 to 5 cm, with or without shielding, and can treat a portion of or the entire vagina. Distal vaginal recurrences or metastases are rare after radiation and occurred in 0.5% to 1% of patients when the upper vagina was treated. It is therefore not recommended to treat more than the upper half of the vagina routinely. Typically, the length of vagina treated with vaginal cylinders is between 3 and 5 cm, depending on risk factors. Due to the longer length of vagina treated and the lack of packing, a larger volume of rectum and bladder will be treated with cylinders.

Most vaginal brachytherapy for endometrial cancer is performed with vaginal cylinders using HDR techniques. Ideally, the dose distribution should conform to the shape of the cylinder, and dose is typically specified either at the vaginal applicator (mucosal surface) surface or at a depth of 0.5 cm from the applicator or vaginal mucosal surface. For LDR insertions, vaginal surface doses of 50 to 80 Gy are reported most frequently in the literature. When used with external beam, cumulative doses of 60 to 100 Gy at the vaginal surface are reported in the literature. For a vaginal recurrence of endometrial cancer, doses of 80 Gy and higher may be needed when combining external beam and brachytherapy.

Vaginal brachytherapy alone is generally considered an option for patients treated with hysterectomy with either no or selective lymph node sampling who are thought to be at low risk for lymph node metastases. It is also used in the setting of a negative pelvic lymph node dissection, even when high-risk factors such as high-grade or deep myometrial invasion are present.

There is debate about whether a vaginal cuff boost is routinely necessary in addition to external beam irradiation for early-stage endometrial cancer; there are few data to support it. Practice patterns are based more on institutional tradition and individual preference rather than prospective randomized trials; however, doses in excess of the 45 to 50 Gy typically delivered with external beam may be necessary if there are microscopic tumor cells embedded in the hypoxic vaginal cuff.

Medically inoperable endometrial cancer is an unusual situation in the current era. When encountered, it can require the use of sophisticated radiation techniques. Either external beam alone or brachytherapy alone, or a combination of the two, may be appropriate for some patients.

Patients with recurrent endometrial cancer usually benefit from both external beam and brachytherapy. Doses in excess of 80 Gy may lead to better local control in these patients. In patients with residual vaginal disease less than 0.5 cm in maximum thickness, vaginal cylinders or ovoids can be used, whereas in patients with thicker lesions following external beam, interstitial techniques are needed.

EXTERNAL BEAM IRRADIATION FOR GYNECOLOGIC CANCERS

KEY POINTS
- In cervical and vaginal cancers, the role of external beam irradiation is to shrink bulky tumor to bring it within range of the high-dose portion of the intracavitary dose distribution and improve tumor geometry by shrinking tumor that may distort anatomy and prevent optimal brachytherapy.
- In cervical, endometrial, and vaginal cancers, external beam additionally sterilizes paracentral and nodal disease.

Cervical and Vaginal Cancers

In cervical and vaginal cancers, the role of external beam irradiation is to shrink bulky tumor prior to implantation to bring it within range of the high-dose portion of the intracavitary dose distribution, improve tumor geometry by shrinking tumor that may distort anatomy and prevent optimal brachytherapy, and sterilize paracentral and nodal disease that lies beyond reach of the intracavitary system. For endometrial cancer, many of the same nodes are at risk as in cervical cancer, but the spread of disease is not as predictable with the paraaortic nodes independently at risk. The presacral nodes are also not at risk unless there is cervical involvement. Both the pelvic and paraaortic nodes are at risk in all sites of uterine involvement, and grade, myometrial invasion, and lymphatic vascular space invasion are more predictive of risk than location. For all gynecologic cancers, patterns of lymphatic spread influence the external beam field borders. For specifics on external beam doses and techniques, please refer to the respective chapters on cervical, endometrial, vulvar, and vaginal cancer.

Radiation-Induced Tissue Effects

The response of a tissue or organ to radiation depends on two factors: (i) the inherent sensitivity of the individual cells and (ii) the kinetics of the population as a whole of which the cells are a part. These factors combine to account for the substantial variation in response to radiation characteristic of different tissues. Additionally, the volume of tissue irradiated as well as the dose, dose rate, and fractionation scheme will affect both acute and late toxicities. The addition of chemotherapy or other systemic agents may impact on toxicity as may other medical comorbidities such as diabetes, hypertension, collagen vascular diseases, Crohn disease, and ulcerative colitis, as well as social risk factors such as smoking. The tolerance doses for tissues are described by the TD 5/5 or the probability of a 5% risk of complications within 5 years of the completion of radiation and TD 5/50 or the probability of a 50% risk of complications within 5 years.

Skin

When treating the vulvar and inguinal regions, there can be marked skin reactions. Erythema is the first visible skin reaction and is usually seen about the third week of radiation. Other skin reactions include dry desquamation and moist desquamation occurring after the fourth week of radiation. Return of the epidermis can take 10 to 14 days. Late manifestations of radiation on the skin include depigmentation, subcutaneous fibrosis, dryness and thinning with the loss of apocrine and sebaceous glands, thinning or loss of hair, and telangiectasias. Necrosis of the skin is rare and generally occurs only with doses of radiation in excess of 60 Gy.

Vagina

There are few noticeable acute reactions when treating the upper two thirds of the vagina with radiation. Some patients may notice a white-yellow vaginal discharge, which is due to mucositis of the vaginal mucosa. This can be evident during radiation and continue for several weeks after radiation. The lower third of the vagina, however, is less tolerant of radiation than the proximal, and the tolerance doses are in the range of 80 to 90 Gy versus 120 to 150 Gy, respectively. Vaginal narrowing and shortening are late sequelae of radiation, which can alter and impede sexual function. Combined brachytherapy and external beam irradiation will cause more late effects than either modality alone. The uterus is very resistant to high doses of radiation as is evident in patients treated with external beam and brachytherapy for cervical cancer. Rare cervical necrosis can occur.

Bladder/Ureters/Urethra

Acute and transient radiation cystitis may be observed with moderate doses of irradiation (>30 Gy). Patients will report urinary frequency and urgency as well as mild dysuria and decreased bladder capacity. Higher radiation doses may cause more severe symptoms of cystitis and spasms of the bladder musculature. It is important to rule out the presence of a concomitant bacterial infection. Radiation cystitis is characterized by the presence of white cells and red cells without bacteria on urinalysis.

Doses above 60 Gy can cause chronic cystitis, telangiectasias, hematuria, fibrosis, and decreased bladder capacity. Rarely, bladder neck contractures as well as fistulas may occur. Fistulas are more likely to occur if there is invasion of the bladder wall by tumor or in the setting of interstitial implants. Studies have demonstrated that with doses below 75 to 80 Gy to limited volumes of the bladder, the incidence of grade 3 or 4 complications is 5% or less, whereas with higher doses, a greater incidence of sequelae is noted. The ureters are quite resistant to radiation, and rare ureteral stenosis is reported in some series. Interstitial implants are more likely to cause this than intracavitary. Urethral stenosis is also rare.

Small Intestine, Large Intestine, and Stomach

It is common to observe watery diarrhea with intermittent abdominal cramping starting in the second or third week of abdominal or pelvic irradiation. Increased peristalsis, disturbance of the absorption mechanisms, and a decreased transit time also occur. Patients may also report increased flatulence and gas pain. Rarely, patients will report nausea. Concurrent 5-fluorouracil (5-FU), taxanes, or gemcitabine can worsen small bowel toxicity. The late effects of radiation on the small bowel can be a continuation of the acute effects. Some patients will experience chronic diarrhea. Small bowel obstructions occur in approximately 5% of irradiated patients, and the ileum is the most common loop of bowel involved.

When the rectum is included in the irradiated volume, there is rectal discomfort with tenesmus, and mucous production, sometimes mixed with blood in the stools. Hemorrhoids may worsen during radiation. This constellation of symptoms is termed "proctitis."

Late radiation effects with high enough doses include temporary or permanent ulceration and bleeding due to telangiectasias. Fibrosis, stenosis, perforation, and fistula formation are rarer. In general, doses in excess of 60 Gy are necessary to produce this more advanced radiation damage to the small bowel and rectosigmoid.

Acute effects involving the stomach, like the small and large bowel reactions, include erosions and thinning and subsequent edema and ulceration. Symptoms can include nausea, vomiting, reflux, and pain. Late effects can include gastritis and ulceration with associated bleeding. Progressive fibrosis can lead to gastric outlet obstruction and rarely perforation, all of which are dose and volume dependent.

Ovaries

In premenopausal patients treated with definitive irradiation, the ovaries will be irradiated incidentally and ovarian failure will occur. Hot flashes and other menopausal symptoms can begin to develop during radiation. Alternatively, the ovaries can also be elevated out of the radiation field and placed above the true pelvis to attempt to avoid them when treating cervical cancer. The dose necessary to castrate a woman depends on her age: a larger dose is required during the period of more active follicular proliferation. A single dose of 4.0 to 8.0 Gy or fractionated doses of 12 to 20 Gy (depending on age) are known to produce permanent castration and sterility in most patients.

Bone Marrow/Pelvic Bones

The lymphocytes are the most radiosensitive cells in the bone marrow. The rate of fall of the various components of the marrow is a function of the half-lives of the mature cells. These half-lives are as follows: erythrocytes—120 days, granulocytes—6.6 hours, platelets—8 to 10 days. Pelvic irradiation may cause transient lymphopenia. This is even more of an issue when whole abdominal or extended field irradiation is used due to the increased bone marrow in the radiation fields. Prior or concurrent chemotherapy will also lead to increased bone marrow toxicity. The frequent monitoring of the CBC is considered standard of care with pelvic or abdominal irradiation.

Insufficiency fractures can also develop in irradiated pelvic bones. These most commonly involve the sacrum and ileum, followed by the pubic bones and, rarely, the acetabulum. MRI is the best imaging modality to detect them and rule out recurrent disease. Symptoms from these changes in the pelvic bones will often improve over time, but patients may also suffer future symptoms from the exacerbation of these fractures or the development of new fractures over time. Femoral neck complications can include avascular necrosis as well as fracture. This is a rare complication following the irradiation of the inguinal nodes.

Liver

Venoocclusive disease is the pathologic entity caused by radiation to the liver, resulting in necrosis and atrophy of the hepatic cells. During radiation, the liver enzymes may be elevated and can continue following completion of radiation. Signs of radiation hepatitis can include a marked elevation of alkaline phosphatase (3 to 10 times normal) with much less elevation of the transaminases (normal to 2 times normal). The TD 5/5 for whole liver is 30 Gy. Small portions of the liver can receive up to 70 Gy.

Kidney

The kidneys are very sensitive to small doses of radiation, and a common goal is to avoid greater than 18- to 20-Gy whole kidney dose. When delivering whole abdominal or paraaortic irradiation, the kidneys are at risk and the equivalent of one kidney must be spared. Functional changes have been described after exposure of the kidney to more than 20 Gy, and signs and symptoms of renal dysfunction can follow; these include hypertension, leg edema, and a urinalysis showing albuminuria and low specific gravity. A normocytic, normochromic anemia may also appear.

Doses to Bladder and Rectosigmoid—LDR

The bladder and rectosigmoid are the organs of concern in the setting of combined external beam irradiation and brachytherapy. Maximum bladder doses of 75 to 80 Gy and rectal doses of 70 to 75 Gy are guidelines. Small bowel doses should be limited to 45 to 50 Gy with 60 Gy maximum. The volume of rectum and bladder irradiated is an important variable in the development of complications in addition to the cumulative dose.

Doses to Bladder and Rectosigmoid—HDR

Rectal and sigmoid complications occur earlier than bladder complications. Rectal bleeding is the most frequent rectal morbidity, occurring in approximately 30% of patients. Fowler has speculated that if only 80% of the tumor dose is received by the critical normal tissues, then 4 to 6 HDR fractions can be used safely.

When possible, the doses to the normal critical structures should be less than the dose at point A, perhaps in the range of 50% to 80%. CT scanning after applicator placement is exceedingly helpful and much more reliable in assessing the proximity of the sigmoid to the tandem and in manipulating the dose distribution.

FUTURE FOCUS

Reducing treatment-related morbidity while improving local control and cure rates continues to be the primary goal in the treatment of patients with gynecologic cancer. Stereotactic body radiation treatment (SBRT), a relatively novel advancement in radiation delivery technique, has proven to be a clinical success in the treatment of early-stage non–small cell lung cancers, renal cell carcinoma, hepatocellular carcinoma, prostate cancer, as well as lung, spine, and liver metastases. In the setting of gynecologic cancers, SBRT has recently been used to treat macroscopic pelvic and periaortic nodes and oligometastatic disease. More prospective trials with long-term follow-up data are needed to fully evaluate the potential benefit of SBRT for gynecologic cancers.

SUGGESTED READINGS

Brown JM, Carlson DJ, Brenner DJ. The tumor radiobiology of SRS and SBRT: Are more than the 5 Rs involved? *Int J Radiat Oncol Biol Phys.* 2014;88:254–262.

Delclos L, Fletcher GH, Moore EB, et al. Minicolpostats, dome cylinders, other additions and improvements of the Fletcher-Suit afterloadable system: Indications and limitations of their use. *Int J Radiat Oncol Biol Phys.* 1980;6:1195–1206.

Erickson B, Eifel P, Moughan J, et al. Patterns of brachytherapy practice for patients with carcinoma of the cervix (1996–1999): A patterns of care study. *Int J Radiat Oncol Biol Phys.* 2005;63:1083–1092.

Ferrigno R, Nishimoto IN, Dos Santos Novaes PE, et al. Comparison of low and high dose rate brachytherapy in the treatment of uterine cervix cancer. Retrospective analysis of two sequential series. *Int J Radiat Oncol Biol Phys.* 2005;62:1108–1116.

Grigsby P, Russell A, Bruner D, et al. Late injury of cancer therapy on the female reproductive tract. *Int J Radiat Oncol Biol Phys.* 1995;31(5):1289–1299.

Haas JS, Dean RD, Mansfield CM. Dosimetric comparison of the Fletcher family of gynecologic colpostats 1950–1980. *Int J Radiat Oncol Biol Phys.* 1985;11:1317–1321.

Higginson DS, Morris DE, Jones EL, et al. Stereotactic body radiotherapy (SBRT): Technological innovation and application in gynecologic oncology. *Gynecol Oncol.* 2011;120:404–412.

Klopp AH, Moughan J, Portelance L, et al. Hematologic toxicity in RTOG 0418: a phase 2 study of postoperative IMRT for gynecologic cancer. *Int J Radiat Oncol Biol Phys.* 2013;86:83–90.

Lanciano RM, Won M, Coia LR, et al. Pretreatment and treatment factors associated with improved outcome in squamous cell carcinoma of the uterine cervix: A final report of the 1973 and 1978 Patterns of Care Studies. *Int J Radiat Oncol Biol Phys.* 1991;20:667–676.

Lim K, Small W Jr, Portelance L, et al. Consensus guidelines for delineation of clinical target volume for intensity-modulated pelvic radiotherapy for the definitive treatment of cervix cancer. *Int J Radiat Oncol Biol Phys.* 2011;79:348–355.

Nag S, Chao C, Erickson B, et al. The American Brachytherapy Society recommendations for low-dose-rate brachytherapy for carcinoma of the cervix. *Int J Radiat Oncol Biol Phys.* 2002;52:33–48.

Perez CA, Breaux S, Madoc-Jones H, et al. Radiation therapy alone in the treatment of carcinoma of the uterine cervix I. Analysis of tumor recurrence. *Cancer.* 1983; 51:1393–1402.

Potter R, Haie-Meder C, Van Limbergen E, et al. Recommendations for Gynecological (GYN) GEC ESTRO Working Group (II): Concepts and terms in 3D image-based treatment planning in cervix cancer brachytherapy—3D volume parameters and aspects of 3D image-based anatomy, radiation physics radiobiology. *Radiother Oncol.* 2006;78:67–77.

Pötter R, Georg P, Dimopoulos JC, et al. Clinical outcome of protocol based image (MRI) guided adaptive brachytherapy combined with 3D conformal radiotherapy with or without chemotherapy in patients with locally advanced cervical cancer. *Radiother Oncol.* 2011;100:116–123.

Small W, Erickson B, Kwakwa F. American Brachytherapy Society survey regarding practice patterns of post-operative irradiation for endometrial cancer: Current status of vaginal brachytherapy. *Int J Radiat Oncol Biol Phys*. 2005;63(5):1502–1507.

Small W, Mundt A. *Gynecologic Pelvis Atlas*. RTOG Radiation Therapy Oncology Group; 2007. Available at: http://www.rtog.org/gynatlas/main.html

Viswanathan AN, Moughan J, Miller BE, et al. A phase 2 study of postoperative intensity modulated radiation therapy (IMRT) with concurrent cisplatin and bevacizumab (Bev) followed by carboplatin and paclitaxel for patients with endometrial cancer: One-year results from RTOG 0921. *Int J Radiat Oncol Biol Phys*. 2013;87:S4–S5.

Clinical Genetics of Gynecologic Cancer

GENETICS IN CLINICAL PRACTICE OF GYNECOLOGY ONCOLOGY

The identification of *BRCA1* in 1994 and *BRCA2* in 1995 has introduced a new component to the practice of gynecologic oncology. Genetic testing for predisposition to ovarian cancer became available by 1996 and is now well established. There are six genes for ovarian cancer susceptibility now in clinical use (*BRCA1*, *BRCA2*, *MLH1*, *MSH2*, *PMS2*, and *MSH6*). *BRCA1* and *BRCA2* are responsible for the hereditary breast–ovarian cancer syndrome (10% to 15% of all ovarian cancers) and *MLH1*, *MSH2*, *PMS2*, and *MSH6* are responsible for Lynch syndrome (2% of ovarian cancers, also referred to as hereditary nonpolyposis colon cancer [HNPCC]) (Tables 3.1 and 3.2). Current strategies for prevention include prophylactic surgery and chemoprevention with oral contraceptives. Screening for ovarian cancer is widespread, but its utility is unproven.

OVARIAN CANCER

KEY POINTS
- Fifteen to twenty percent of all ovarian cancer is associated with a *BRCA1* or *BRCA2* mutation.
- Risk-reducing bilateral salpingo-oophorectomy is an effective method of ovarian cancer risk reduction for mutation carriers.
- Ovarian cancer screening remains unproven.

Genetic Epidemiology

Approximately 15% to 20% of all women with invasive ovarian cancer carry a *BRCA1* or *BRCA2* mutation, and several national groups suggest offering genetic testing to all woman diagnosed with invasive epithelial ovarian cancer (with the exception of mucinous cancers). In the event of a positive genetic test, testing is extended to unaffected female relatives. However, if there is no living affected relative, then testing may begin with an unaffected woman.

The frequency of *BRCA* mutations among ovarian cancer patients is not the same for all ethnic groups. In some populations, there are recurrent (founder) mutations. In these populations, the overall frequency of *BRCA* mutations tends to be high and one, or a small number, of specific mutations, will account for a large proportion of mutations. For example, approximately 30% to 40% of Jewish women with ovarian cancer carry

Table 3.1	Lifetime Risks of Cancers Associated with Specific Genes		
	BRCA1	*BRCA2*	*MMR*[a]
Breast	50%–85%	50%–85%	NI
Ovarian	30%–40%	15%–25%	5%–10%
Endometrial	NI	NI	40%–60%

[a]Mismatch repair genes *MLH1*, *MSH2*, *MSH6*, and *PMS2*.
NI, not increased.

one of the three founder mutations (two in *BRCA1* and one in *BRCA2*). The frequency of *BRCA* mutations has been estimated at 1 in 12 cases of ovarian cancer in French-Canadians and 1 in 6 cases in Pakistan. In these populations, it may be possible to offer testing for a limited number of mutations. The excess risk of ovarian cancer in Jewish families with multiple cases of breast or ovarian cancer appears to be almost entirely due to the three Jewish founder mutations. Among women with a *BRCA* mutation, the ovarian cancer incidence is much greater than expected. If a founder mutation is not identified through screening of a Jewish family, a different (nonfounder) mutation will be found in approximately 2% to 4%.

In the ethnically mixed populations of North America, approximately 15% to 20% of all patients with invasive ovarian cancer carry a mutation in *BRCA1* or *BRCA2*. However, the range of mutations is wide, and genetic testing must be comprehensive (full genomic screening with rearrangement testing). Among *BRCA1* carriers, the risk of ovarian cancer is significant in women above the age of 35 (approximately 1% per year) and preventive measures must be initiated early. Women who carry a pathogenic mutation in the *BRCA1* gene have a lifetime risk of approximately 40% for developing invasive ovarian cancer. Among *BRCA2* carriers, the risk is lower and is less likely to occur below age 50. A meta-analysis estimated the risk of

Table 3.2	Genes Associated with Common Cancers		
Breast	Ovary	Colon	Endometrial
BRCA1	*BRCA1*		
BRCA2	*BRCA2*	*APC*	*PMS2*
RAD51C	*MSH2*	*MSH2*	*MSH2*
CHEK2	*MLH1*	*MLH1*	*MLH1*
TP53	*MSH6*	*MSH6*	*MSH6*
PALB2	*PMS2*	*PMS2*	*PTEN*

ovarian cancer to be 16%. Also, among *BRCA2* carriers, the risk of ovarian cancer may vary with the position of the mutation. Other genes that have been implicated in breast cancer risk may increase the risk of ovarian cancer; these include *CHEK2, PALB2, BARD1, BRIP1, RAD50, RAD51C, NBN,* and *MRE11.* Though germline mutations in these genes can be identified in up to 5% of women with ovarian cancer, the actual increase in ovarian cancer risk associated with these genes is unknown at present. These preliminary research findings have led some experts to suggest multigene panel testing in women who do not have mutations in *BRCA1* or *BRCA2.*

Pathology and Surgical Presentation of Hereditary Ovarian Cancer

Ovarian cancers that occur in women with a *BRCA* mutation appear to be similar to their sporadic counterparts with the exception that mucinous tumors and tumors of low malignant potential (or "borderline" tumors) are rarely observed in women with a *BRCA* mutation. The great majority of *BRCA*-linked ovarian cancers show moderate to poor differentiation. In most of the studies to date, the proportion of endometrioid and clear cell carcinomas associated with *BRCA* mutations may be overrepresented due to inaccurate historical diagnoses. Most hereditary ovarian tumors present at an advanced surgical stage, but stage I or stage II tumors are now being discovered in the context of high-risk screening programs, or as an incidental finding associated with a risk-reducing salpingo-oophorectomy (RRSO) in an asymptomatic woman. Several studies have reported on the presence of early ovarian cancers among pathology specimens obtained at the time of risk-reducing surgery. The frequency of occult malignancy ranges between 2% and 10%. Some of these early tumors are identified in the distal fallopian tube, supporting the hypothesis that this may be a site of origin for most ovarian/fallopian tube cancers in high-risk women. It is necessary that the fallopian tube be completely removed and serially sectioned when a RRSO is performed.

Clinical Outcome and Treatment Effects

A number of studies have reported that the survival of patients with *BRCA*-associated ovarian cancer is improved, compared to women with sporadic ovarian cancer. A study of consecutive cases of ovarian cancers that compared *BRCA*-associated cancer to sporadic ovarian cancers from the same institution found that *BRCA* mutation status was a favorable and independent predictor of survival for women with advanced disease. It is clear that improved survival rate is most likely the result of a better response of *BRCA*-associated tumors to current DNA damaging therapies and less likely a factor of improved surgical outcomes as a result of different patterns of tumor invasion.

Risk-Reducing Bilateral Salpingo-Oophorectomy

In 1995, a consensus panel of the NIH recommended RRSO for high-risk women at age 35 years, or after childbearing is complete. It seems logical that this procedure should eliminate the incidence of ovarian cancer, but there are two reasons for the potential failure of RRSO. First, it is possible that the removed ovaries or fallopian tubes contain foci of occult carcinoma and that the cancer had spread locally to the peritoneum at the time of the resection. Secondly, it is possible that *de novo* cancer arises in the peritoneum after salpingo-oophorectomy. The peritoneum is derived from coelomic epithelium, of the same embryologic origin as the surface epithelium of the ovary. Despite the recent understanding that high-grade serous ovarian cancer likely originates in the distal fallopian tube, it is becoming increasingly difficult to justify a *de novo* origin for high-grade serous carcinoma in the peritoneum.

It is difficult to measure the risk of peritoneal cancer in women with intact ovaries. Peritoneal, fallopian, and serous ovarian cancers are histologically indistinguishable, and symptomatic women often present with multiple foci of cancer involving the peritoneum, tubes, omentum, and ovary. Tubal cancer is also difficult to discriminate from ovarian cancer and may be classified as ovarian cancer. New serous cancers that arise in the abdominal peritoneum, following a salpingo-oophorectomy, are considered primary peritoneal cancers, even though they may have a biologic relationship to the distal fallopian tube.

Piver et al. reported that 6 of 324 women who underwent RRSO experienced primary peritoneal cancer. The mutation status of these women was unknown, and there was no standard period of follow-up. Kauff et al. followed 170 *BRCA* carriers for an average of 2 years. They observed 1 peritoneal cancer among 98 women who chose RRSO, versus 5 ovarian/peritoneal cancers in 72 women with intact ovaries. In a historical cohort study of 551 *BRCA1* and *BRCA2* carriers, Rebbeck et al. reported that the incidence of ovarian or peritoneal cancer was diminished by 96% (95% confidence interval [CI]: 84% to 99%) in women who underwent risk-reducing oophorectomy, compared to those with intact ovaries.

Finch et al. followed 1,045 women with a mutation who underwent a bilateral RRSO and compared the cancer risk with that in 783 women who did not undergo the procedure. The overall reduction in cancer risk associated with bilateral salpingo-oophorectomy was 80% (hazard ratio = 0.20; 95% CI: 0.07 to 0.58; $p = 0.003$). The estimated cumulative incidence of peritoneal cancer was 4.3% at 20 years after salpingo-oophorectomy.

An additional benefit of risk-reducing oophorectomy is a marked reduction in the risk of breast cancer. Oophorectomy performed at a relatively early age (<40) is associated with a greater degree of protection than is surgery performed near the age of menopause, and the protective effect is evident for 15 years post-oophorectomy. Eisen et al. found that oophorectomy was associated with a significant reduction in breast cancer risk: 56% for *BRCA1* carriers and of 46% for *BRCA2* carriers. Reductions of similar magnitude have been reported in other studies.

Hormone Replacement Therapy

Premenopausal oophorectomy is associated with the induction of acute menopause. There is concern that the use of hormone replacement therapy in these women may be associated with an increased risk of breast cancer, or may offset the protective effect of the oophorectomy itself. Rebbeck et al. estimated the effect of oophorectomy on breast cancer risk in a study of 462 *BRCA1* and *BRCA2* carriers. They found that the odds ratio for breast cancer associated with oophorectomy in the entire study group was 0.40 (95% CI: 0.18 to 0.92) and was 0.37 (95% CI: 0.14 to 0.96) in the subgroup of women with oophorectomy who used hormone replacement therapy. Hormone replacement therapy is likely safe in mutation carriers and may slightly reduce the breast cancer protection offered by premenopausal oophorectomy.

Oral Contraceptives and Tubal Ligation

A protective effect of oral contraceptives against ovarian cancer has been reported in BRCA carriers. In a matched case–control study of 799 ovarian cancer cases and 2,424 controls, 3 to 5 years of oral contraceptive use was associated with a 64% reduction in the risk of ovarian cancer ($p = 0.0001$). In a second, smaller study, 6 or more years of use of oral contraceptives was associated with a decreased in risk of 38% (OR = 0.62; 95% CI: 0.35 to 1.09). Tubal ligation has been found to be protective against ovarian cancer in the general population. There is some evidence that it is also effective among BRCA1 carriers. Oral contraceptives should be considered in mutation carriers who have not undergone RRSO.

Screening for Hereditary Ovarian Cancer

Screening for ovarian cancer using serial CA-125 levels and transvaginal ultrasound has been proposed as a method of reducing mortality through early detection. There have been no randomized trials of screening in BRCA1 carriers, but observational cohort studies have been disappointing. Neither CA-125 nor ultrasound have proven to be sensitive means of detecting stage I and stage II ovarian cancers. Until an effective early detection method has been identified for hereditary ovarian cancer, risk-reduction methods should be recommended (Table 3.3).

ENDOMETRIAL CANCER

KEY POINTS

- Lynch syndrome (also known as hereditary nonpolyposis colon cancer [HNPCC] syndrome) increases the risks of both endometrial and colon cancer in women.
- Prophylactic hysterectomy is an effective method of endometrial cancer risk reduction for mutation carriers.
- Endometrial cancer screening remains unproven in patients with Lynch syndrome.
- Risk-reducing bilateral salpingo-oophorectomy should be performed at the time of prophylactic hysterectomy in Lynch syndrome patients.

Genetic Epidemiology

The most important factor in the etiology of endometrial cancer is prolonged estrogen exposure, but inherited factors are important for a small proportion of cases (approximately 5%). Susceptibility genes for endometrial cancer include BRCA1, PTEN, and four mismatch repair

Table 3.3	Risk-Reduction Recommendations for Carriers of *BRCA1* and *BRCA2* Mutations

Breast
- Annual mammography and annual breast MRI starting by age 30
- RRSO to reduce breast cancer risk between age 35 and 40 and when child-bearing is complete
- Consider chemoprevention with tamoxifen, raloxifene, or an aromatase inhibitor
- Consider risk-reducing mastectomy

Ovary/Fallopian Tube
- RRSO to reduce ovarian and fallopian tube cancer risk between age 35 and 40 and when childbearing is complete
- Consider chemoprevention with oral contraceptives
- Consider ovarian cancer screening with q6 month transvaginal ultrasound and CA-125 from age 30 to 35 until definitive risk-reduction with RRSO

Adapted from National Comprehensive Cancer Network: NCCN Clinical Practice Guidelines in Oncology—Genetic/Familial High-Risk Assessment: Breast and Ovarian. Version 2.2014. http://www.nccn.org. 2014.

genes (*MSH2*, *MLH1*, *PMS2*, and *MSH6*). These genes are responsible for the hereditary breast–ovarian cancer syndrome, Cowden syndrome, and Lynch syndrome, respectively (discussed below).

The Breast Cancer Linkage Consortium reported that some endometrial cancers were due to mutations in *BRCA1* but none were due to mutations in *BRCA2*. However, two smaller studies (one on patients with serous endometrial tumors and one on patients with endometrial carcinomas in general) concluded that the risk of endometrial carcinoma in women with a germ-line *BRCA1* mutation was not increased. These findings suggest that it is likely that some cases of endometrial carcinoma are due to an inherited *BRCA1* mutation, but the penetrance of *BRCA1* mutations for endometrial carcinoma is low and the hereditary fraction is small. Data suggest that the excess risk of endometrial cancer among *BRCA* carriers can be attributed to past tamoxifen use and not to the effect of the gene.

Somatic mutations in *PTEN* are common in endometrial cancers, and rare inherited constitutional mutations in *PTEN* are present in women with endometrial cancer. In the latter case, endometrial cancer is seen in the context of Cowden syndrome—a rare dominant disease of the skin that is associated with increased risks of cancer of the breast, thyroid gland, and the endometrium.

Women in families with Lynch syndrome are at elevated risk for both endometrial and ovarian cancers. This syndrome is characterized by an autosomal dominant inherited tendency to develop colon and other cancers. The colon cancers tend to be of young onset and right sided and are often multicentric. Individuals in families with Lynch syndrome are at risk for a range of cancer types, and endometrial cancer is also a common site of cancer among women. Genes that are responsible for the repair of mismatched DNA (mismatch repair) are defective in families with this syndrome. *MSH2*, *MLH1*, *PMS2*, and *MSH6* are the four major genes responsible for it. The risk of colon cancer is high in families with a mutation in any of these genes, and the lifetime risk for endometrial cancer in women from these families is reported to be from 40% to 60%. The risk of endometrial cancer also depends on which gene carries the mutation. Mutations in *MSH2* and *MSH6* have been implicated in most Lynch syndrome families with endometrial cancer, but families with *MLH1* mutations have been reported as well. Germ-line mutations in *MSH6* are relatively rare in Lynch syndrome but are overrepresented in families with multiple cases of endometrial cancer. Goodfellow et al. reported that an inactivating germ-line *MSH6* mutation was present in 7 of 441 women with unselected endometrial cancer (1.6%). Cancers were diagnosed in women with mutations on average 10 years earlier than in women without mutations.

Most Lynch syndrome endometrial cancers have endometrioid histology, though 15% or more will be serous carcinoma, clear cell carcinoma, and carcinosarcomas. In one study, all of the nonendometrioid tumors occurred in patients with *MSH2* mutations. Lynch syndrome endometrial cancers are most commonly stage I and frequently have lower uterine segment involvement and tumor-infiltrating lymphocytes. Women with Lynch syndrome also have an approximate 5% to 10% lifetime risk for developing ovarian cancer. The ovarian cancers seen in Lynch syndrome are more likely to present at stage I and less likely to be of serous histology.

Clinical Care and Treatment

The majority of tumors from individuals from Lynch syndrome families demonstrate microsatellite instability (MSI). MSI is a feature of tumors that are genetically unstable, associated with error-prone DNA replication during cell division. Approximately one-quarter of women with nonhereditary endometrial cancer (sporadic cancer) have tumors that demonstrate MSI. If the mutation is present in the germline, it may be transmitted from parent to child. In this case, genetic counseling is warranted. It is not necessary that genetic counseling be undertaken when the mutation is limited to the tumor tissue only, as this situation does not pose a risk to relatives. Individuals with an inherited mutation in one of the mismatch repair genes are also at risk for additional cancers, including ovarian, gastric, urologic tract, and small bowel cancers, but the risk for these is much less than the risk of colon or endometrial cancer. In a study that examined 101 women with Lynch syndrome who had developed both GI cancer and gynecologic cancer, half of the women presented first with their gynecologic cancer.

While family history remains an important component in identifying individuals who may be at risk for Lynch syndrome, tumor testing for evidence of mismatch repair defects can be useful for triaging which patients may be at risk for having one of the germ-line DNA mismatch repair mutations. These tumor tests include immunohistochemistry (IHC) for one of the four mismatch repair proteins (*MLH1*, *MSH2*, *MSH6*, and *PMS2*) and MSI analysis. Although it has been suggested that it may be cost-effective to do these tests on all endometrial cancers, this approach has not yet been widely adopted. For IHC tests, the absence of a specific mismatch repair protein can focus sequencing efforts to a particular gene, which may reduce costs. Other screening approaches that are being employed at some centers include routine IHC testing of tumors in women who are under age 50 or who have tumors with morphologic features of DNA mismatch repair deficiency such as tumor infiltrating lymphocytes, lower uterine segment involvement, or dedifferentiated histology. As our understanding of the genomic and pathogenic manifestations of Lynch syndrome tumors expands, the system of screening will evolve.

There is currently no consensus on the screening and management of women with inherited mutations in the mismatch repair genes. No studies have examined the mortality impact of annual endometrial sampling in women with Lynch syndrome. Consensus guidelines currently recommend consideration of annual surveillance with endometrial biopsy for evaluation of the uterus, and transvaginal ultrasound for evaluation of the ovaries. The data to support these recommendations are limited. Because of the high lifetime risk of endometrial cancer in women with mutations in the mismatch repair genes, preventive hysterectomy should be considered. A multi-institutional retrospective study of women with Lynch syndrome demonstrated that the incidence of endometrial cancer fell from 33% to 0% in women who underwent hysterectomy, and the incidence of ovarian cancer fell from 5.4% to 0% in women who underwent salpingo-oophorectomy.

SUGGESTED READINGS

Boyd J, Sonoda Y, Federici MG, et al. Clinicopathologic features of *BRCA*-linked and sporadic ovarian cancer. *JAMA*. 2000;283:2260–2265.

Eisen A, Lubinski J, Klijn J, et al. Breast cancer risk following bilateral oophorectomy in *BRCA1* and *BRCA2* mutation carriers: An international case–control study. *J Clin Oncol*. 2005;23:7491–7496.

Finch A, Beiner M, Lubinski J, et al. Salpingo-oophorectomy and the risk of ovarian, fallopian tube and peritoneal cancers in women with a *BRCA1* or *BRCA2* mutation. *JAMA*. 2006;296:185–192.

Goodfellow PJ, Buttin BM, Herzog TJ, et al. Prevalence of defective DNA mismatch repair and MSH6 mutation in an unselected series of endometrial cancers. *Proc Natl Acad Sci U S A*. 2003;100:5908–5913.

Kauff ND, Mitra N, Robson ME, et al. Risk of ovarian cancer in BRCA1 and BRCA2 mutation-negative hereditary breast cancer families. *J Natl Cancer Inst*. 2005;97:1382–1384.

Kauff ND, Satagopan JM, Robson ME, et al. Risk-reducing salpingo-oophorectomy in women with a BRCA1 mutation. *N Engl J Med*. 2002;346:1609–1615.

Levine DA, Lin O, Barakat RR, et al. Risk of endometrial carcinoma associated with *BRCA* mutation. *Gynecol Oncol*. 2001;80:395–398.

Liede A, Karlan BY, Baldwin RL, et al. Cancer incidence in a population of Jewish women at risk of ovarian cancer. *J Clin Oncol*. 2002;20:1570–1577.

Moslehi R, Chu W, Karlan B, et al. *BRCA1* and *BRCA2* mutation analysis of 208 Ashkenazi Jewish women with ovarian cancer. *Am J Hum Genet*. 2000;66:1259–1272.

Narod SA, Risch H, Mosleh R, et al. Oral contraceptives and the risk of hereditary ovarian cancer. *N Engl J Med*. 1998;339:424–428.

Phelan CM, Kwan E, Jack E, et al. A low frequency of non-founder mutations in Ashkenazi Jewish breast-ovarian cancer families. *Hum Mutat*. 2002;20:352–357.

Piver MS, Jishi MF, Tsukada Y, et al. Primary peritoneal carcinoma after prophylactic oophorectomy in women with a family history of ovarian cancer. A report from the Gilda Radner Family Ovarian Cancer Registry. *Cancer*. 1993;71:2751–2755.

Powell CB, Kenley E, Chen LM, et al. Risk-reducing salpingo-oophorectomy in BRCA muta-tion carriers: Role of serial sectioning in the detection of occult disease. *J Clin Oncol.* 2005;23:127–132.

Rebbeck TR, Lynch HT, Neuhausen SL, et al. Prophylactic oophorectomy in carriers of *BRCA1* and *BRCA2* mutation. *N Engl J Med.* 2002;346:1616–1622.

Risch HA, McLaughlin JR, Cole DEC, et al. Prevalence and penetrance of germline BRCA1 and BRCA2 mutations in a population series of 649 women with ovarian cancer. *Am J Hum Genet.* 2001;68:700–710.

Thompson D, Easton D; Breast Cancer Linkage Consortium. Variation in cancer risks, by muta-tion position, in BRCA2 mutation carriers. *Am J Hum Genet.* 2001;68:410–419.

Whittemore AS, Balise RR, Pharoah PD, et al. Oral contraceptive use and ovarian cancer risk among carriers of BRCA1 or BRCA2 mutations. *Br J Cancer.* 2004;91:1911–1915.

4

Preinvasive Lesions of the Genital Tract

PATHOGENESIS AND DIAGNOSIS OF PREINVASIVE LESIONS OF THE LOWER GENITAL TRACT

The high level of public and professional interest in various aspects of preinvasive lesions of the lower genital tract is due to the increased knowledge surrounding pathogenesis and the availability of preventative vaccination. Perhaps, the most important is the marked increase over the last four decades in the number of patients in North America and Western Europe diagnosed with human papillomavirus (HPV)-associated disease. This increase is due partly to a heightened awareness of various clinical and pathologic manifestations of HPV infections and the increased use of highly sensitive tests for the detection of HPV infections and cervical cancer precursors. In addition, a real increase in the prevalence of HPV infections appears to have taken place during this time. Over half of men and women who are sexually active will be infected at some point in their lives.

Cervix—Squamous Lesions

For more than a century, it has been recognized that invasive squamous cell carcinomas of the cervix are associated with lesions that are histologically and cytologically identical to invasive cervical carcinoma but lack the capacity to invade the subepithelial stroma. These intraepithelial lesions were referred to as *carcinoma in situ*. It also became clear that there were squamous epithelial abnormalities whose histologic and cytologic features were less severe than carcinoma *in situ*. These lesions were referred to as *dysplasia* and were often divided into three grades: *mild*, *moderate*, or *severe*. Dysplastic lesions, carcinoma *in situ*, and invasive carcinoma form a continuum rather than a series of discrete steps. In 1973, based on follow-up studies of patients with cervical cancer precursor lesions and studies of the biology of these lesions, Richart proposed that the term *cervical intraepithelial neoplasia* (CIN) be used to encompass all forms of cervical cancer precursor lesions, including dysplasia and carcinoma *in situ*.

Cervix—Glandular Lesions

Interest in glandular lesions of the cervix has been stimulated by an apparent increase in the number of women, especially those under the age of 35, who are being diagnosed with invasive adenocarcinoma of the cervix and glandular precursor lesions. However, the absolute number of invasive adenocarcinomas has not actually increased when women of all age groups are combined. Instead, the number of women with invasive squamous cell carcinomas has decreased, producing a relative increase. It is important to note that although there is considerable evidence indicating that adenocarcinoma *in situ* (AIS) is a precursor for invasive adenocarcinoma of the cervix, there is little evidence to support such a role for the lower-grade glandular abnormalities. Though multifocal preinvasive glandular lesions or "skip lesions" do occur in 10% to 15% of cases, the majority are solitary.

Vulva and Vagina

The nomenclature used for preinvasive lesions of the vulva and vagina has tended to parallel that used for the cervix. In the 1980s, many clinicians and pathologists began to apply the intraepithelial neoplasia terminology widely used for describing cervical cancer precursors to the vulva. Thus, the term *vulvar intraepithelial neoplasia* (VIN), together with a grade of 1 to 3, was adopted. More recently, a two-category system has been adopted, with usual-type VIN being associated with HPV infection and generally less aggressive than differentiated VIN, which is not associated with HPV infection and more likely to progress to invasive carcinoma. Similarly, the term *vaginal intraepithelial neoplasia* (VAIN), together with a grade of 1 to 3, is widely used to describe preinvasive lesions of the vagina. It should be pointed out, however, that data that suggest a continuum between all grades of vaginal preinvasive lesions and invasive squamous cell carcinoma at these sites are significantly less compelling than that for the cervix.

NATURAL HISTORY OF PREINVASIVE LESIONS OF THE LOWER GENITAL TRACT

KEY POINTS
- Dysplasia is a precursor to invasive squamous cell carcinoma of the cervix.
- The time required for progression from dysplasia to carcinoma is controversial.
- A smaller portion of vulvar carcinomas arise from precursor lesions.

Cervix

A variety of epidemiologic and long-term follow-up studies support the concept that certain epithelial lesions are precursors of invasive squamous cell carcinoma of the cervix. A number of follow-up studies clearly demonstrate that, once established, carcinoma *in situ* has a significant potential for progression to invasive cancer (estimated at 30% if untreated), and progression is a slow process that usually requires a decade or more. Whether carcinoma *in situ*, once established, can spontaneously regress in the absence of therapy is controversial.

Many prospective studies have also followed the transitions between different grades of CIN. These studies have obtained quite different estimates of the frequency of mild dysplasia, the likelihood of progression from low-grade to high-grade precursors, and the time required for this progression. Until recently, it was generally believed that it took many years for a low-grade lesion to progress to a high-grade lesion. Mathematical modeling studies based on the prevalence of cytologic abnormalities in an unscreened

Table 4.1	Natural History of CIN Is Dependent on Lesional Grade		
	% Regression	% Persist	% Progress to CIS
CIN 1	57	32	11
CIN 2	43	35	22
CIN 3	32	56	12

population suggested that it takes on average almost 5 years for a mild dysplasia to progress to carcinoma *in situ*. More recent studies indicate, however, that high-grade lesions can develop quite rapidly after an incident HPV infection. A prospective study of college students found that the median length of time from the first detection of an HPV infection to the detection of CIN 2,3 was only 14.1 months. The finding that CIN 2,3 lesions can develop quite rapidly after initial HPV infections has been confirmed in the HPV vaccine trials. A systematic review of the different studies investigating the natural history of untreated biopsy-confirmed CIN, most of which were conducted in the 1970s and 1980s, found that the higher the grade of lesion, the more likely it is to persist and the less likely it is to regress (Table 4.1).

Vulva

Studies on the natural history of VIN lesions are much fewer than for CIN. Partly because of the paucity of studies, the relationships between VIN and invasive squamous cell carcinoma of the vulva appear to be less straightforward than those documented between CIN and invasive squamous cell carcinoma of the cervix. Unlike the cervix, in which the majority of carcinomas are associated with a CIN lesion, only a third of invasive vulvar squamous carcinomas have a coexisting VIN 3 lesion. A review of six published follow-up studies found that only 16 of 330 patients (4.8%) with VIN progressed to invasive cancer. What is generally not emphasized when the data are discussed is that most of the patients in these follow-up studies were treated for their VIN or followed for relatively short periods of time.

RISK FACTORS FOR THE DEVELOPMENT OF LOWER GENITAL TRACT CANCERS AND PREINVASIVE LESIONS OF THE LOWER GENITAL TRACT

KEY POINTS
- Smoking and number of sexual partners are the greatest risk factors for cervical cancer and its precursors.
- HPV infection is acquired through sexual contact and is necessary for the development of cervical cancer and its precursors.
- The majority of HPV-infected women spontaneously clear their infections within 1 to 2 years.

Cervix

Risk Factors

A large number of epidemiologic studies have analyzed risk factors for the development of cervical cancer and its precursors. Although the risk factors are similar for both cervical cancer and its precursors, the association with the risk factors is generally much stronger for cervical cancer than for precursor lesions. The major risk factors found in most studies are markers of sexual behavior such as number of sexual partners, early age of first pregnancy and first intercourse, sexually transmitted diseases, and parity. In addition, lower socioeconomic class, cigarette smoking, oral contraceptive use, specific HLA-DR haplotypes, and immunosuppression from any cause are associated with both cervical cancer and its precursors.

Human Papillomavirus

Over the last 15 years, considerable evidence has been accumulating rapidly to implicate HPV in the pathogenesis of cervical cancer and its preinvasive precursors. Epidemiologic and molecular studies have found that there is a consistent and strong relationship between HPV infection and cervical neoplasia, that the temporal sequence between the infection and the development of cancer is correct, that the association between HPV and cervical cancer is relatively specific, and that the epidemiologic findings are consistent with the natural history and biologic behavior of HPV infections and cervical cancer.

Epidemiologic studies clearly demonstrate that there is a strong and consistent association between specific types of HPV DNA and invasive cervical cancer and its precursor lesions and that exposure to HPV precedes the development of cervical disease. When combined with the enormous body of molecular evidence demonstrating a role for HPV in the development of cervical cancer and CIN, these findings clearly indicate that HPV infection, acquired through sexual contact, is a "necessary cause" of both CIN and invasive cervical cancer. Based on these data, the International Agency for Research on Cancer of the World Health Organization has classified HPV 16 and 18 and all of the other "high-risk" types of HPV as carcinogens in humans.

Smoking and Oral Contraceptives

In addition to risk factors associated with sexual behavior, several other risk factors such as low socioeconomic class and cigarette smoking have also been associated with the development of cervical cancer. The use of combined oral contraceptives has also been found to be a risk factor for the development of cervical cancer and its precursors in some studies. A recent reanalysis of epidemiologic studies involving over 50,000 women confirmed an increase risk of cervical cancer in oral contraceptive users, though the confounding effects of sexual behavior may not have been fully considered.

Immunosuppression

Immunosuppression is another risk factor for the development of both CIN and cervical cancer. In studies of patients with renal transplants, transplant recipients have a relative risk of 13.6 for the development of cervical carcinoma *in situ* compared to women in the general population. Over the last decade, it has become widely accepted that there is also an association between cervical disease and infection with the human immunodeficiency virus (HIV). Among women in New York City, the standardized incidence ratio for cervical cancer is 9.2 times higher in HIV-infected women compared to noninfected women. It is clear that the invasive cervical cancers that do develop in HIV-infected women act aggressively and respond poorly to standard forms of therapy. Invasive cervical cancer was designated in 1993 as an AIDS case–defining illness by the Centers for Disease Control and Prevention.

HUMAN PAPILLOMAVIRUS

Classification

Papillomaviruses are a diverse group of viruses that are widely distributed in mammals and birds. Papillomavirus isolates are traditionally described as *types*. The characteristic features of papillomaviruses are a double-stranded, circular DNA genome of about 8,000 base pairs, a nonenveloped virion, and an icosahedral capsid. To date, 118 papillomavirus types have been completely described. Over 30 types of HPV that infect the anogenital tract have been described. These different types of HPV tend to be associated with different types of lesions. HPV 6 and 11 are the most common HPV types found in association with exophytic condylomas of the male and female anogenital tracts in adults.

Almost half of all CIN 2,3 lesions are associated with HPV 16. A meta-analysis of the distribution of HPV types in CIN 2,3 lesions recently concluded that HPV 16 is identified in 45.3%, HPV 18 in 6.9%, and HPV 31 in 8.6%. Based on their associations with benign epithelial proliferations, high-grade cancer precursors, or invasive cancers of the vulva, vagina, anus, and cervix, HPVs can been categorized into "high risk" or "low risk" based on the relative risk of being associated with cancer (Table 4.2).

Table 4.2	Classification of Anogenital HPV Types
"Low-risk" types	6, 11, 40, 42, 43, 44, 53[a], 54, 61, 72, and 81
"High-risk" types	16, 18, 31, 33, 35, 39, 45, 51, 52, 56, 58, 59, 68, and 82
Possible high-risk types	26, 66, and 73

[a]Classified as "low risk" based on other data.
Reprinted with permission from: Munoz N, Bosch FX, de Sanjose S, et al. Epidemiologic classification of human papillomavirus types associated with cervical cancer. *N Engl J Med.* 2003;348:518.

PREVALENCE AND TRANSMISSION OF HPV INFECTIONS

The prevalence of genital tract HPV infections and the frequency of exposure to HPV in the general population vary widely in different studies. The recent National Health and Nutrition Examination Study (NHANES) found that the overall prevalence of HPV infection was 42.5% in women aged 14 to 49 years. The prevalence is highest in college-age women (Fig. 4.1). It is clear that the prevalence of HPV infection in the general population is consistently higher than the prevalence of CIN, by about one order of magnitude. The majority of women who are infected with HPV will never develop CIN 2,3 or cancer.

Both genital and nongenital HPV appear to be transmitted predominately through close "skin-to-skin" or "mucosa-to-mucosa" contact, and transmission is facilitated by minor trauma at the site of inoculation. The importance of sexual transmission is highlighted by studies of young women initiating sexual activity. In a study of 604 women attending a university, HPV DNA was detected by PCR in only 3% of women reporting no prior vaginal intercourse, 7% of women with 1 male sexual partner, 33% of women with 2 to 4 partners, and 53% of women with 5 or more male partners.

OUTCOME AFTER EXPOSURE TO HPV

Infection with a high-risk anogenital HPV in most women leads to a transient productive viral infection that lasts for a period of months to years. Approximately one third of these women develop low-grade cytologic or histologic changes. Nevertheless, the vast majority of HPV-infected women spontaneously clear their infections within 1 to 2 years. Clearance appears to be mediated by cellular immune responses. Prospective follow-up studies

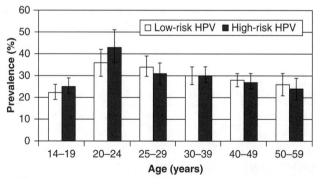

FIGURE 4.1 US prevalence of HPV infections in women. *Source:* Reprinted with permission from Harir S, Unger ER, Sternberg M, et al. Prevalence of genital human papillomavirus in the United States, the National Health and Nutrition Examination Survey, 2003–2006. *J Infect Dis.* 2011;204:566–573.

Table 4.3		**HPV Persistence**			
Study	Year	Average Age	Type of Infection	HPV Persistence at 1 year	HPV Persistence at ~2 years
Richardson et al.	2003	23	Incident, high risk	61%	X
Ho et al.	1998	20	Incident, high and low risk	30%	9%
Dalstein et al.	2003	32	Prevalent, high risk	60%	50%
Bae et al.	2009	48	Prevalent, high risk	X	41%

Sources: Richardson H, et al. The natural history of type-specific human papillomavirus infections in female university students. *Cancer Epidemiol Biomarkers Prev.* 2003;12:485–490; Ho GY, et al. Natural history of cervicovaginal papillomavirus infection in young women. *N Engl J Med.* 1998;338:423–428; Dalstein V, et al. Persistence and load of high-risk HPV are predictors for development of high-grade cervical lesions: A longitudinal French cohort study. *Int J Cancer.* 2003;106:396–403; Bae J, et al. Natural history of persistent high-risk human papillomavirus infections in Korean women. *Gynecol Oncol.* 2009;115:75–80.

report that less than 20% of women remain DNA positive after 24 months of follow-up (Table 4.3).

It is currently unknown what proportion of women who appear to spontaneously clear their HPV infections and become HPV DNA negative truly clear the infection from the anogenital tract and what proportion continue to have a latent, undetectable HPV infection.

Reactivation of latent infections could explain the increase in the prevalence of HPV among cytologically negative older women (Fig. 4.2).

Although spontaneous clearance can continue to occur even after 24 months, clinically significant persistent infections should probably be defined as infections that last at least 2 years. Long-term, stable persistent infections appear to occur in only about 10% of infected individuals. Although newer studies suggest that CIN 2,3 lesions can develop within a relatively short period of time after initial infection, lesions that do not persist for at least 2 years are unlikely to have clinical significance.

CYTOLOGIC SCREENING FOR CERVICAL CANCER AND ITS PRECURSORS

KEY POINTS
- Cervical cytology has reduced the incidence of cervical cancer by almost 80% in the United States.
- Cervical screening should begin at age 21 years regardless of age at first sexual intercourse.
- Liquid-based Pap smears have the advantage of providing reflex HPV testing in women with atypical squamous cells of undetermined significance (ASCUS).

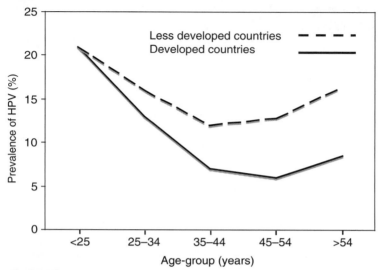

FIGURE 4.2 Estimate of prevalence of HPV DNA positivity in women with normal cervical cytology. The estimate is based on a meta-analysis that included published studies from all regions of the world. *Source:* Adapted with permission from de Sanjose S, Diaz M, Casellsague X, et al. Worldwide prevalence and genotype distribution of cervical HPV DNA in women with normal cytology: A metaanalysis. *Lancet Infect Dis.* 2007;7(7): 453–459.

Cytology-based cervical cancer screening programs were first introduced in the mid-20th century and are now widely recognized as being able to reduce both the incidence of, and mortality from, invasive cervical cancer. Strong evidence for their effectiveness comes from a comparison of incidence and mortality trends of invasive cervical cancer with screening activity in a given country or region.

Accuracy of Cervical Cytology

Despite the proven effectiveness of cervical cytology in reducing the incidence of cervical cancer, over the last several years, the accuracy of cervical cytology has been questioned. However, when the cytologic cutoff is low-grade squamous intraepithelial lesion (LSIL) and the end point is biopsy-confirmed CIN 2,3 or worse, the average sensitivity is 81% and the specificity is 77%.

A number of factors influence the false-negative rate of cervical cytology. Since the majority of CIN and cancers involve the transformation zone, sampling devices have been specifically designed to sample this area. Sampling the endocervical canal reduces the false-negative rate. This sample can be taken with an endocervical brush (e.g., cytobrush) or one of the newer collection devices such as a cell broom. Saline-moistened cotton-tipped applicators should not be used. Other important factors for reducing the false-negative rate are the rapid fixation of cells to prevent artifactual changes secondary to air-drying and the use of a cytology laboratory with stringent quality control standards.

The use of cervical cytology has reduced the incidence of cervical cancer by almost 80% in the United States over the last three decades. The effectiveness of cervical cytology is attributable to the fact that invasive cervical cancer requires many years to develop from a CIN 2,3 lesion. If cervical cytology is performed on a routine basis, it is unlikely that a CIN 2,3 lesion will remain undetected, although such cases do rarely occur. The current unified screening recommendation from various professional societies including the American Cancer Society, the American College of Obstetricians and Gynecologists and the American Society for Colposcopy and Cervical Pathology is that cervical cancer screening should be initiated at age 21 years regardless of the age at first sexual intercourse or other risk factors. Screening should occur every three years if normal without HPV co-testing until age 30. After 30 years of age, the interval between cervical cytology examinations can be extended to 5 years with co-testing including both cytology and HPV. There is general consensus that screening may stop after age 65 in women with adequate negative prior screens. Routine screening is not recommended for women who have undergone a hysterectomy for benign indications and who have no prior history of CIN 2,3.

Liquid-Based Cytology

Liquid-based cytology (LBC) is now widely used in the United States for cervical cytology. A major reappraisal of the performance of LBC is under way in the screening community. When it was first introduced, LBC was believed to provide a significant advantage compared to conventional cervical cytology with respect to sensitivity for the identification of women with CIN 2,3 or cancer. However, most of the studies that compared LBC with conventional cytology had methodologic problems. When all of the studies are taken into account and combined, there is no evidence that LBC reduced the proportion of unsatisfactory slides nor that it has better performance than conventional cytology with respect to the identification of women with CIN 2,3.

There is no evidence that LBC is either more sensitive or more specific than conventional cytology. However, there are other advantages of LBC. The greatest of these appears to be the availability of residual fluid for "reflex" HPV testing in women with ACS of undetermined significance (ASC-US) as well as testing for other pathogens such as *Chlamydia*. Moreover, almost all cytologists agree that it is easier to evaluate LBC specimens than conventional cytology specimens and it is unlikely that cytology laboratories will want to switch back to conventional cytology now that the conversion to LBC has taken place.

HPV Testing Alone

Cotesting is a recommended approach to cervical cancer screening using a combination of Pap smear and HPV testing. The use of HPV testing alone, without concurrent Pap, has been demonstrated to have slightly better detection rates and associations with future development of CIN.

In 2012, the American Society for Colposcopy and Cervical Pathology (ASCCP) did not endorse HPV testing alone since the sensitivity is only slightly better than cotesting, the specificity is not clear, and an assessment of specimen adequacy is not possible. However, in April 2014, the FDA approved HPV testing alone as a screening method to determine which women require additional diagnostic testing. The press release indicates that women with HPV 16 or 18 subtypes should be referred for immediate colposcopy, women with other high-risk subtypes should have a Pap smear performed, and women with negative HPV testing can have routine screening.

Terminology of Cytology Reports

The Bethesda system terminology is used for reporting cervical cytology results in the United States. The Bethesda system underwent significant modifications in 2001 (Table 4.4). The major features of the 2001 Bethesda system are that it requires (i) an estimate of the adequacy of the specimen for diagnostic evaluation; (ii) a general categorization of the specimen as being "negative for intraepithelial lesion or malignancy," as having an "epithelial cell abnormality," or as "other" (i.e., having endometrial cells in a woman 40 years of age and older); and (iii) a descriptive diagnosis that includes a description of epithelial cell abnormalities. The terms LSIL and *high-grade squamous intraepithelial lesion* (HSIL) are used to designate cytologic changes that correlate with CIN 1 and CIN 2,3, respectively. In addition, the Bethesda system attempts to separate epithelial changes secondary to inflammation or repair from those associated with cervical cancer precursors whenever possible. Nondiagnostic squamous cell abnormalities are included in a category of *atypical squamous cells* (ASC). ASC is used when a specimen has features suggestive, but not diagnostic, of an SIL. This category is further subdivided into two subcategories: ASC-US and ASC—cannot exclude HSIL (ASC-H). The risk of a woman with ASC-US having biopsy-confirmed CIN 2,3 is approximately 7% to 17%, and the risk for a woman with ASC-H is approximately 40%. Nondiagnostic glandular cell abnormalities are included in a category of *atypical glandular cells* (AGC). This category is further subdivided into either *not otherwise specified* or *AGC—favor neoplasia*.

USE OF COLPOSCOPY

Over the last 25 years, colposcopy combined with colposcopically directed cervical biopsies have become the primary modality by which women with abnormal Pap smears are evaluated. Colposcopic examination consists of viewing the cervix with a long-focal-length, dissecting-type microscope after a solution of dilute (4%) acetic acid has been applied to the cervix. The acetic acid solution acts to remove and dissolve the cervical mucus and causes CIN lesions to become whiter than the surrounding epithelium (acetowhite) by dehydrating the cells. This coloration allows the colposcopist to identify and biopsy epithelial lesions. In addition to allowing the detection of acetowhite areas, colposcopy also allows for the detection of blood

Table 4.4	The 2001 Bethesda System

SPECIMEN ADEQUACY

Satisfactory for evaluation (*note presence/absence of endocervical transformation zone component*)
Unsatisfactory for evaluation (*specify reason*)
Specimen rejected/not processed (*specify reason*)
Specimen processed and examined but unsatisfactory for evaluation of epithelial abnormality because of (*specify reason*)

GENERAL CATEGORIZATION (OPTIONAL)

Negative for intraepithelial lesion or malignancy
Epithelial cell abnormality
Other

INTERPRETATION/RESULT

Negative for intraepithelial lesion or malignancy
Organisms
    Trichomonas vaginalis
    Fungal organisms morphologically consistent with *Candida* species
    Shift in flora suggestive of bacterial vaginosis
    Bacteria morphologically consistent with *Actinomyces* species
    Cellular changes consistent with herpes simplex virus
    Other nonneoplastic findings (*optional to report; list not comprehensive*)
    Reactive cellular changes associated with inflammation (includes typical repair)
    Radiation
    Intrauterine contraceptive device
    Glandular cells status posthysterectomy
    Atrophy

Epithelial cell abnormalities
Squamous cell
    ASC-US; cannot exclude HSIL (ASC-H)
    LSIL
    HSIL
    Squamous cell carcinoma

Glandular cell
    AGC (*specify endocervical, endometrial, or not otherwise specified*)
    AGCs, favor neoplastic (*specify endocervical or not otherwise specified*)
    Endocervical AIS
    Adenocarcinoma

Other (*list not comprehensive*)
    Endometrial cells in a woman ≥40 y of age

Reprinted with permission from Solomon D, Davey D, Kurman R, et al. The 2001 Bethesda System: Terminology for reporting results of cervical cytology. *JAMA.* 2002;287:2114.

vessel patterns that can indicate high-grade CIN lesions and the detection of invasive cancers. Colposcopy and appropriately directed biopsy have greatly facilitated the management of patients with preinvasive lesions of the cervix because it allows the clinician to rule out invasive cancer and determine the limits of preinvasive disease.

MANAGEMENT OF CYTOLOGIC ABNORMALITIES AND CIN

KEY POINTS

- Complete recommendations and management algorithms are available at www.asccp.org.
- Over 90% of LSIL will spontaneously clear in adolescents.
- A diagnosis of HSIL confers a significant risk for CIN 2,3 and invasive cervical cancer.

In 2006, the ASCCP sponsored a consensus workshop to update the 2001 Consensus Guidelines for the Management of Women with Cytological Abnormalities and Cervical Cancer Precursors. In 2012, the ASCCP worked with 23 other national organizations on a revision of the 2006 guidelines for management of abnormal screening tests and CIN/AIS. These guidelines are widely used in the United States and are evidence based, with each recommendation accompanied by a grading of both the strength of the recommendation and the strength of the data supporting the recommendation. The complete recommendations and management algorithms are available at www.asccp.org.

Atypical Squamous Cells of Undetermined Significance

A vexing group of patients for both clinicians and cytologists are those whose cervical cytology is atypical (i.e., not normal) but lack the characteristic features of SIL or cancer. Clinicians need to be aware that a cytologic result of ASC-US is the least reproducible cytologic category. Overall, it appears that approximately one half of all women diagnosed as having CIN 2,3 have ASC-US as their initial abnormal cervical cytology result due to the high prevalence of this diagnostic category. Although the risk that a woman with ASC-US has invasive cervical cancer is quite low (about 1/1,000), the very large number of women with this cytology interpretation (2.3 million annually) guarantees that each year approximately 2,300 women with invasive cervical cancer will have only equivocal results on their cervical cytology (Fig. 4.3). Therefore, women with ASC-US need to receive some form of follow-up evaluation, but consideration should be given to preventing unnecessary inconvenience, anxiety, cost, and discomfort.

Two methods are recommended for the management of women with ASC-US. These are HPV DNA testing or repeat cervical cytology. The option of immediate colposcopy is no longer recommended. A number of studies have directly compared the sensitivity and specificity of repeat cervical cytology and HPV DNA testing for identifying women with CIN 2,3. In every single study, HPV DNA testing identified more cases of CIN 2,3 than did a single repeat cervical cytology but referred approximately equivalent numbers of women for colposcopy. The 2012 ASCCP Consensus Conference concluded that HPV DNA testing is the preferred approach to managing women with ASC-US. Figure 4.4 provides the algorithm recommended for the management of women in the general population with ASC-US. For women aged 21 to 24 years, repeat cytology at 12 months is recommended over reflex HPV testing.

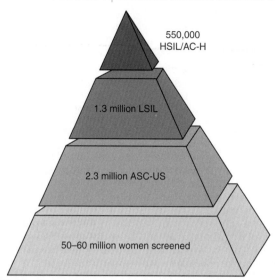

FIGURE 4.3 Distribution of abnormal cervical cytology. *Source:* Adapted with permission from Davey DD, Neal MH, Wilbur DC, et al. Bethesda 2001 implementation and reporting rates: 2003 practices of participants in the College of American Pathologists Interlaboratory Comparison Program in Cervicovaginal Cytology. *Arch Pathol Lab Med.* 2004;128:1224–1229.

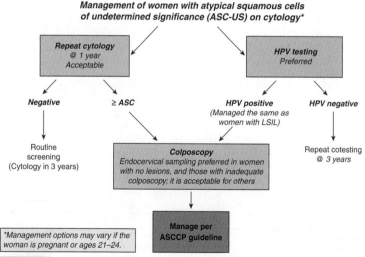

FIGURE 4.4 ASCCP guidelines for the management of women with atypical squamous cells of undetermined significance (ACS-US) on cytology. *Source:* Reprinted with permission from Massad LS, Einstein MH, Huh WK, et al. 2012 updated consensus guidelines for the management of abnormal cervical cancer screening tests and cancer precursors. *J Low Genit Tract Dis.* 2013;17(5 suppl 1):S1–S27.

The prevalence of HPV DNA positivity is much higher in young women with ASC-US than in older women. Therefore, the 2012 Consensus Guidelines do not recommend the use of HPV DNA testing in women aged 21 to 29 years. The recent guidelines also do not recommend screening in women under 21 years regardless of sexual activity or other risk factors. Management options for pregnant patients with ASC-US are identical to those for nonpregnant patients with the exception that it is acceptable to defer the colposcopic examination until the patient is 6 to 8 weeks postpartum and endocervical curettage (ECC) is unacceptable.

Atypical Squamous Cells—Cannot Exclude HSIL

The prevalence of biopsy-confirmed CIN 2,3 is considerably higher among women referred for the evaluation of an ASC-H cervical cytology than it is for women referred for the evaluation of ASC-US. Therefore, for the purposes of management, colposcopy is recommended regardless of HPV status, which is not necessary or useful. If CIN is not identified following an adequate colposcopy with negative ECC, follow-up utilizing repeat cytology with HPV testing at 6 and 12 months or an excisional procedure are recommended. For women aged 21 to 24 years, adequate colposcopy with cytology is recommended every 6 months for 2 years.

Low-Grade Squamous Intraepithelial Lesions

As with ASC-US, there is considerable variation between populations and laboratories in the rate at which LSIL is reported. A cytologic result of LSIL is a very specific indicator of the presence of high-risk types of HPV. In ALTS, approximately 80% of the women referred for the evaluation of LSIL were high-risk HPV DNA positive. However, a cytologic result of LSIL is a poor predictor of the grade of CIN that will be identified at colposcopy. CIN 2,3 is identified at colposcopy in approximately 25% of women with LSIL on cervical cytology. Therefore, the 2012 Consensus Guidelines recommend that all women in the general population with a cytologic result of LSIL be referred for a colposcopic evaluation (Fig. 4.5). This allows women with significant disease to be rapidly identified and reduces the risk of women being lost to follow-up. A diagnostic excisional procedure is not required when a woman with LSIL cytology is found to have an unsatisfactory colposcopic examination. For women with LSIL who have had cotesting as part of standard screening and are found to be HPV negative, repeat cotesting at 1 year is preferred.

The risk of invasive cervical cancer is very low in young women, and prospective studies have shown that over 90% of LSIL will spontaneously clear over a period of years. Therefore, women aged 21 to 29 years with LSIL are considered to be a "special population," and it is now recommended that they should have repeat cotesting yearly for a period of 2 years. Another "special population" is postmenopausal women with LSIL. In some studies, the prevalence of HPV DNA in postmenopausal women with LSIL is lower than in premenopausal women, and the prevalence of CIN 2,3 also declines in postmenopausal women with LSIL. Therefore, the 2012 Consensus Guidelines indicate that postmenopausal women with LSIL without HPV testing can have repeat cytology at 6 and 12 months

Management of women with low-grade squamous intraepithelial lesions (LSIL)*

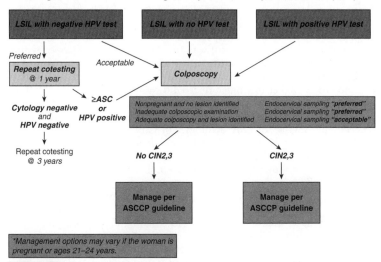

FIGURE 4.5 ASCCP guidelines for the management of women with low-grade squamous intraepithelial lesions (LSIL). *Source:* Reprinted with permission from Massad LS, Einstein MH, Huh WK, et al. 2012 updated consensus guidelines for the management of abnormal cervical cancer screening tests and cancer precursors. *J Low Genit Tract Dis.* 2013;17(5 suppl 1):S1–S27.

or HPV testing. For pregnant women with LSIL, colposcopy is preferred without ECC unless the woman is aged 21 to 24 years.

High-Grade Squamous Intraepithelial Lesions

The cytologic result of HSIL is uncommon, accounting for only about 0.7% of all cervical cytology results, but the prevalence varies with age. A diagnosis of HSIL confers a significant risk for CIN 2,3 and invasive cervical cancer. CIN 2,3 or cancer has been identified at a single colposcopic examination in approximately 60% of women with HSIL and in approximately 90% of those evaluated using a loop electrosurgical excisional procedure (LEEP). Invasive cervical cancer is identified in approximately 2% of women with HSIL. Therefore, women with a cytologic result of HSIL should be referred for either a colposcopic evaluation or an immediate LEEP. Subsequent management depends on whether or not the patient is pregnant, aged 21 to 24 years, and whether the colposcopic examination is satisfactory.

Biopsy-Confirmed CIN 1

Women with a histologically confirmed CIN 1 lesion represent a heterogeneous group. A number of studies have clearly demonstrated a high level of variability in the histologic diagnosis of CIN 1. In ALTS, only 43% of biopsies that were originally diagnosed as CIN 1 at the clinical centers were subsequently classified as CIN 1 by the reference pathology committee. Forty-one percent were downgraded to normal, and 13% were upgraded to CIN 2,3. There is a very high rate of spontaneous regress of CIN 1 in the absence of treatment. One prospective Brazilian study found that 90% of women with a cytologic diagnosis of LSIL spontaneously regressed within 24 months. Recent studies indicate that CIN 1 only rarely progresses to CIN 2,3. Since the risk of an undetected CIN 2,3 or glandular lesion is expected to be higher in women referred for the evaluation of an HSIL or AGC on cytology, women with CIN 1 preceded by ASC-H or HSIL cervical cytology can be managed more aggressively than women with CIN 1 preceded by ASC-US or LSIL cytology. For CIN 1 preceded by ASC-H or HSIL, cotesting at 12 and 24 months or a diagnostic excision procedure is recommended. For CIN 1 preceded by ASC-US or LSIL, cotesting at 12 months can be followed by return to routine screening if both tests are normal.

If CIN 1 persists for at least 2 years, either continued follow-up or treatment is acceptable. Randomized controlled clinical trials comparing cryotherapy, laser ablation, and LEEP for treating biopsy-confirmed CIN have reported no significant differences in either complication rates or success rates. Before treating any grade of CIN using an ablative modality such as cryotherapy, it is important to perform an endocervical sampling in order to assure that an unsuspected lesion is not present in the endocervical canal. Cryotherapy can make subsequent monitoring more challenging.

Biopsy-Confirmed CIN 2,3

Women with an untreated histologically confirmed CIN 2,3 lesion are felt to have a significantly high risk of progressing to invasive cervical cancer to warrant routine treatment. Initial treatment may involve an excisional or ablative procedure. In patients with recurrent CIN (either CIN 1 or CIN 2,3), it is preferred that an excisional treatment modality be used. A diagnostic excisional procedure is recommended for all women with biopsy-confirmed CIN 2,3 and an unsatisfactory colposcopic examination. The risk of recurrent CIN 2,3 or invasive cancer after treatment remains elevated for many years after treatment. The 2012 Consensus Guidelines recommend that after treatment for CIN 2,3, women be followed up using cotesting at 12 and 24 months. If any test is abnormal, colposcopy with ECC is recommended. After two negative cytology results are obtained, repeat testing at 3 years followed by routine screening is recommended. When CIN is identified at the margins of a diagnostic excisional procedure, a 4- to 6-month follow-up visit with cytology with endocervical sampling is recommended.

Atypical Glandular Cells and Adenocarcinoma *In Situ*

Patients with AGC are at risk for both cervical and endometrial abnormalities. For women under age 35, colposcopy with ECC should be performed. For women older than 35 or any women with abnormal vaginal bleeding in the setting of AGC, an endometrial biopsy should also be performed. For women with AGC–NOS, who are not found to have high-risk findings, cotesting at 12 and 24 months is recommended. For high-grade (CIN 2+)

squamous lesions, standard recommendations can be followed. For negative findings after AGC favor neoplasia or AIS on Pap smear, a diagnostic excisional procedure is recommended.

Patients with biopsy-proven AIS are known to have both multifocal disease and a risk of invasive adenocarcinoma when thoroughly sampled. Therefore, excision is required for all patients, and due to the risk of invasive disease and an average failure rate of 8% for conservative treatment, failure is defined as recurrent AIS or invasive disease. Hysterectomy is the preferred treatment of choice but must be preceded by an excisional biopsy that can reasonably exclude invasion that might require a more radical procedure. For women desiring fertility preservation, a cold knife cone biopsy with negative margins is an acceptable alternative, though other forms of excision procedures may be considered as long as they produce a specimen that is not fragmented.

Vulvar and Vaginal Intraepithelial Neoplasia

VIN and VAIN require more individualization and creativity in treatment. Most VIN is detected at the time of biopsy for a suspicious lesion; therefore, definitive treatment should be complete excision, although positive margins for a low-grade lesion could be observed. Higher-grade VIN should be completely excised with negative margins; however, laser ablation would be an acceptable alternative. VAIN treatment must be more tailored to the disease location and patient. In general, VAIN should be treated, though low-grade lesions could be followed akin to biopsy-proven CIN 1. VAIN 2,3 should be treated, and simple excision is the preferred method as it provides a specimen in which to rule out invasive disease. Topical treatment with intravaginal 5-FU has been used; however, it is associated with serious adverse events and is not recommended as an initial choice of therapy. Laser ablation is a reasonable alternative to excision for diffuse lesions or lesions in regions that are challenging to resect.

HPV VACCINATION

KEY POINTS
- Prophylactic vaccination is an important element in cervical cancer prevention.
- HPV vaccination is recommended in girls between ages 9 and 26 and boys ages 9 and 22.
- HPV vaccination is nearly 100% effective against target subtypes and has cross-coverage against some off-target subtypes.
- HPV vaccination, at present, is not therapeutic and is much less effective in people with preexisting infection.

Infection with HPV is necessary for the development of almost all preinvasive cervical and vaginal lesions, and it is present in roughly half of preinvasive vulvar disease. It is the most commonly diagnosed sexually transmitted disease, with an overall lifetime prevalence of 80% and a point prevalence of 40%. With our current understanding of the role of HPV in preinvasive and invasive disease, prophylactic vaccination has emerged as an important element in cervical cancer prevention. Currently, two vaccines are approved in the United States for the prevention of cervical cancer. The quadrivalent vaccine (Merck & Co., Inc., Whitehouse Station, NJ, USA) contains virus-like particles (VLPs) to HPV types 6, 11, 16, and 18. The bivalent vaccine (GlaxoSmithKline, Rixensart, Belgium) contains VLPs to HPV types 16 and 18.

The FDA originally approved the quadrivalent vaccine in 2006 for girls and women aged between 15 and 25 years for the prevention of cervical cancer caused by HPV types 16 and 18; precancerous genital lesions caused by HPV types 6, 11, 16, and 18; and genital warts caused by HPV types 6 and 11. The federal advisory committee on immunization practices (ACIP) recommends routine vaccination of all 11- and 12-year-old girls. The three-shot vaccination series can begin as young as age 9 and can be given to women up to age 26. In 2008, the quadrivalent vaccine was also approved for the prevention of vaginal and vulvar cancer in this same population. The following year, its use was expanded to the prevention of genital warts due to HPV type 6 and 11 in boys and men aged between 15 and 25. The FDA further expanded the indications to include the prevention of anal cancer and associated premalignant lesions caused by these same HPV types. The ACIP recommends routine vaccination of all 11- and 12-year-old boys. The ACIP recommendations for the bivalent vaccine mirror those for the quadrivalent vaccine, except the bivalent vaccine is not approved for use in males.

In an international trial, the quadrivalent vaccine was 99% effective in preventing HPV 16 and 18 preinvasive or invasive lesions in women who were HPV naive at baseline. In the 4-year follow-up of a bivalent HPV vaccine trial, efficacy against HPV 16– and HPV 18–mediated CIN 3 lesions was 100% in women who were HPV negative at the time of vaccination. The vaccine was also effective against other lesions caused by HPV types 31, 33, and 45, which are closely related to HPV 16 and 18. Specifically, in women who were HPV negative at the time of vaccination, there was 93% efficacy against all CIN 3, irrespective of HPV type, as well as 100% efficacy against all AIS. High rates of efficacy even in non–HPV 16– or non–HPV 18–mediated lesions suggest that the vaccine's effects may be more far-reaching. HPV vaccination has not been shown to be therapeutic against preexisting HPV infections. Therefore, the HPV vaccine is most effective if it is administered prior to the onset of sexual activity.

SUGGESTED READINGS

Appleby P, Beral V, Berrington de Gonzalez A, et al. Cervical cancer and hormonal contraceptives: Collaborative reanalysis of individual data for 16,573 women with cervical cancer and 35,509 women without cervical cancer from 24 epidemiological studies. *Lancet.* 2007;370:1609.

Arbyn M, Bergeron C, Klinkhamer P, et al. Liquid compared with conventional cervical cytology: A systematic review and meta-analysis. *Obstet Gynecol.* 2008;111:167.

de Sanjose S, Diaz M, Castellsague X, et al. Worldwide prevalence and genotype distribution of cervical human papillomavirus DNA in women with normal cytology: A meta-analysis. *Lancet Infect Dis.* 2007;7:453.

Massad LS, Einstein MH, Huh WK, et al. 2012 updated consensus guidelines for the management of abnormal cervical cancer screening tests and cancer precursors. *J Low Genit Tract Dis.* 2013;17(5, suppl 1):S1–S27.

Munoz N, Bosch FX, de Sanjose S, et al. Epidemiologic classification of human papillomavirus types associated with cervical cancer. *N Engl J Med.* 2003;348:518.

Richardson H, Kelsall G, Tellier P, et al. The natural history of type-specific human papillomavirus infections in female university students. *Cancer Epidemiol Biomarkers Prev.* 2003;12:485.

Saslow D, Solomon D, Lawson HW, et al. American Cancer Society, American Society for Colposcopy and Cervical Pathology, and American Society for Clinical Pathology screening guidelines for the prevention and early detection of cervical cancer. *J Low Genit Tract Dis.* 2012;16(3):175–204.

Sideri M, Jones RW, Wilkinson EJ, et al. Squamous vulvar intraepithelial neoplasia; 2004 modified terminology. ISSVD Vulvar Oncology Subcommittee. *J Reprod Med.* 2005;50:807.

Solomon D, Davey D, Kurman R, et al. The 2001 Bethesda System: Terminology for reporting results of cervical cytology. *JAMA.* 2002;287:2114.

Solomon D, Schiffman M, Tarrone R. Comparison of three management strategies for patients with atypical squamous cells of undetermined significance: Baseline results from a randomized trial. *J Natl Cancer Inst.* 2001;93:293.

Stoler MH, Schiffman M. Interobserver reproducibility of cervical cytologic and histologic interpretations: Realistic estimates from the ASCUS-LSIL Triage Study. *JAMA.* 2001;285:1500.

The Atypical Squamous Cells of Undetermined Significance/Low-Grade Squamous Intraepithelial Lesions Triage Study (ALTS) Group. Human papillomavirus testing for triage of women with cytologic evidence of low-grade squamous intraepithelial lesions: Baseline data from a randomized trial. *J Natl Cancer Inst.* 2000;92:397.

Winer RL, Hughes JP, Feng Q, et al. Condom use and the risk of genital human papillomavirus infection in young women. *N Engl J Med.* 2006;354:2645.

Winer RL, Kiviat NB, Hughes JP, et al. Development and duration of human papillomavirus lesions, after initial infection. *J Infect Dis.* 2005;191:731.

5 The Vulva

Malignant tumors of the vulva account for 5% of all cancers of the female genital tract, with an estimated 4,700 new cases and 990 deaths occurring in 2013. The majority of women with vulva cancer initially present with symptoms most commonly reported as irritation, pruritus, pain, or a mass lesion that does not resolve. Less common symptoms include vulvar bleeding or discharge, dysuria, or an enlarged groin lymph node. Diagnosis is frequently delayed due to a combination of patient and physician factors, with one report noting 88% of patients had experienced symptoms for more than 6 months prior to diagnosis. While the traditional therapeutic approach to vulva cancer has been radical surgical excision of the primary tumor and inguinal femoral lymph nodes, a more tailored individualized approach to vulva cancer management, often employing multiple modalities in an effort to achieve excellent disease control with better cosmetic results and sexual function, is now the norm.

HISTOLOGY

The majority (>90%) of malignant vulva tumors are squamous cell carcinomas (SCC), with malignant melanoma being the second most common histology. Basal cell carcinoma, adenocarcinomas (derived from the Bartholin gland, eccrine sweat glands, Paget disease, or ectopic breast tissue), and a host of very rare soft tissue sarcomas including leiomyosarcomas, malignant fibrous histiocytomas, liposarcomas, angiosarcomas, rhabdomyosarcomas, epithelioid sarcomas, and Kaposi sarcomas may also arise on the vulva. Finally, the vulva may be secondarily involved with malignant disease originating in the bladder, anorectum, or other genital organs.

ANATOMY

The vulva consists of the external genital organs including the mons pubis, labia minora and majora, clitoris, vaginal vestibule, perineal body, and their supporting subcutaneous tissues. The Bartholin glands, two small mucus-secreting glands, have ducts opening onto the posterolateral portion of the vestibule. The perineal body is a 3- to 4-cm band of skin and subcutaneous tissue located between the posterior extensions of the labia majora and the anus; it forms the posterior margin of the vulva.

The vulva has a rich blood supply derived primarily from the internal pudendal artery and the superficial and deep external pudendal arteries. The innervation of the vulva is derived from L1 (ilioinguinal nerve), L1–2 (genitofemoral nerve), and S2–4 (pudendal nerves). The vulva lymphatics run anteriorly through the labia majora, turn laterally at the mons pubis,

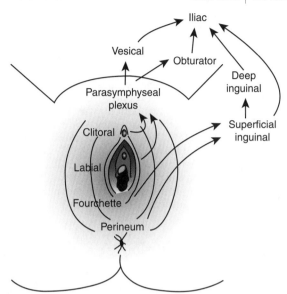

FIGURE 5.1 The lymphatic drainage of the vulva initially flows to the superficial inguinal nodes and then to the deep femoral and iliac groups. Drainage from midline structures may flow directly beneath the symphysis to the pelvic nodes. *Source*: Modified from DiSaia PJ, Creasman WT, Rich WM. An alternative approach to early cancer of the vulva. *Am J Obstet Gynecol.* 1979;133:825.

and drain primarily into the superficial inguinal lymph nodes. The vulva lymphatic channels do not cross the midline, unless the site of dye injection is in midline structures (the clitoris or perineal body). Drainage from midline lesions could be bilateral. Several small lymphatics may drain from the clitoris under the pubic symphysis directly into the pelvic nodes. The superficial inguinal lymph nodes are located within the femoral triangle, which is formed by the inguinal ligament superiorly, the border of the sartorius muscle laterally, and the border of the adductor longus muscle medially. Lymphatic drainage proceeds from the superficial to the deep inguinal (or femoral) nodes and then into the pelvic lymph node basin (Fig. 5.1). There are usually three to five deep nodes, the most superior of which is Cloquet node located under the inguinal ligament.

EPIDEMIOLOGY

KEY POINTS
- Vulvar cancer is more common in menopausal women.
- Human papillomavirus (HPV) is found in 55% to 60% of invasive tumors.
- All suspicious lesions should be biopsied in the office.
- Vulvar dystrophies may be precursor lesions of invasive disease.

Most vulvar cancers occur in postmenopausal women, although more recent reports suggest a trend toward younger age at diagnosis. Risk factors for vulvar cancer include a history of genital condylomata, a previously abnormal Papanicolaou smear, a history of smoking, and chronic immunosuppression. Both chronic vulvar inflammatory lesions, such as vulvar dystrophy or lichen sclerosus, and squamous intraepithelial lesions, particularly *carcinoma in situ*, have been suggested as precursors of invasive squamous cancers.

HPV DNA has been isolated from both invasive and carcinoma *in situ* lesions, with HPV type 16 being the most common subtype. Insinga and colleagues have reported that HPV DNA can be identified in approximately 80% to 90% of intraepithelial lesions, and 50% to 60% of invasive lesions. The rising incidence of HPV-related vulvar intraepithelial neoplasia (VIN) among young women may explain the trend toward younger age at diagnosis of invasive vulvar cancers. Other infectious agents that have been proposed as possible etiologic agents in vulvar carcinoma include granulomatous infections and herpes simplex virus.

CLINICAL PRESENTATION

Most women with vulvar cancer present with pruritus and a recognizable lesion. Optimal management for any patient presenting with a suspicious lesion is to proceed directly to biopsy under local analgesia. Tissue biopsies should include the cutaneous lesion in question and contiguous underlying stroma so that the presence and depth of invasion can be accurately assessed. The goals of immediate evaluation with outpatient biopsy are to avoid delay in the planning of appropriate therapy. The presentation in advanced disease is generally dominated by local pain, bleeding, and surface drainage from the tumor.

DIAGNOSTIC EVALUATION

Initial evaluation should include a detailed physical examination with measurements of the primary tumor, assessment for extension to adjacent mucosal or bony structures, and possible involvement of the inguinal lymph nodes. Because neoplasia of the female genital tract is often multifocal, evaluation of the vagina and cervix—including cervical cytologic screening—should always be performed in women with vulvar neoplasms. Fine needle aspiration biopsy from sites of suspected metastases may eliminate the need for surgical exploration in some patients with advanced tumors.

STAGING SYSTEMS

The International Federation of Gynecology and Obstetrics (FIGO) adopted a modified surgical staging system for vulvar cancer in 1989, which was most recently modified in 2009 (Table 5.1). The TNM classification scheme is correlated with the updated FIGO staging system (Table 5.2). Nodal status is determined by the surgical evaluation of the groin. The presence or absence of distant metastases is based on an unspecified diagnostic workup tailored to the patient's clinical presentation.

Table 5.1	FIGO Staging of Carcinoma of the Vulva (Updated 2009)
I	Tumor confined to the vulva
IA	Lesions ≤2 cm in size, confined to the vulva or perineum and with stromal invasion ≤1.0 mm*, no nodal metastasis
IB	Lesions >2 cm in size or with stromal invasion >1.0 mm*, confined to the vulva or perineum, with negative nodes
II	Tumor of any size with extension to adjacent perineal structures (1/3 lower urethra, 1/3 lower vagina, anus) with negative nodes
III	Tumor of any size with or without extension to adjacent perineal structures (1/3 lower urethra, 1/3 lower vagina, anus) with positive inguinofemoral lymph nodes
IIIA	1. With one lymph node metastasis (≥5 mm), or 2. One to two lymph node metastasis(es) (<5 mm)
IIIB	1. With two or more lymph node metastases (≥5 mm), or 2. Three or more lymph node metastases (<5 mm)
IIIC	With positive nodes with extracapsular spread
IV	Tumor invades other regional (2/3 upper urethra, 2/3 upper vagina) or distant structures
IVA	Tumor invades any of the following: 1. Upper urethral and/or vaginal mucosa, bladder mucosa, rectal mucosa, or fixed to pelvic bone, or 2. Fixed or ulcerated inguinofemoral lymph nodes
IVB	Any distant metastasis including pelvic lymph nodes

*The depth of invasion is defined as the measurement of the tumor from the epithelial–stromal junction of the adjacent most superficial dermal papilla to the deepest point of invasion.
Source: Reprinted with permission from Pecorelli S. Revised FIGO staging for carcinoma of the vulva, cervix, and endometrium. *Int J Gynaecol Obstet.* 2009;105:103–104.

PATTERNS OF SPREAD

Vulvar cancers metastasize in three ways: (i) local growth and extension into adjacent organs; (ii) lymphatic embolization to regional lymph nodes in the groin; and (iii) hematogenous dissemination to distant sites. Descriptive definitions of local extension are clinically useful in that local surgical resection with a wide margin is almost universally feasible in women with T1 or T2 tumors, occasionally possible in those with T3 lesions and impossible in those with T4 tumors without resorting to an exenterative operation. More recent experience with intraoperative mapping has demonstrated that lymphatic drainage from most vulvar sites proceeds initially to a "sentinel" node located within the superficial inguinal group.

Inguinal node metastasis can be predicted by the presence of certain parameters, including lesion diameter greater than 2 cm, poor differentiation,

Table 5.2	American Joint Committee on Cancer (AJCC) Staging of Vulvar Cancer (7th Edition)

Primary Tumor (T)

TX	Primary tumor cannot be assessed
T0	No evidence of primary tumor
Tis*	Carcinoma *in situ* (preinvasive carcinoma)
T1a	Lesions 2 cm or less in size, confined to the vulva or perineum and with stromal invasion 1.0 mm or less**
T1b	Lesions more than 2 cm in size *or* any size with stromal invasion more than 1.0 mm, confined to the vulva or perineum
T2***	Tumor of any size with extension to adjacent perineal structures (lower/distal 1/3 urethra, lower/distal 1/3 vagina, anal involvement)
T3****	Tumor of any size with extension to any of the following: upper/proximal 2/3 of urethra, upper/proximal 2/3 vagina, bladder mucosa, rectal mucosa, or fixed to pelvic bone

Regional Lymph Nodes (N)

NX	Regional lymph nodes cannot be assessed
N0	No regional lymph node metastasis
N1	One or two regional lymph nodes with the following features
N1a	1 lymph node metastasis 5 mm or less
N1b	1 lymph node metastasis 5 mm or greater
N2	Regional lymph node metastasis with the following features
N2a	Three or more lymph node metastases each <5 mm
N2b	Two or more lymph node metastases 5 mm or greater
N2c	Lymph node metastasis with extracapsular spread
N3	Fixed or ulcerated regional lymph node metastasis (*An effort should be made to describe the site and laterality of lymph node metastases.*)

Distant Metastasis (M)

M0	No distant metastasis
M1	Distant metastasis (including pelvic lymph node metastasis)

Anatomic Stage/Prognostic Groups

Stage 0*	Tis	N0	M0
Stage I	T1	N0	M0
Stage IA	T1a	N0	M0
Stage IB	T1b	N0	M0
Stage II	T2	N0	M0
Stage IIIA	T1, T2	N1a, N1b	M0
Stage IIIB	T1, T2	N2a, N2b	M0
Stage IIIC	T1, T2	N2c	M0
Stage IVA	T1, T2	N3	M0
	T3	Any N	M0
Stage IVB	Any T	Any N	M1

*FIGO no longer includes Stage 0 (Tis).
**The depth of invasion is defined as the measurement of the tumor from the epithelial–stromal junction of the adjacent most superficial dermal papilla to the deepest point of invasion.
***FIGO uses the classification T2/T3. This is defined as T2 in TNM.
****FIGO uses the classification T4. This is defined as T3 in TNM.
Source: Reprinted with permission from Byrd SB, Compton DR, Fritz CC, et al., eds. *AJCC Cancer Staging Manual Edge*, 7th ed.; New York, NY: Springer, 2010:383–384.

increasing depth of stromal invasion, and invasion of lymphovascular spaces. Clinically important observations regarding nodal metastases include the following: (i) the superficial inguinal nodes are the most frequent site of lymphatic metastasis; (ii) in-transit metastases within the vulvar skin are exceedingly rare, suggesting that most initial lymphatic metastases represent embolic phenomena; (iii) metastasis to the contralateral groin or deep pelvic nodes is unusual in the absence of ipsilateral groin metastases; and (iv) nodal involvement generally proceeds in a stepwise fashion from the superficial inguinal to the deep inguinal and then to the pelvic nodes. Spread beyond the inguinal lymph nodes is considered distant metastasis.

PATHOLOGY

KEY POINTS
- Squamous cell carcinoma is the most common histologic subtype.
- Melanoma is the second most common subtype, and 25% may be nonpigmented.
- The risk of lymph node metastases is negligible when the depth of invasion is less than or equal to 1 mm.
- Paget disease of the vulva has a high likelihood of recurrence and may be associated with underlying adenocarcinoma.

Most vulvar squamous carcinomas arise within areas of epithelium involved by some recognized epithelial cell abnormality. Approximately 60% of cases have adjacent VIN. In cases of superficially invasive squamous carcinoma of the vulva, the frequency of adjacent VIN approaches 85%. Lichen sclerosus, usually with associated squamous cell hyperplasia, and/or VIN, can be found adjacent to vulvar squamous cell carcinoma in 15% to 40% of the cases.

Vulvar squamous cell carcinoma precursors can be considered in two distinct groups: those associated with HPV, usually associated VIN, and those that are not (e.g., those associated with lichen sclerosus, chronic granulomatous disease).

Vulvar Carcinomas

Squamous Cell Carcinomas
The term microinvasive carcinoma is not recognized as meaningful in reference to the vulva because there are no commonly agreed upon pathologic criteria established for this term. However, a substage of FIGO stage I, stage IA, is defined as a solitary squamous carcinoma of the vulva measuring 2 cm or less in diameter with clinically negative nodes, with depth of tumor invasion 1 mm or less. Tumors with a depth or thickness of 1 mm or less carry little or no risk of lymph node metastasis. Stage I squamous carcinomas of the vulva, with a reported depth or thickness of 5 mm or more, have a lymph node metastasis rate of 15% or higher. In addition to tumor stage and depth or thickness, other pathologic features include lymphovascular space invasion, growth pattern of the tumor, grade of the tumor, and tumor type.

In a multivariable retrospective analysis of 39 cases of vulvar squamous carcinoma, in addition to clinical stage, and when corrected for treatment modality, pattern of tumor invasion, depth of tumor invasion, and lymph node status were all found to be significant prognostic factors. In addition, desmoplasia (a fibroblastic stromal tumor response) has been correlated with a higher risk of lymph node metastasis and poorer survival.

Verrucous carcinoma of the vulva is an exophytic-appearing growth that can be locally destructive. Clinically, it may resemble condyloma acuminatum. Because of its excellent prognosis, strict histologic criteria should be used in the diagnosis of verrucous carcinoma. Verrucous tumors may be associated with HPV type 6 or its variants.

Adenocarcinoma and Carcinoma of Bartholin Gland
Most primary adenocarcinomas of the vulva arise within Bartholin glands. Invasive vulvar Paget disease has been associated with underlying adenocarcinoma. Primary malignant tumors arising within Bartholin glands include adenocarcinoma and squamous cell carcinoma, which occur with approximately equal frequency. Carcinoma of Bartholin glands generally occurs in older women and is rare in women younger than 50. In clinical practice, it is generally advisable to excise an enlarged Bartholin gland in a woman 50 years of age or older, especially if there is no known history of prior Bartholin cyst. If a cyst is drained and a palpable mass persists, excision is also indicated.

Primary carcinomas within Bartholin glands are characteristically deep in location and difficult to detect in their early growth. Approximately 20% of women with primary carcinoma of Bartholin glands have metastatic tumor to the inguinofemoral lymph nodes at the time of primary tumor diagnosis.

Vulvar Paget Disease and Paget-Like Lesions
Vulvar Paget disease typically presents as an eczematoid, red, weeping area on the vulva, often localized to the labia majora, perineal body, clitoral area, or other sites. This disease typically occurs in older, postmenopausal Caucasian women and may be associated with an underlying primary adenocarcinoma. Invasive Paget disease 1 mm or less in depth of invasion has reportedly little risk for recurrence.

Vulvar Malignant Melanoma
Malignant melanoma of the vulva accounts for approximately 9% of all primary malignant neoplasms on the vulva, and vulvar melanoma accounts for approximately 3% of all melanomas in women. This tumor occurs predominantly in Caucasian women, and the mean age at diagnosis is 55 years. Although usually pigmented, approximately one fourth are nonpigmented, amelanotic melanomas.

The level of invasion and tumor thickness are essential measurements in evaluating malignant melanoma. Malignant melanomas that have a thickness of less than 0.75 mm have little or no risk for metastasis and tumors up to 1 mm in thickness are generally considered to have minimal risk of recurrence. Melanomas of 1.49 mm thickness or less also correlate with good prognosis. A poor prognosis is correlated with thickness greater than 2 mm, or mitotic count exceeding 10/mm^2. Other poor prognostic factors include minimal or nil inflammatory reaction and surface ulceration.

Metastatic Tumors to the Vulva

Most metastatic tumors to the vulva involve the labia majora or Bartholin glands. Metastatic tumors account for approximately 8% of all vulvar tumors, and in approximately one half of the cases, the primary tumor is in the lower genital tract, including the cervix, vagina, endometrium, and ovary. In approximately 10% of the cases, the primary site of the metastatic tumor cannot be identified.

PROGNOSTIC FACTORS

Prognosis has been most extensively evaluated in women with SCC. The major prognostic factors in vulvar cancer—tumor diameter, depth of tumor invasion, nodal spread, and distant metastasis—have been incorporated into the current FIGO staging system. Risk of local recurrence, although clearly associated with tumor size and extent, is also related to the adequacy of the surgical resection margins. Several retrospective studies have confirmed an increased incidence of local recurrence in patients with microscopic margins less than 8 mm in formalin-fixed tissue specimens.

The single most important prognostic factor in women with vulvar cancer is metastasis to the inguinal lymph nodes, and most recurrences will occur within 2 years of primary treatment. The presence of inguinal node metastases portends a 50% reduction in long-term survival. Because the clinical prediction of lymph node spread is inaccurate, node status is best determined via surgical biopsy. Prognostic issues that appear to be important in evaluating lymphatic involvement are (i) whether nodal spread is bilateral or unilateral, (ii) the number of positive nodes, (iii) the volume of tumor in the metastasis, and (iv) the level of the metastatic disease. Multiple positive nodes, bilateral metastases, involvement beyond the groin, and bulky disease are associated with poor prognosis.

TREATMENT

KEY POINTS
- Treatment should be individualized based on lesion location.
- Partial radical vulvectomy with inguinal lymphadenectomy through separate incisions is the treatment of choice for stage IB and some stage II tumors.
- Combined chemotherapy and radiation therapy is indicated for more advanced lesions and those that involve vital structures where primary resection would be morbid.
- Postoperative inguinal and pelvic irradiations are indicated for most patients with positive nodes.

The development of the radical vulvectomy with bilateral inguinofemoral lymphadenectomy during the 1940s and 1950s was a dramatic improvement over prior surgical options and greatly enhanced survival, particularly for women with smaller tumors and negative lymph nodes. Long-term survival of 85% to 90% can now be routinely obtained with radical surgery.

However, radical surgery can be associated with postoperative complications such as disfigurement, wound breakdown, and lymphedema.

More recently, surgical emphasis has evolved to an individualized approach for tumors at either end of the spectrum. Many gynecologic oncologists believe that smaller vulvar tumors can be acceptably managed by less radical surgical approaches and have proposed more limited resections for certain subsets considered to represent early or low-risk disease. The obvious advantages of such an approach are retention of a significant portion of the uninvolved vulva, less operative morbidity, and fewer late complications. In contrast, radical surgery is frequently ineffective in curing patients with bulky tumors or positive groin nodes. Multimodality programs that incorporate radiation, surgery, and chemotherapy are now being investigated in women with these high-risk tumors based upon success with similar approaches in women with squamous cancers of the cervix.

Early Tumors

Tumors demonstrating early invasion of the vulvar stroma (≤ 1 mm) have minimal risk for lymphatic dissemination. Excisional procedures that incorporate a 1-cm unfixed normal tissue margin are likely to provide a curative result. Patients in this category represent the only subset for whom evaluation of the groin lymph nodes is unnecessary. After primary therapy, these patients should undergo frequent follow-up examinations.

Stage I and II Cancers

Traditional management of stage I and II vulvar cancers has been radical vulvectomy with bilateral inguinofemoral lymphadenectomy. The operation removes the primary tumor with a wide margin of normal skin, along with the remaining vulva, dermal lymphatics, and regional nodes. This approach provides excellent long-term survival and local control in approximately 90% of patients. Disadvantages of radical surgery include the loss of normal vulvar tissue with alterations in appearance and sexual function, a 50% incidence of wound breakdown, a 30% incidence of groin complications (breakdown, lymphocyst, and lymphangitis), and a 10% to 15% incidence of lower extremity lymphedema. Additional postoperative therapy, primarily irradiation, should be considered in the 10% to 20% of patients with positive nodes with the understanding that this will further increase the incidence of lymphedema.

In an effort to reduce morbidity and enhance psychosexual recovery, several groups have espoused a more limited surgical approach for women with small vulvar cancers. The most frequent recommendation is to resect the primary lesion with a 1- to 2-cm margin of normal tissue and to carry the dissection to the deep perineal fascia. This partial radical vulvectomy should not be confused with the concept of excisional biopsy, which is used primarily as a diagnostic procedure.

Limited resection of the primary tumor is combined with a more conservative surgical approach to the groin, in which the ipsilateral groin nodes are used as the sentinel group for lymphatic metastases. Bilateral dissections are performed in patients whose tumors encroach on midline structures (within 1 cm of midline or involvement of midline structures such as the clitoris or perineal body). In patients with negative inguinal nodes, no further dissection or postoperative therapy is used. Patients with positive nodes can undergo additional nodal dissection of the contralateral groin or be treated with postoperative irradiation, or both. Patients with deep lymphadenectomy followed by irradiation have the greatest likelihood of lymphedema.

With limited resection, survival of 90% or better is attainable for patients with stage I vulva carcinoma with acceptable anatomic appearance and function. In an attempt to reduce treatment-related morbidity, the classic radical operation has been replaced by the use of "triple incision" techniques that separate the vulvectomy incision from the groin incisions.

Another surgical concept, which was the subject of evaluation in the recent Gynecologic Oncology Group (GOG) 137 study, is the potential for cutaneous lymphatic mapping to define and target the true sentinel groin nodes. In this study, which examined 452 patients with clinically negative groin lymph nodes and T2 (primary 2 to 6 cm) SCC of the vulva with at least 1 mm invasion, the sensitivity of the sentinel lymph node biopsy (SLNB) was 92% and the negative predictive value was 96%. In patients with tumors less than 4 cm, the negative predictive value was even higher at 98%. Supported by similar results of the GROINS V study, the GOG 137 data offer convincing evidence that assessment of lymphatic metastases may ultimately be reduced to the biopsy of 1 or 2 identifiable nodes in well-selected patients.

In summary, therapy for women with stage I and II cancers must be individualized to the patient and her tumor. Radical vulvectomy provides excellent local control and long-term survival but has significant morbidity and detrimental sexual function effects. More conservative approaches appear safe in most stage I settings and may be applicable in some stage II patients. The surgical approach to the groin nodes is evolving with recent publications supporting the feasibility of the "sentinel" node identified by intraoperative mapping as predictors of nodal spread in well-selected patients.

Stage III and IV Cancers

By definition, stage III tumors extend to adjacent mucosal structures or the inguinal lymph nodes. Many are bulky, but some are of limited volume but considered high stage because of proximity to critical central structures. Some of these primary tumors can be curatively resected by radical operations, such as radical vulvectomy or some variation of the pelvic exenteration and vulvectomy. Recent therapeutic efforts have focused on combined modality treatment programs involving sequenced radiation therapy or chemoradiation therapy and radical surgery. There are now ample data from retrospective series, and a few prospective trials, from which to conclude that vulvar cancers are radioresponsive and that function-sparing operations are feasible in selected patients with advanced disease who receive combined modality treatment (see Radiation Therapy section). A similar experience has been reported for patients with stage IVA tumors. Ultraradical (exenteration) resection may also be considered for selected patients.

Node-Positive Cancers

Patients who undergo bilateral inguinofemoral lymphadenectomy as initial therapy and are found to have positive nodes—particularly more than one positive node—are likely to benefit from postoperative irradiation to the groin and lower pelvis. Radiation therapy was demonstrated to be superior to surgery in the postoperative management of patients with positive pelvic nodes through the GOG 37 study. This trial randomized patients with groin node-positive vulvar cancer to postoperative radiation (45 to 50 Gy) versus ipsilateral pelvic node resection after radical vulvectomy and inguinal lymphadenectomy. At a median survivor follow-up of 74 months, the relative risk of progression was 39% in the radiation arm. The 6-year cancer-related death rate was significantly higher for pelvic node resection compared with radiation, 51% and 29%, respectively. In a recent update, there was a persistent 6-year overall survival benefit for the radiation arm in patients with clinically suspected or fixed ulcerated nodes, as well patients with 2 or more positive groin nodes. Several management options are available for patients found to have positive nodes; however, if postoperative radiotherapy to the inguinal nodes is deemed necessary, it would be reasonable to limit resection to grossly positive nodes. Excellent local control and minimal morbidity have been achieved when selective inguinal lymphadenectomy and tailored postoperative adjuvant therapy were administered to carefully selected patients.

Recurrent Cancer

Regardless of initial treatment, vulvar cancer recurrences can be categorized into three clinical groups: local (vulva), groin, and distant. The reported experience with local recurrence on the vulva is surprisingly good. Recurrence-free survival can be obtained in up to 75% of cases when the recurrence is limited to the vulva and can be resected with a gross clinical margin. Recurrences in the groin have, in the past, been deemed to be universally fatal; however, a few patients may be salvaged by combined modality therapy utilizing chemoradiation ± surgical resection of residual bulky disease (Table 5.3). Patients who develop distant metastases are candidates for systemic cytotoxic therapy, which is largely palliative.

Table 5.3	Unanticipated Groin Failure in Patients with Negative Superficial Lymphadenectomy	
Investigators	No.	%
Burke et al.	4/76	5.2
Berman et al.	0/50	0
Stehman et al.	6/121	5.0
Gordinier	9/104	8.6
Total	19/351	5.4

Source: Moroney JW, Kunos C, Wilkinson EJ, et al. Chapter 19: Vulva. In: *Principles and Practices of Gynecologic Oncology*, 6th ed. Philadelphia, PA: Lippincott Williams & Wilkins; 2013:543.

SURGICAL TECHNIQUES

Radical Vulvectomy and Bilateral Inguinofemoral Lymphadenectomy

The traditional incisions for radical vulvectomy and bilateral lymphadenectomy described as a "butterfly" or a "longhorn" approach have largely been abandoned.

Partial Radical Vulvectomy

In procedures used to resect small vulvar cancers, incisions are devised to allow for at least a 2-cm resection margin encompassing the primary lesion (Fig. 5.2). Dissection is carried to the deep perineal fascia. Recent data suggest that a 1-cm unfixed tissue margin may be adequate for some tumors. Most radical wide excision sites can be closed primarily. Some form of

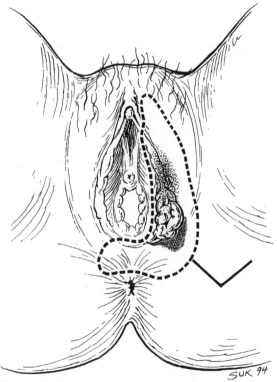

FIGURE 5.2 Planned resection of a left labial squamous carcinoma and adjacent carcinoma *in situ* by radical wide excision. A 2-cm margin is outlined. Rhomboid flap repair using a V-incision is anticipated. **Source**: Reprinted with permission from Burke TW, Morris M, Levenback C, et al. Closure of complex vulvar defects using local rhomboid flaps. *Obstet Gynecol.* 1994;84:1044.

inguinal lymphadenectomy, performed through a separate incision, is generally combined with radical hemivulvectomy. The necessary extent of the groin dissection is an area of current investigation. Wound breakdown, usually of minor degree, is reported in approximately 15% of cases.

Triple Incision Techniques

This resection allows complete removal of the vulvar skin in a manner identical to that achieved with radical vulvectomy; however, bilateral inguino-femoral lymphadenectomy is accomplished via separate incisions parallel to the inguinal ligaments. The three incision concept preserves the radicality of the vulvar resection while retaining skin over the groin and the incidence of major wound breakdown is reduced.

Management of the Groin

Excisional Biopsy

Most preoperative diagnostic dilemmas related to enlarged groin nodes can be resolved simply and accurately using fine needle aspiration biopsy. However, selective excision of groin lymph nodes may be considered when fine needle aspiration biopsy results are negative or equivocal or to remove bulky positive nodes before beginning a course of combined modality therapy.

Superficial Inguinal Lymphadenectomy

Superficial inguinal lymphadenectomy involves the removal of the eight to ten lymph nodes that lie superficial to the cribriform fascia and surrounding the branches of the saphenous vein. This is a more meticulous and complete lymphatic dissection than that described for excisional biopsy.

Deep Inguinal (Femoral) Lymphadenectomy

The deep inguinal (femoral) lymph nodes lie medial to the femoral vein beneath the cribriform fascia. This space contains three to five nodes, the channels of which course beneath the inguinal ligament and continue in the pelvis as the external iliac nodal chain. The most superior deep inguinal node is known as Cloquet node.

Surgical removal of the deep nodes is performed as an extension of a superficial lymphadenectomy rather than as an isolated procedure. The usual approach is to open the cribriform fascia along the sartorius muscle at the time of the superficial lymphadenectomy. Because all of the deep nodes are consistently located medial to the femoral vein, some surgeons have recommended eliminating the removal of the entire cribriform fascia.

Sentinel Lymph Node Mapping and Biopsy

The concept of a "sentinel lymph node" suggests that the sentinel lymph node (SLN) is the first lymph node in the lymphatic pathway and the initial site of metastasis. The use of an intraoperative blue dye staining technique along with lymphoscintigraphy (LSG) using radioactive ^{99m}Tc administered shortly before surgery, combined with the intraoperative use of a handheld gamma probe, produces the highest sensitivity of SLN identification.

Because SLNs are subjected to a more rigorous pathologic (ultrastaging) examination, SLNB can allow for the detection of smaller tumor foci compared to complete groin node dissection and traditional pathologic examination. Factors that may contribute to the failure of SLN identification include the following: midline location for the primary tumor and/or stasis of lymph flow from a node completely replaced by tumor. On a subset analysis of 234 patients in the GOG 137 study who underwent SLN localization with both blue dye and LSG, LSG demonstrated bilateral lymphatic draining in 22% of patients with lateral tumors (>2 cm from midline) versus 69% with midline tumors. None of the 64 patients with lateral tumors had contralateral groin lymph node involvement, whereas 12% of patients with midline tumors had contralateral groin lymph node metastases despite unilateral lymphatic drainage detected by LSG. These findings suggest that unilateral SLN localization can only be safely utilized in patients with lateral primaries and unilateral drainage on LSG. Given the poor prognosis associated with groin relapse, selection of patients who are appropriate candidates for SLN identification and biopsy should be conducted carefully by experienced, well-trained gynecologic oncologists.

Surgical Resection for Recurrent Disease

The site, extent, and volume of recurrent vulvar cancer have important implications for both resectability and potential for cure. Surgical therapy plays a curative or palliative role in selected subsets of patients with recurrent disease.

Radical Wide Excision

As many as 75% of patients with recurrent disease limited to the vulva can be salvaged by radical wide excision or reexcision of the tumor. Surgical principles for recurrent vulvar tumors are identical to those for primary tumors: wide excision with a measured normal tissue margin of at least 2 cm. Particular attention is also focused on obtaining a clear deep margin.

Pelvic Exenteration

Selected patients have achieved long-term survival after pelvic exenteration for vulvar recurrences extending to the vagina, proximal urethra, or anus. The surgical approach in these cases should be individualized to the size and location of the recurrent tumor, prior therapies, and the age and overall health of the patient. Patients considered for pelvic exenteration should have a thorough preoperative evaluation to exclude the presence of regional and/or distant metastases.

Resection of Groin Recurrence

Surgical resection should be viewed with caution in the previously irradiated patient. Cure is unlikely with resection alone, and wound healing is impaired. The debility caused by a combination of unresolved recurrence and surgical wound breakdown is worse than that of progressive recurrence alone. Patients who develop groin recurrence without a history of prior irradiation should be considered for surgical resection in combination with preoperative or postoperative radiation therapy ± concurrent chemotherapy. Isolated groin recurrence is a rare event, so the data to support the efficacy of this treatment are anecdotal.

RADIATION THERAPY

Treating Locally Advanced Disease in the Vulva

Following initial resection of a vulvar primary, various surgicopathologic features have been identified that are associated with a higher risk of local recurrence. Tumor size, nodal status, margin status (<8 mm on fixed tissue), lymphovascular space invasion, and deep tumor penetration have all been associated with an increased risk of recurrence. Although many local recurrences are controlled with additional surgery or irradiation, salvage surgery is often morbid, and local recurrences may provide additional opportunity for regional and distant tumor spread. While no prospective trials of postoperative vulvar site radiotherapy have been completed, adjuvant radiation of the primary tumor bed in selected patients with close margins or with other high-risk features does improve local tumor control.

Alternatively, in patients who present with more advanced primary tumors, radiation therapy may be delivered preoperatively. Several investigators have reported excellent responses and high local control rates after preoperative treatment of advanced tumors with relatively modest doses of radiation therapy followed by local resection. More recently, a number of published series have suggested the therapeutic benefit of concurrent chemoradiation, typically followed by limited surgical resection, in addressing locally advanced disease (Table 5.4). Randomized trials of the role of chemoradiation have not been done in vulvar cancer. However, recent trials that demonstrated improved local control and survival when concurrent cisplatin-containing chemotherapy was added to radiation treatment of cervical cancers suggest that this approach may also be useful for women with other locally advanced lower genital tract neoplasms.

Table 5.4	Concurrent Chemoirradiation in the Management of Locally Advanced or Recurrent Carcinoma of the Vulva				
Investigators	No.	Chemotherapy	RT Dose (Gy)	No. with Recurrent or Persistent Local Disease after RT Surgery	Follow-Up (months)
Moore	73	5-FU + CDDP	47.6	15 (21%)	22–72
Lupi	31	5-FU + Mito	54	7 (23%)	22–73
Scheistroen and Trope	42	Bleomycin	45	39 (93%)	7–60
Han	14	5-FU + CDDP or Mito	40–62	6 (43%)	4–273

5-FU, 5-fluorouracil; Mito, mitomycin C; CDDP, cisplatin; RT, radiation therapy.
Source: Adapted from Moroney JW, Kunos C, Wilkinson EJ, et al. Chapter 19: Vagina. In: *Principles and Practices of Gynecologic Oncology*, 6th ed. Baltimore, MD: Lippincott Williams & Wilkins; 2013:547.

The most compelling initial data in support of concurrent chemora-diation in the management of locally advanced disease come from a large prospective phase II trial performed by the GOG. In the GOG 101 study, 71 evaluable patients with locally advanced T3 or T4 disease who were deemed not resectable by standard radical vulvectomy underwent preoperative chemoradiation. Chemotherapy consisted of 2 cycles of 5-fluorouracil and cisplatin. Radiation was delivered to a dose of 47.6 Gy, using a planned split-course regimen, with part of the radiation given twice daily during the 5-fluorouracil infusion. Patients underwent planned resection of the residual vulvar tumor, or incisional biopsy of the original tumor site in the case of complete clinical response, 4 to 8 weeks after chemoradiotherapy. A complete clinical tumor response was noted in 33/71 (47%) patients. Following vulvar excision or biopsy, 22 patients (31%) were found to have no residual tumor in the pathologic specimen. With a median follow-up interval of 50 months, 11 patients (16%) have developed locally recurrent disease in the vulva.

Encouraged by the impressive outcome of their initial chemoradiation protocol, the GOG conducted a second phase II prospective trial to examine a more intensive chemoradiation regimen. In the GOG 205 study, the total radiation dose was increased to 57.6 Gy at 1.8 Gy daily over 32 fractions. Chemotherapy consisted of weekly cisplatin (40 mg/m^2). As with the GOG 101 study, patients underwent a planned surgical resection of residual tumor or biopsy to confirm complete clinical response 6 to 8 weeks after completion of chemoradiation. Out of 58 evaluable patients, 37 patients achieved a complete clinical response (64%), and 29 of these 37 patients (78%) also demonstrated a complete pathologic response. Among all evaluable patients, the complete pathologic response rate was 50% (29/58). With a median follow-up of 24.8 months, 4 patients (7%) have developed recurrent or persistent disease in the vulva. The superior results of this study compared to that of GOG 101 supports a dose–response curve for SCC of the vulva to radiotherapy. As a follow-up to the GOG 205 study, the ongoing GOG 279 protocol is investigating an even more intensive chemoradiation regimen, consisting of radiation to a total boost dose of 64 Gy with weekly cisplatin and gemcitabine.

Treatment of Regional Disease

Although radical inguinal lymphadenectomy has historically been considered the treatment of choice for regional management of invasive vulvar carcinoma, a number of retrospective studies have suggested that regional prophylactic radiation therapy is an effective method of preventing groin recurrences with minimal morbidity. The GOG tried to define the optimal approach to clinically negative inguinal nodes in a trial that randomized patients between inguinal node irradiation and radical lymphadenectomy (followed by inguinopelvic irradiation in patients with positive nodes) after resection of the primary tumor. This study was closed after entry of only 58 patients when there appeared to be a higher rate of groin recurrence in the radiation treatment arm. However, this study has been criticized because the treatment protocol was not CT based, recommended combination photon and electron dosing was to a depth of 3 to 4 cm, and likely delivered an inadequate dose to the inguinal nodes.

While the role of prophylactic radiotherapy in the undissected but high-risk groin remains controversial, there is strong evidence that adjunctive radiation therapy improves regional tumor control and survival in patients who have documented nodal metastases following inguinal node dissection. The critical role of radiation therapy was not appreciated until 1986, when results of a prospective GOG trial in 114 patients with inguinal metastases were published. In that study, all patients underwent radical vulvectomy and inguinal lymphadenectomy. Patients who had positive inguinal nodes were randomized intraoperatively to receive either pelvic node dissection or postoperative irradiation to the pelvis and inguinal nodes. This trial was closed before the projected accrual goal because an interim analysis revealed a statistically significant overall survival advantage for the radiation treatment arm ($p = 0.03$). The differences between the 2-year survival rates of patients treated with radiation therapy or pelvic dissection were most marked for patients presenting with clinically positive nodes (59% and 31%, respectively) and for those with two 2 or more positive groin nodes (63% and 37%, respectively). There was no significant difference in survival between the treatment groups for patients with only one microscopically positive node, although the authors commented that the number of patients in this subset was insufficient for reliable analysis. The most striking difference in the patterns of recurrence for the two treatment groups was the much larger number of inguinal failures among patients who were treated with surgery alone (Fig. 5.3). These groin recurrences were rarely if ever salvageable. The vulva, regardless of tumor pathologic risk factors, was not included in the radiation treatment fields

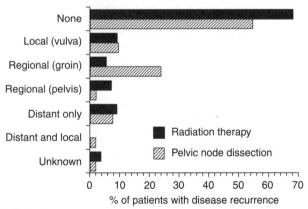

FIGURE 5.3 Sites of disease recurrence in patients treated with adjuvant radiation therapy to the pelvis and inguinal region or with pelvic node dissection following radical vulvectomy and bilateral inguinal lymphadenectomy. *Source*: Modified from Homesley HD, Bundy BN, Sedlis A, et al. Radiation therapy versus pelvic node resection for carcinoma of the vulva with positive groin nodes. *Obstet Gynecol*. 1986;68:733, with permission.

in this study, and approximately 9% of patients in both treatment arms had recurrences at the primary site at the time of the analysis, raising the question of whether selective radiation to the vulva may have decreased local recurrences. The role of adjuvant radiation for patients with a single positive groin node following inguinal node dissection remains unresolved.

Successful use of concurrent chemoradiation following radical hysterectomy in cervical cancer patients with positive lymph nodes suggests that concurrent chemoradiotherapy might be valuable for patients with node-positive vulvar cancer. The GOG opened a phase III, prospective, randomized study (GOG 185) to compare inguinofemoral irradiation alone or in combination with weekly cisplatin for 6 weeks in patients with vulvar cancer and positive groin nodes. Unfortunately, this study was closed due to lack of accrual.

The role of preoperative chemoradiation has been assessed in patients who present with bulky, unresectable inguinal adenopathy. In the GOG 101 study of preoperative chemoradiation for locoregionally advanced vulvar cancer, there was a cohort of 42 evaluable patients with N2 or N3 nodal disease that were deemed initially unresectable. In only two patients (5%) did nodal disease remain unresectable after combined chemotherapy and radiation therapy. The surgical specimen showed histologic clearance of nodal disease in 15 patients (36%). At a median follow-up of 78 months, only 1/37 (3%) patients relapsed in the groin. This study, while nonrandomized, provides further evidence of the efficacy of combined chemoradiotherapy in the management of locoregionally advanced vulvar cancer and in patients with significant regional adenopathy. Given the high risk of distant relapse with node-positive vulvar cancer, especially in those with greater than or equal to two involved nodes, it seems reasonable to consider adjuvant chemoradiation for such high-risk patients. In patients with positive inguinal nodes, the risk of pelvic node involvement is approximately 30%.

Radiation Therapy Technique

Techniques commonly used for the treatment of vulvar carcinoma reflect the need to encompass the lower pelvic and inguinal nodes as well as the vulva while minimizing the dose to the femoral heads. One approach is to treat with an anterior field that encompasses the inguinal regions, lower pelvic nodes, and vulva and a more narrow posterior field that encompasses the lower pelvic nodes and vulva but excludes the majority of the femoral heads. CT scans are used to determine the appropriate electron energy to supplement the nodes covered only in the anterior field and to detect enlarged nodes that may not be appreciated on clinical exam. Gross disease in the groins or vulva may be boosted with *en face* electron fields. In some cases, interstitial implants or *en face* electron fields may be used to boost the dose to the primary site. If radiation is directed to the regional nodes only, with intentional sparing of the vulva, care must be taken to avoid a large "midline" block, which may lead to higher medial groin and vulvar failures.

The complex anatomy of the vulva and its regional lymphatics, interwoven with adjacent critical normal tissues, has led some investigators to advocate for the use of intensity modulated radiation therapy (IMRT) in the management of vulvar cancer. Compared to conventional three-dimensional conformal therapy, IMRT can achieve a more conformal and homogenous dose distribution, resulting in decreased toxicity to normal tissue. Initial single-institution experience with preoperative IMRT in conjunction with chemotherapy for locally advanced vulvar cancer has been positive, with no documented grade 3 or higher gastrointestinal or genitourinary toxicity and excellent rates of pathologic response (48.5% with complete pathologic response). A potential drawback of IMRT is that this technique relies heavily on precise and reproducible target delineation in order to obtain safe and effective outcomes. The RTOG is currently developing an expert consensus contouring atlas and guidelines for vulva IMRT. In addition, the GOG is currently conducting a phase II trial examining the efficacy of cisplatin and gemcitabine with concurrent IMRT for the primary treatment of locally advanced squamous cell carcinoma of the vulva.

Acute Complications of Radiation Therapy

Acute radiation reactions are brisk, and doses of 35 to 45 Gy routinely induce confluent moist desquamation. However, with adequate local care, this acute reaction usually heals within 3 to 4 weeks. Sitz baths, steroid cream, and treatment of possible superimposed *Candida* infection all help to minimize the discomfort. If the patient is sufficiently flexible, she may be placed in a frog-leg position during treatment to minimize the dose and ensuing skin reaction on the medial thighs; care must then be taken, however, to deliver an adequate dose to the vulvar skin, especially when using IMRT. Dose verification strategies, such as thermolucent dosimeters, should be routinely used. Although most patients will develop confluent mucositis by the fourth week of treatment, this is usually tolerated if the patient is warned in advance and assured that the discomfort will resolve after treatment is completed. Although a treatment break is occasionally required, delays should be minimized because they may allow time for the repopulation of tumor cells.

Late Complications of Radiation Therapy

Many factors add to the late morbidity of radiation treatment in patients with vulvar carcinoma. Patients with advanced vulvar carcinomas often are treated with radiation therapy following radical surgery, which may include extensive dissection of the inguinal and possibly pelvic nodes. Large ulcerative cutaneous lesions frequently have superimposed infection. If the vulva is treated, late complications on the underlying bladder and rectum would mirror complications seen with postoperative radiation for endometrial or cervical carcinoma. Irradiation to the vagina during vulvar irradiation can lead to shortening, narrowing, decreased lubrication, and sexual dysfunction. Use of a vaginal dilator, especially in younger patients, should be considered posttreatment. Patients are often elderly and may have complicating medical conditions, such as diabetes, multiple prior surgeries, and osteoporosis. The contribution of concurrent chemotherapy to local morbidity is not yet clearly defined but may contribute to bowel and bone complications.

The incidence of lower extremity edema after inguinal irradiation alone is negligible. Although radiation therapy probably contributes to the incidence of peripheral edema following radical node dissection, no difference was evident in a GOG randomized study. In general, with careful treatment planning technique, the risk of major late complications following regional nodal radiation, either electively or adjuvant to lymph node dissection, is low.

CHEMOTHERAPY

Squamous Cell Carcinoma

Squamous carcinoma is the only cell type for which reproducible information exists on the value of cytotoxic therapy. Several drugs have undergone phase II testing in squamous vulvar cancer. Only doxorubicin and bleomycin appear to have activity as single agents. Cisplatin has notably little activity in vulvar and vaginal squamous tumors. This lack of activity, however, is based on the treatment of refractory patients only. No trials of this agent as a presurgical cytoreductive regimen have been attempted. With the impressive results obtained with concurrent cisplatin-based chemotherapy and radiation therapy in locally advanced squamous cancer of the cervix, one must consider a similar approach in the patient with locally advanced squamous cancer of the vulva. Several drug combinations have also been used in squamous vulvar cancer. Toxicity with these regimens has been reported as tolerable.

There are some increasing reports of the concomitant use of cytotoxic therapy with irradiation, usually as primary therapy in advanced and inoperable disease. Cisplatin-based combination therapy with agents such as 5-fluorouracil and, in the current GOG study, gemcitabine has been used to good effect. The largest experience in vulvar cancer was recently reported by the GOG and is noted above.

RESULTS OF THERAPY

The overall results of therapy for women with squamous cancers of the vulva are excellent. Approximately two thirds of patients present with early-stage tumors. Five-year survival rates of 80% to 90% are routinely reported for stage I and II diseases, respectively. As anticipated, survival rates for patients with advanced disease are poor: 60% for stage III cases and 15% for stage IV (Fig. 5.4). The survival rate for women with nodal spread is one half that of women without nodal disease who have similarly sized primary tumors (Fig. 5.5).

MANAGEMENT OF OTHER VULVAR MALIGNANCIES

Malignant Melanoma

Malignant melanoma is the second most common vulvar malignancy. The primary treatment modality for vulvar melanoma is radical surgical excision. Because most failures are distant, ultraradical local resection does not

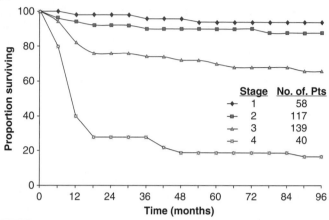

FIGURE 5.4 Invasive squamous vulvar carcinoma. Survival by FIGO stage. *Source*: Patients treated at M. D. Anderson Cancer Center 1944–1990; data courtesy of F. N. Rutledge.

appear to enhance survival. Depth of invasion and the presence of ulceration are significant prognostic factors and should be considered in treatment planning. Look et al. reported that none of the patients with lesion depth of less than or equal to 1.75 mm experienced a recurrence and suggested that these patients could be treated with wide local excision. In contrast, all patients with lesion depth of greater than 1.75 mm recurred despite radical tumor excision. Lymphadenectomy can be avoided in patients with superficial melanomas for whom the risk of metastatic disease is negligible. SLN identification and biopsy may have a role, although data regarding SLNB for vulvar melanomas are limited. Radiation therapy may be useful in enhancing local and regional control for some high-risk patients.

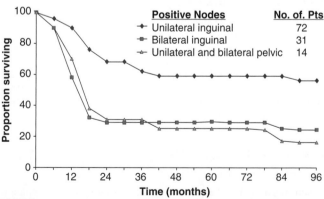

FIGURE 5.5 Invasive squamous vulvar carcinoma. Survival of patients with positive nodes. *Source*: Data courtesy of F. N. Rutledge.

Systemic chemotherapy, in either an adjuvant or salvage setting, is considered palliative, but responses are truly rare, and adverse effects may be significant. Biologic and immunologic approaches to the treatment of malignant melanoma are currently being evaluated.

Overall survival rates in women with vulvar melanoma are approximately 50%. Patients with superficial lesions have an excellent chance for cure after surgical resection, but patients with deeper lesions or metastases at the time of diagnosis have a more dismal prognosis.

Verrucous Carcinoma

Verrucous carcinomas are locally invasive and rarely metastasize. Consequently, treatment by radical wide excision is usually curative. Local recurrence can occur, especially when the tumor has been inadequately resected. Radiation therapy is generally not recommended due to published reports of anaplastic transformation and widespread metastases following radiotherapy.

Basal Cell Carcinoma

Basal cell carcinomas should be removed by excisional biopsy using a minimum surgical margin of 1 cm. Lymphatic or distant spread is exceedingly rare. In patients who are poor surgical candidates or with lesions where resection would cause undue morbidity, consideration can be given to primary radiation therapy. Large retrospective reviews demonstrate 5-year local control rates of over 90% in previously untreated lesions.

Adenocarcinoma

Despite the paucity of data regarding the evaluation and treatment of vulva adenocarcinoma, resection of localized disease by radical wide excision, hemivulvectomy, or radical vulvectomy seems appropriate. The incidence of groin node metastases is approximately 30%. Some form of inguinal lymphadenectomy should be included with primary surgical resection. Radiation therapy may have a role in enhancing local control for women with small margins, unresectable disease, large primary tumors, or inguinal metastases.

Paget Disease

Paget disease should be resected with a wide margin, but recurrences are common. If underlying invasion is suspected, the deep margins should be extended to the perineal fascia. Repeat local excision of recurrent disease is usually effective in the absence of invasion.

Vulvar Sarcomas

All types of vulva sarcoma are rare, but leiomyosarcoma, malignant fibrous histiocytoma, and rhabdomyosarcoma predominate. Cures have occasionally been obtained with aggressive resection of either primary or locally recurrent disease. The results of regional and systemic therapy for leiomyosarcoma are disappointing; however, rhabdomyosarcoma seems to be more responsive to both chemotherapy and radiation than other soft tissue sarcomas. The current treatment of choice is to combine chemoradiation with limited surgical resection of residual disease.

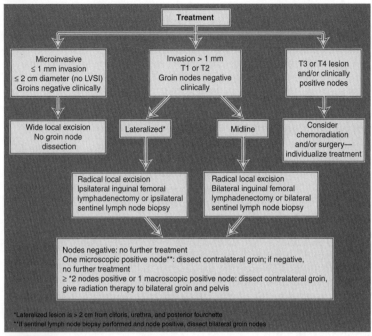

FIGURE 5.6 Management of invasive vulvar cancer. *Source:* Reprinted with permission from Markman M, ed. *Atlas of Cancer,* 2nd ed. Philadelphia, PA: Springer; 2008.

FUTURE DIRECTIONS

Vulvar cancer is an uncommon neoplastic disease, and its relative rarity is a major obstacle in designing prospective randomized trials. Current trends in its management are focusing on a more individualized approach that emphasizes conservative vulva surgical resection when feasible, the use of reconstructive procedures to preserve or restore vulva function, potential reduction in groin complications through SLNB, and multimodality therapy for advanced or disseminated disease (Fig. 5.6).

SUGGESTED READINGS

Beriwal S, Shukla, G, Shinde A, et al. Preoperative intensity modulated radiation therapy and chemotherapy for locally advanced vulvar carcinoma: Analysis of pattern of relapse. *Int J Radiat Oncol Biol Phys.* 2013;85(5):1269–1274.

Coleman RL, Ali S, Levenback CF, et al. Is bilateral lymphadenectomy for midline squamous carcinoma of the vulva always necessary? An analysis from Gynecologic Oncology Group (GOG) 173. *Gynecol Oncol.* 2013;128:155–159.

Insinga RP, Liaw KL, Johnson LG, et al. A systematic review of the prevalence and attribution of human papillomavirus types among cervical, vaginal, and vulvar precancers and cancers in the United States. *Cancer Epidemiol Biomarkers Prev.* 2008;17:1611.

Kunos C, Simpkins F, Gibbons H, et al. Radiation therapy versus pelvic node resection for carcinoma of the vulva with positive groin nodes: An update of a Gynecologic Oncology Group study. *Obstet Gynecol*. 2009;114(3):537–546.

Levenback CF, Ali S, Coleman RL, et al. Lymphatic mapping and sentinel lymph node biopsy in women with squamous cell. Carcinoma of the vulva: a Gynecologic Oncology Group study. *J Clin Oncol*. 2012;30:3786–3791.

Locke J, Karimpour S, Young G, et al. Radiotherapy for epithelial skin cancer. *Int J Radiat Oncol Biol Phys*. 2001;51(3):748.

Monk BJ, Burger RA, Lin F, et al. Prognostic significance of human papillomavirus DNA in vulvar carcinoma. *Obstet Gynecol*. 1995;85:709.

Siegel R, Naishadham D, Jemal A. Cancer statistics, 2013. *CA Cancer J Clin*. 2013;63:11.

Silverman MK, Kopf AW, Gladstein AH, et al. Recurrence rates of treated basal cell carcinomas. Part 4: X-ray therapy. *Dermatol Surg Oncol*. 1992;18(7):549.

6 The Vagina

ANATOMY

The vagina is a muscular dilatable tubular structure averaging 7.5 to 8.5 cm in length that extends from the cervix to the vulva. It lies dorsal to the bladder and urethra, and ventral to the rectum. The upper portion of the posterior wall is separated from the rectum by a reflection of peritoneum, the pouch of Douglas. The vaginal wall is composed of three layers: the mucosa, muscularis, and adventitia. The inner mucosal layer is formed by a thick, nonkeratinizing, stratified squamous epithelium.

The lymphatics in the upper portion of the vagina drain primarily via the lymphatics of the cervix; the upper anterior vagina drains along cervical channels to the internal iliac and parametrial nodes; the posterior vagina drains into the inferior gluteal, presacral, and anorectal nodes. The distal vaginal lymphatics follow drainage patterns of the vulva into the inguinal and femoral nodes and from there to the pelvic nodes. Bilateral pelvic nodes should be considered to be at risk in any invasive vaginal carcinoma, and bilateral groin nodes should be considered to be at risk in those lesions involving the distal third of the vagina.

EPIDEMIOLOGY AND ETIOLOGIC RISK FACTORS

KEY POINTS
- Eighty to ninety percent of vaginal neoplasms represent metastases from other primary gynecologic (cervix or vulva) sites, involving the vagina by direct extension or lymphatic routes.
- Peak incidence of vaginal carcinoma is in the sixth and seventh decades of life; however, it is increasingly seen in younger women, possibly due to human papillomavirus (HPV) infection.

Primary vaginal cancer, defined as a lesion arising in the vagina without involvement of the cervix or vulva, is a rare entity, representing only 1% to 2% of all female genital neoplasias. In 2014, an estimated 3,000 new cases of primary vaginal cancer will be identified and almost 900 deaths are expected to occur from this disease. Most vaginal neoplasms, 80% to 90%, represent metastases from other primary gynecologic (cervix or vulva) and nongynecologic sites, involving the vagina by direct extension or lymphatic or hematogenous routes.

Carcinoma of the vagina is considered to be associated with advanced age, with the peak incidence occurring in the sixth and seventh decades of life. However, vaginal cancer is increasingly being seen in younger women, possibly due to HPV infection or other sexually transmitted diseases. Only about 10% of patients are 40 years of age or younger. A decrease in the incidence of primary vaginal tumors has been noted in recent years, possibly because of early detection with cervical cytology or more rigid diagnostic criteria, which have eliminated from this category primary cancers arising from adjacent organs, such as the cervix, vulva, or endometrium.

Vaginal Intraepithelial Neoplasia and Squamous Cell Carcinoma

Approximately 80% to 90% of vaginal neoplasias are squamous cell carcinomas (SCC), and the incidence of this histology increases with age. Potential risk factors for vaginal SCC include prior history of HPV infection, cervical intraepithelial neoplasia (CIN), vulvar intraepithelial neoplasia (VIN), immunosuppression, and possibly previous pelvic irradiation. HPV is the likely etiologic agent of SCC and its precursor lesion, vaginal intraepithelial neoplasia (VAIN). One population-based case–control study of 156 women with SCC *in situ* or invasive vaginal cancer demonstrated the presence of HPV DNA in over 80% and 60% of these two respective patient groups.

In studies reporting on groups of women with VAIN and SCC of the vagina, the following risk factors have been identified: five or more sexual partners, first sexual intercourse before age 17, smoking, low socioeconomic status, a history of genital warts, prior abnormal cytology, and prior hysterectomy. There is also evidence that *in utero* exposure to diethylstilbestrol (DES) doubles the risk of development of VAIN. The putative mechanism is an enlargement of the transformation zone at risk, which is then at risk for infection with HPV.

Patients with previous cervical carcinoma have a substantial risk of developing vaginal carcinoma, presumably because these sites share exposure and/or susceptibility to endogenous or exogenous carcinogenic stimuli. About 10% to 50% of patients with VAIN–carcinoma *in situ* (CIS) or invasive carcinoma of the vagina have undergone prior hysterectomy or radiotherapy (RT) for CIS or invasive carcinoma of the cervix. The interval from therapy for cervical cancer or preinvasive disease to the development of carcinoma of the vagina averages nearly 14 years.

Clear Cell Adenocarcinoma

An increased incidence of clear cell adenocarcinoma (CCA) of the vagina in young women related to *in utero* exposure to DES during the first 16 weeks of pregnancy was first reported in 1971. Specific suggested mechanisms of carcinogenesis focus on the retention of nests of abnormal cells of müllerian duct origin, which, after stimulation by endogenous hormones during puberty, are promoted into adenocarcinomas. The median age at diagnosis in the DES-exposed patients is 19 years, whereas prior to this report, most patients with CCA of the vagina were elderly. Hicks and Piver noted that 60% of CCA patients had been exposed to DES or similar agents *in utero*, that most cases involved the anterior upper third of the vaginal wall, and that DES-associated CCA cases had been reported from ages

7 to 34 (median, 19 years). Fortunately, the incidence of this tumor has decreased in recent years and may decrease even more since the practice of prescribing DES during pregnancy has been discontinued.

Melanoma

Malignant melanoma is a very rare cancer of the vagina with less than 300 cases reported to date. Primary vaginal malignant melanoma accounts for less than 3% of all vaginal neoplasms and has known risk factors. The mean age of diagnosis is approximately 60 years, and these cases are reported predominantly in Caucasian women. The most common location is the lower third and the anterior vaginal wall, although often times it is multifocal.

Sarcomas

Sarcomas represent 3% of primary vaginal cancers and are most common in adults, with leiomyosarcoma representing 50% to 65% of vaginal sarcomas. Malignant mixed müllerian tumor (carcinosarcoma), endometrial stromal sarcoma, and angiosarcoma are less common. Embryonal rhabdomyosarcoma (RMS)/sarcoma botryoides is a rare, malignant pediatric tumor, and RMS arising in the female genital tract accounts for less than 4% of all pediatric RMS. Prior pelvic RT is a risk factor, particularly for mixed mesodermal tumors and vaginal angiosarcomas. Histopathologic grade appears to be the most important predictor of outcome.

NATURAL HISTORY

KEY POINTS

- The majority of vaginal primaries occur in the upper third or at the apex of the vault, most commonly in the posterior wall. (Note: if the examiner is not careful, this area can be excluded by the posterior blade of the speculum.)
- If positive biopsies of the cervix or the vulva return at the time of initial diagnosis, the tumor cannot be considered to be a primary vaginal lesion.
- There is a significant risk of nodal metastasis for patients with disease beyond stage I.

The majority (57% to 83%) of vaginal primaries occur in the upper third or at the apex of the vault, most commonly in the posterior wall; the lower third may be involved in as many as 31% of patients. Lesions confined to the middle third of the vagina are uncommon. The location of the vaginal carcinoma is an important consideration in planning therapy and determining prognosis. Vaginal tumors may spread along the vaginal walls to involve the cervix or the vulva. However, if biopsies of the cervix or the vulva are positive at the time of initial diagnosis, the tumor cannot be considered a primary vaginal lesion. A lesion on the anterior wall may infiltrate the vesicovaginal septum and/or the urethra; those on the posterior wall may eventually involve the rectovaginal septum and subsequently infiltrate the rectal mucosa. Lateral extension toward the parametrium and paracolpal tissues is not uncommon in more advanced stages of the disease.

There is a significant risk of nodal metastasis for patients with disease beyond stage I. Although data on staging lymphadenectomy are sparse, two studies reported a significant incidence of nodal disease in early-stage vaginal carcinoma. In the series by Al-Kurdis and Monaghan, the incidence of pelvic nodal metastasis was 14% and 32% for stages I and II, respectively, whereas in the series by Davis et al., the incidence was 6% and 26% for stages I and II, respectively. The incidence is expected to be higher for stage III, although no substantial data are available. The incidence of clinically positive inguinal nodes at diagnosis reported by several authors ranges from 5.3% to 20%.

Distant metastasis may occur, primarily in patients with advanced disease at presentation, or those who recurred after primary therapy. In the series by Perez et al. (1999), the incidence of distant metastasis was 16% in stage I, 31% in stage IIA, 46% in stage IIB, 62% in stage III, and 50% in stage IV.

CLINICAL PRESENTATION

Vaginal Intraepithelial Neoplasia—Carcinoma *In Situ*

VAIN most often is asymptomatic. In modern practice, VAIN is usually detected by cytologic evaluation performed following hysterectomy as part of a surveillance strategy in patients with a history of CIN or invasive cervical carcinoma. In these cases, VAIN has a predilection for involvement of the upper vagina, likely secondary to a "field effect." It should be noted that evidence-based guidelines do not support routine cytologic studies following hysterectomy for noncervical pathology. Rather, surveillance cytology post hysterectomy should be limited to those patients with a prior history of CIN or invasive cervix cancer.

Invasive Squamous Cell Carcinoma

In patients with invasive disease, irregular vaginal bleeding, often postcoital, is the most common presenting symptom, followed by vaginal discharge and dysuria. Pelvic pain is a relatively late symptom generally related to tumor extent beyond the vagina.

Other Histologies

The most common presenting symptom in patients with CCA is vaginal bleeding (50% to 75%) or abnormal discharge. More advanced cases may present with dysuria or pelvic pain.

Embryonal RMS, the most common malignant vaginal tumor in children, presents as a protruding, edematous grapelike mass. Ninety percent of these sarcomas present before the age of 5 years.

DIAGNOSTIC WORKUP

In general, in patients with suspected vaginal malignancy, thorough physical examination with detailed speculum inspection, digital palpation, colposcopic and cytologic evaluation, and biopsy constitutes the most effective procedure for diagnosing primary, metastatic, or recurrent carcinoma of the vagina. In order to obtain a biopsy, examination under anesthesia is recommended for the thorough evaluation of all of the vaginal walls and local extent of the disease, primarily if the patient is in great discomfort because of advanced disease. Biopsies of the cervix, if present, are recommended to rule out a primary cervical tumor. The speculum must be rotated as it is slowly withdrawn from the vaginal fornix so that the total vaginal mucosa may be visualized, and, in particular, so that posterior wall lesions, which occur frequently, are not overlooked.

The patient with a history of preinvasive or invasive carcinoma of the cervix found to have abnormal cytology following prior hysterectomy or RT should be offered vaginoscopy with the application of acetic acid to the entire vault, followed by biopsies as indicated by areas of white epithelium ("acetowhite" areas), mosaicism, punctation, or atypical vascularity. Application of half-strength Schiller iodine following the application of acetic acid to determine if the Schiller-positive (nonstaining) areas correspond with the acetowhite areas is another method of identifying high-risk regions requiring biopsy.

STAGING

At present, primary malignancies of the vagina are all staged clinically. In addition to a complete history and physical examination, routine laboratory evaluations including complete blood cell count with differential and platelets and assessment of renal and hepatic function should be undertaken. In order to determine the extent of disease, the following tests are allowed by International Federation of Gynecology and Obstetrics (FIGO) criteria: chest and skeletal radiograph, a thorough bimanual and rectovaginal examination, cystoscopy, proctoscopy, and intravenous pyelogram. It can be difficult even for the experienced examiner to differentiate between disease confined to the mucosa (stage I) and disease spread to the submucosa (stage II).

Pelvic computed tomography (CT) scan is generally performed to evaluate inguinofemoral and/or pelvic lymph nodes, as well as extent of local disease. In patients with vaginal melanoma or sarcoma, chest, abdomen, and pelvic CT scans are often part of the workup. Magnetic resonance imaging (MRI) has emerged as a potentially important imaging modality in the evaluation of vaginal cancers, predominantly the T1-weighted images with contrast and T2-weighted images. Because it offers superior soft tissue resolution, it is particularly helpful for evaluation of extent of invasion. Radiation oncology is particularly interested in this evaluation so determination can be made on the appropriateness of interstitial or intracavitary boost. Positron emission tomography (PET) is evolving as a modality of potential use in the evaluation of vaginal cancer for it can detect the extent of the primary as well as abnormal lymph nodes more often than CT scan. In modern practice, for the majority of patients with disease volume and/or location requiring definitive RT to achieve cure, therapeutic planning will be guided by disease volume assessment utilizing CT, MRI, and/or PET/CT, even though such radiologic modalities are not "allowed" for purposes of staging.

The two commonly used staging systems for carcinoma of the vagina are the FIGO (Table 6.1) and the American Joint Commission on Cancer (TNM) (Table 6.2) classifications. According to FIGO guidelines, patients

Table 6.1 FIGO Staging System for Carcinoma of the Vagina

Stage	Description
I	Limited to the vaginal wall
II	Involvement of the subvaginal tissue but without extension to the pelvic sidewall
III	Extension to the pelvic sidewall
IV	Extension beyond the true pelvis or involvement of the bladder or rectal mucosa. Bullous edema as such does not permit a case to be allotted to stage IV
IVA	Spread to adjacent organs and/or direct extension beyond the true pelvis
IVB	Spread to distant organs

Source: From FIGO Committee on Gynecologic Oncology. Current FIGO staging for cancer of the vagina, fallopian tube, ovary, and gestational trophoblastic neoplasia. *Int J Gynaecol Obstet*. 2009;105(1):3–4, with permission.

Table 6.2 American Joint Commission on Cancer (AJCC, 7th Edition) Staging of Vaginal Cancer

Primary Tumor (T)

Tx	Primary tumor cannot be assessed
T0	No evidence of primary tumor
Tis/0	Carcinoma *in situ* (preinvasive carcinoma)
T1/I	Tumor confined to the vagina
T2/II	Tumor invades paravaginal tissues but not to the pelvic wall
T3/III	Tumor extends to the pelvic wall
T4/IVA	Tumor invades mucosa of the bladder or rectum and/or extends beyond the pelvis (bullous edema is not sufficient to classify a tumor as T4)

Regional Lymph Nodes (N)

Nx	Regional lymph nodes cannot be assessed
N0	No regional lymph nodes
N1/IVB	Pelvic or inguinal lymph node metastasis

Distant Metastasis (M)

Mx	Distant metastasis cannot be assessed
M0	No distant metastasis
M1/IVB	Distant metastasis

AJCC Stage Groupings

Stage 0	Tis N0 M0
Stage I	T1 N0 M0
Stage II	T2 N0 M0
Stage III	T1–3 N1 M0, T3 N0 M0
Stage IVA	T4, any N, M0
Stage IVB	Any T, any N, M1

Source: Edge SB, Byrd DR, Compton CC, et al. *American Joint Committee on Cancer, American Cancer Society. AJCC Cancer Staging Manual*, 7th ed. New York: Springer; 2010:388.

with tumor involvement of the cervix or vulva should be classified as primary cervical or vulvar cancers, respectively.

PATHOLOGIC CLASSIFICATION

Squamous Cell Carcinoma

The most common malignant tumor of the vagina is SCC, representing about 80% to 90% of primary vaginal cancers. These tumors occur in older women and are most often located in the upper, posterior wall of the vagina. For a neoplasm to be considered a vaginal primary, there must not be involvement of the cervix or vulva or a history of cervical cancer for 5 years prior to the diagnosis. Histologically, keratinizing, nonkeratinizing, basaloid, warty, and verrucous variants have been described. Tumors may also be graded as well, moderately, or poorly differentiated, based on a combination of cytologic and histologic features. However, there is little correlation between tumor grade and survival.

Verrucous carcinoma is a rare distinct variant of well-differentiated SCC, usually with the appearance of a large, well-circumscribed, soft, cauliflower-like mass. Verrucous carcinoma may recur locally after surgery but rarely, if ever, metastasizes.

VAIN is a precursor of SCC and is graded from 1 to 3, based on the thickness of epithelial involvement. Alternatively, VAIN can be classified as low or high grade. High-grade lesions indicate involvement of the outer third of the mucosa and include CIS, which encompasses the entire thickness of the epithelium. The true incidence of VAIN and its rate of progression to invasive carcinoma are unknown, ranging in several series from 9% to 28%. High-risk HPV was noted in 35% of VAIN 1 and 94% of VAIN 3 lesions. Comparison of the distribution of HPV types in the vagina, vulva, and cervix suggests that VAIN is more closely related to CIN than to VIN.

Clear Cell Adenocarcinoma and Vaginal Adenosis

DES-associated CCA has a predilection for the upper third of the vagina and the exocervix. It is frequently located at or near the lower margin of the zone of glandular tissue in the vagina or cervix. Most CCAs are exophytic and superficially invasive. About 97% will be associated with mucosal adenosis. CCA is mainly composed of clear and hobnail-shaped cells. The major determinant of outcome in CCA is stage, but some pathologic features are statistically associated with better outcome, including a tubulocystic growth pattern, size less than 3 cm^2, and less than 3 mm of stromal invasion.

Vaginal adenosis is a condition in which müllerian-type glandular epithelium is present after vaginal development is complete. Although adenosis is the most common histologic abnormality in women exposed to DES *in utero*, it is not strictly confined to this population. Atypical adenosis of tuboendometrial type appears to be a precursor lesion of CCA.

Other Adenocarcinomas

Primary adenocarcinoma of the vagina is rare and occurs predominantly in postmenopausal women.

Melanoma

Malignant melanoma of the vagina accounts for less than 3% of vaginal neoplasms. In contrast to SCC, the most common locations of vaginal melanoma are the lower third and the anterior vaginal wall. Grossly, these tumors are typically pigmented and show considerable variation in size, color, and growth patterns, being polypoid or nodular in the majority of cases. Immunohistochemical stains are frequently positive for S100 protein, HMB-45, and melan-A. Tyrosinase and MART-1 are useful markers when S100 is negative or only focally positive. Tumor thickness correlates with prognosis and may be measured by the method of Breslow.

Mesenchymal Tumors

Embryonal RMS is a rare pediatric tumor. The botryoid variant, or sarcoma botryoides, is the most common malignant vaginal tumor in infants and children. Ninety percent of cases occur in children younger than 5 years of age. Sarcoma botryoides has a characteristic macroscopic appearance consisting of multiple gray-red, translucent, edematous, grapelike masses that fill the vagina and may protrude from it.

Leiomyosarcoma is the most common vaginal sarcoma in adults. Smooth muscle tumors 3 cm or greater in diameter have an increased risk of recurrence. Although they may originate in any part of the vagina, most are submucosal.

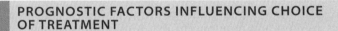

PROGNOSTIC FACTORS INFLUENCING CHOICE OF TREATMENT

KEY POINTS

- Primary malignancies of the vagina are all staged clinically.
- The most common malignant tumor of the vagina is SCC.
- VAIN is a precursor of SCC.
- Exposure to DES *in utero* is associated with the development of clear cell adenocarcinoma.
- Stage of disease is the dominant prognostic factor in terms of outcome.
- Vaginal melanoma has a higher propensity for the development of distant metastases, and these patients do more poorly than patients with SCC.

Invasive Squamous Cell Carcinoma

Stage of disease is the dominant prognostic factor in terms of outcome. In the report by Creasman et al. (1998), the 5-year survival rate was 96% for patients with stage 0, 73% for stage I, 58% for stage II, and 36% for those with stage III and IV diseases, respectively. In Perez's series, including 165 patients with primary vaginal carcinomas treated with definitive RT, the 10-year actuarial disease-free survival (DFS) was 94% for stage 0, 75% for stage I, 55% for stage IIA, 43% for stage IIB, 32% for stage III, and 0% for those with stage IV.

The impact of lesion location has been controversial. Several investigators have shown better survival and decreased recurrence rates for patients with cancers involving the proximal half of the vagina when compared with those in the distal half or those involving the entire length of the vagina. In addition, lesions of the posterior wall have a worse prognosis than those involving other vaginal walls (10-year recurrence rates of 32% and 19%, respectively), which probably reflects the greater difficulty of performing adequate brachytherapy procedures in this location.

The prognostic importance of lesion size has also been controversial. Chyle et al. (1996) noted that lesions measuring less than 5 cm in maximum diameter had a 20% 10-year local recurrence rate compared to 40% for those lesions larger than 5 cm. Similarly, in the Princess Margaret Hospital experience and more recently in the Stanford experience, tumors larger than 4 cm in diameter fared significantly worse than smaller lesions. Other data suggest that disease volume, a likely surrogate for stage or lesion size, adversely impacted survival as well as local control.

Several series have shown histologic grade to be an independent, significant predictor of survival. Chyle et al. (1996) also noted histology was a significant predictor of outcome, with a higher incidence of local recurrence in patients with adenocarcinoma compared with SCC (52% and 20%, respectively, at 10 years), as well as a higher incidence of distant metastases (48% and 10%, respectively) and lower 10-year survival rate (20% vs. 50%).

Other Histologies

An increased propensity for distant metastases to the lung and supraclavicular nodes has been reported in patients with CCA. Stage, tubulocystic pattern, size less than 3 cm, and depth of invasion less than 3 mm were all noted to be associated with superior survival.

Vaginal melanoma has a higher propensity for the development of distant metastases, and affected patients do more poorly than patients with SCC.

Patients with malignant mesenchymal tumors of the vagina do less well than those with invasive SCC. Specific, adverse prognostic factors for vaginal sarcoma identified by Tavassoli and Norris included infiltrative versus pushing borders, high mitotic rate of 5 or more mitoses per 10 HPFs, size greater than 3 cm in diameter, and cytologic atypia.

GENERAL MANAGEMENT: TREATMENT OPTIONS AND OUTCOME BY FIGO STAGES

KEY POINTS

- Treatment options for VAIN range from partial or complete vaginectomy to more conservative approaches such as local excision, electrocoagulation, laser vaporization, topical 5% fluorouracil, or intracavitary brachytherapy.
- Surgery may be preferable in select stage I and II patients with small, superficially invasive SCC lesions at the apex and upper third of the posterior or lateral vagina.

■ External beam radiotherapy (EBRT) is advisable in patients with deeply infiltrating or poorly differentiated stage I and II lesions and in all patients with stage III to IVA disease.

■ Consideration should be given to delivering cisplatin-based chemotherapy concurrently with RT in patients with advanced vaginal cancer.

Vaginal Intraepithelial Neoplasia—Carcinoma *In Situ*

VAIN has been approached both surgically and medically by multiple investigators. Treatment options range from partial or complete vaginectomy to more conservative approaches such as local excision, electrocoagulation, laser vaporization, topical 5% fluorouracil (5-FU) administration, or ICB. For patients in whom invasive disease cannot be ruled out, as well as for those who fail conservative therapy, surgical resection remains the treatment of choice. Overall, the reported control rates are very similar among the different approaches, ranging from 48% to 100% for laser, 52% to 100% for colpectomy, 75% to 100% for topical 5-FU, and 83% to 100% for RT. The degree of VAIN and the age and general health of the patient are important treatment considerations.

Partial colpectomy is favored by many for the treatment of focal VAIN without any prior history of pelvic RT. Patients who have received prior pelvic RT, wherein partial colpectomy would have high risk of fistula formation, may benefit from a medical approach with topical application of 5-FU. This acts by inciting a desquamation of the vaginal squamous epithelium, which later reepithelializes with presumably normal cells. Several schedules of topical 5-FU have been reported; however, one preferred schedule is one third applicator weekly for 10 weeks. Regardless of which 5-FU application schedule is chosen, it is important that the perineal skin be protected with a topical ointment, such as zinc oxide, to prevent painful vulvar erosions. More recently, investigators have demonstrated the feasibility and efficacy of topical imiquimod in the treatment of VAIN, with cure rates of up to 86% reported in small single institution studies. Imiquimod is a heterocyclic imidazoquinoline amine that acts through Toll-like receptor 7 to induce cytokine expression and subsequent activation of both the innate and adaptive immune responses. This topical medication is generally well tolerated with the majority of side effects limited to mild skin reactions, such as redness, swelling, itching/burning, tenderness, and flaking.

Partial or total vaginectomy has been considered by many to be an acceptable treatment for VAIN. However, one of its main drawbacks is shortening or stenosis of the vagina, frequently with poor functional results. Prior RT is probably a contraindication to vaginectomy owing to significantly increased morbidity. Control rates of 66% to 100% following partial colpectomy have been achieved.

RT has a long history of documented efficacy with control rates ranging between 80% and 100%, and a significantly better therapeutic ratio than other modalities. Using conventional low dose rate (LDR) ICB techniques, the entire vaginal mucosa should receive between 50 and 60 Gy, given the high incidence of multicentricity; the area of involvement should receive 70 to 80 Gy, in one or two implants, prescribed to the mucosal surface. Higher doses may cause significant vaginal fibrosis and stenosis. Perez et al. (1999) reported only one distal local failure in the 20 patients treated for CIS. A more recent publication from Blanchard et al. (2011) reported only one "in-field" recurrence in 28 patients treated with LDR brachytherapy for VAIN 3. Pelvic recurrences or distant failures have not been observed in the absence of invasive component after ICB.

There have been some reports in the literature regarding the use of high dose rate (HDR) ICB for patients with VAIN 3; however, data are limited, and there is a lack of consensus regarding fraction schedules. Based on the excellent local control and functional results obtained with LDR-ICB, this remains the treatment of choice when definitive RT is used, unless unavailable.

Invasive Squamous Cell Carcinoma

Surgical Approach and Outcomes

In general, SCC of the vagina has been treated with RT. However, several surgical series have reported acceptable to excellent outcomes in well-selected patients, with survival rates after radical surgery for stage I disease ranging from 75% to 100%. Cases in which surgery may be the preferred treatment include selected stage I and II patients with lesions at the apex and upper third of the posterior or lateral vagina that could be approached with radical hysterectomy, upper vaginectomy, and pelvic lymphadenectomy, providing adequate margins for very superficial lesions. Lesions in the lower third of the vagina would require vulvovaginectomy in addition to dissection of inguinofemoral nodes to achieve negative margins. If the margins are found to be close or positive after resection, adjuvant RT is recommended. However, for lesions at other sites, and those cases requiring more extensive resection, definitive RT is the treatment of choice since it offers excellent results. Exenteration should be reserved for those with central failure after RT or as primary therapy in those with disease not fixed to the bone.

Advanced-stage patients should receive definitive RT, probably in combination with concurrent chemotherapy, although the role of combined modality therapy is unknown and is used as an extrapolation from the cervical data.

Radiation Therapy Techniques and Outcome
Stage I
In patients with stage I lesions, usually 0.5 to 1 cm thick that may involve one or more vaginal walls, it is important to individualize radiation therapy techniques to obtain optimal functional results. Superficial lesions can be adequately treated with ICB alone using afterloading vaginal cylinders. The entire length of the vagina is generally treated to a mucosal dose of 60 to 65 Gy (LDR), and an additional mucosal dose of 20 to 30 Gy is delivered to the area of tumor involvement. For lesions thicker than 0.5 cm at the time of implantation, it is advisable to combine ICB and interstitial brachytherapy (ITB) with a single-plane implant to increase the depth dose

and limit excessive irradiation to the vaginal mucosa. An additional 15 to 20 Gy at a depth of 0.5 cm beyond the plane of the implant will be delivered with the ITB such that the base of the tumor receives between 65 and 70 Gy, with the involved vaginal mucosa receiving an estimated 80 to 100 Gy. The proximal and distal vaginal mucosal doses should be limited to 140 and 100 Gy, respectively. The optimal fractionation schedule and dose for HDR brachytherapy remain to be defined, especially for HDR monotherapy. The HDR dose schedules proposed in the American Brachytherapy Society consensus guidelines are for HDR brachytherapy combined with EBRT and are based on empirical protocols or extrapolated from LDR parameters.

There is general consensus that EBRT is advisable for larger, more infiltrating, or poorly differentiated tumors that may have a higher risk of lymph node metastasis. The whole pelvis is treated to 45 to 50 Gy to the parametria and pelvic sidewalls. Chyle et al. (1996) recommended EBRT in addition to brachytherapy for stage I disease to cover at least the paravaginal nodes and, in larger lesions, to cover the external and internal iliac nodes. About 95% to 100% of local control has been achieved with intracavitary and interstitial techniques, with 5-year survival for patients with stage I disease treated with RT alone ranging from 70% to 95% (Table 6.3).

Stage II
Patients with stage IIA tumors have more advanced paravaginal disease without parametrial infiltration to the sidewall. These patients are uniformly treated with EBRT followed either by ICB and/or ITB. Generally, the whole pelvis receives a total of 45 to 50 Gy to the pelvis. A combination of LDR-ICB, LDR-ITB, HDR-ICB, or HDR-ITB or pulse dose rate may be used depending on institutional preference. The modality used should aim for 25 to 35 Gy (if using HDR, use conversion for equivalent dose at 2 Gy—EQD2) 0.5 cm beyond the deep margin of the tumor in addition to the whole pelvis dose, to a total tumor dose of 70 to 80 Gy, depending on tumor response and vaginal tolerance. The upper vagina has a greater tolerance than the lower vagina. Double-plane or volume implants may be necessary for more extensive disease. Perez et al. (1999) showed that in stage IIA, the local tumor control was 70% (37 of 53) in patients receiving brachytherapy combined with EBRT, compared with 40% (4 of 10) in patients treated with either brachytherapy or EBRT alone. The superiority of the combination of EBRT and brachytherapy over EBRT or brachytherapy alone has been shown in other series as well.

Patients with stage IIB, with more extensive parametrial infiltration, will receive 40 to 50 Gy to the whole pelvis with consideration of a parametrial boost for bulky disease or with a poor response. An additional boost of 30 to 35 Gy EQD2 will be given with LDR or HDR interstitial and ICB, to deliver a total tumor dose of 75 to 80 Gy to the vaginal tumor and 60 to 65 Gy to parametrial and paravaginal extensions. Patients with lesions limited to the upper third of the vagina can be treated with an intrauterine tandem and vaginal ovoids or cylinders. The locoregional control in patients with stage IIB in Perez's series was also superior with combined EBRT and brachytherapy (61% vs. 50%, respectively).

Table 6.3	FIGO Stage I and II Vaginal Cancers: Treatment Approach and Results	

Treatment Modality Author	No. of Patients	Outcome–Survival
Irradiation ± surgery		
Chyle	59 St I	10 y 76%
	104 St II	10 y 69%
Creasman (NCDB)	169 St I	5-year surv. 73%; 79% S + RT (47), 63% RT (122)
	175 St II	5-year surv. 58%; 58% S + RT (39), 57% RT (136)
Davis	19 St I	5-year surv. 100% S + RT (5), 65% RT (14)
	18 St II	5-year surv. 69% S + RT (9), 50% RT (9)
Kirkbride	40 St I	5 y 72%
	38 St II	5 y 70%
Kucera	16 St I	5 y 81%
	23 St II	5 y 43.5%
Perez	59 St I	10 y 80%
	63 St IIA	10 y 55%
	34 St IIB	10 y 35%
Stock	8 St I	5 y 100% S + RT, 80% RT
	35 St II	5 y 69% S + RT, 31% RT
Urbanski	33 St I	5 y 73%
	37 St II	5 year 54%
Frank	50 St I	5-year DSS, 85%
	97 St II	5-year DSS, 78%
Hiniker	38 St I	2-year surv. 96%
Hiniker	28 St II	2-year surv. 92%
Murakami	9 St I	2-year surv. 100%
Murakami	8 St II	2-year surv. 62.5%
Radical surgery		5-year surv.
Ball	19 St I	84%
	8 St II	63%
Creasman (NCDB)	76 St I	90%
	34 St II	70%
Davis	25 St I	85%
	27 St II	49%

Treatment Modality Author	No. of Patients	Outcome–Survival
Rubin	5 St I	80%
	3 St II	33%
Stock	17 St I	56%
	23 St II	68%
Tjalma	26[a]	91%

[a]Four patients received adjuvant irradiation.
St, stage; RT, radiotherapy; S, surgery; surv., survival; DSS, disease-specific survival.
Source: Adapted from Cardenes VR, Schilder JM, Emerson R. Chapter 20: Vagina. In: Barakat RB, Berchuck A, Markman M, et al., eds. *Principles and Practices of Gynecologic Oncology*, 6th ed. Philadelphia, PA: Lippincott Williams & Wilkins; 2013:572.

The 5-year survival for patients with stage II disease treated with RT alone ranges between 35% and 70% for stage IIA and 35% and 60% for stage IIB. The results of several series published in the literature using different treatment approaches for stage I and II vaginal cancers are shown in Table 6.3.

Stages III and IVA
Generally, patients with stage III and IVA diseases will receive 45 to 50 Gy EBRT to the pelvis, and in some cases, additional parametrial dose to deliver up to 60 Gy to the pelvic sidewalls. Ideally, ITB boost is performed, if technically feasible, to deliver a minimum tumor dose of 75 to 80 Gy. If brachytherapy is not feasible, a shrinking field technique can be used, with fields defined using the three-dimensional (3D) treatment planning capabilities to deliver a tumor dose around 65 to 70 Gy. An alternative approach is intensity-modulated RT (IMRT) using multiple beams of varying intensity that conform the high-dose region to the shape of the target tissues, with more adequate sparing of the surrounding normal tissues, primarily the bladder, rectum, and small bowel.

The overall cure rate for patients with stage III disease is 30% to 50%. Stage IVA includes patients with rectal or bladder mucosa involvement, or in most series, positive inguinal nodes. Although some patients with stage IVA disease are curable, many patients are treated palliatively with EBRT only. Pelvic exenteration can also be curative in highly selected stage IV patients with small-volume central disease. Table 6.4 shows the treatment results with different therapeutic modalities, including four series that reported the use of primary surgery in highly selected patients with advanced disease. However, each of these series reported a far greater number of patients with similar stage disease treated with RT, which represents the preferred approach in contemporary practice.

External Beam Radiotherapy
EBRT is advisable in patients with deeply infiltrating or poorly differentiated stage I lesions and in all patients with stage II to IVA diseases. The treatment was traditionally delivered using a two- or four-field technique.

Table 6.4	FIGO Stage III and IV Vaginal Cancers: Outcome with Radiation Therapy with/without Surgery	
Treatment Modality Author	No. of Patients	Outcome–Survival
Irradiation ± surgery		
Chyle	55 St III	10 y 47%
	16 St IV	10 y 27%
Creasman (NCDB)	St III and IV, 180	5-year surv. 36%; 60% S + RT (36), 35% RT (144)
Kirkbride	42[a] St III and IV	5 y 53%
Kucera	46 St III	5 y 35%
	19 St IVA	5 y 32%
Perez	20 St III	10 y 38%
	15 St IV	0%
Stock	9 St III	5 y 0%
	8 St IV	0%
Urbanski	40 St III	5 y 22.5%
	15 St IVA	0%
Frank	46 St III and IVA	5-year DSS, 58%
Hiniker	13 St III	2-year surv. 96%
Hiniker	12 St IV	2-year surv. 25%
Murakami	17 St III	2-year surv. 69.1%
Murakami	2 St IV	2-year surv. 0%
Radical surgery		*5-year surv.*
Ball	2 St III	50%
Creasman (NCDB)	St III and IV, 21	47%
Rubin	2 St III	50%

[a]Twenty patients with stages III and IV were treated with chemotherapy (5-FU ± mitomycin-C) and radiotherapy.
St, stage; RT, radiotherapy; S, surgery; surv., survival; DSS, disease-specific survival.
Source: Adapted from Cardenes VR, Schilder JM, Emerson R. Chapter 20: Vagina. In: Barakat RB, Berchuck A, Markman M, et al., eds. *Principles and Practices of Gynecologic Oncology*, 6th ed. Philadelphia, PA: Lippincott Williams & Wilkins; 2013:573.

More recently, 3D conformal therapy has been used with contouring of target tissues and arrangement of beams/field blocks to cover the proposed targets. Publications on IMRT for vaginal carcinoma are lacking.

The pelvis receives 45 Gy. This will be followed, in some cases, by bilateral pelvic sidewall boosts to a total dose of 55 to 60 Gy. High-energy photons (≥ 10 MV) are usually preferred. CT simulation is highly encouraged since it allows a more accurate delineation of the regional lymph node areas. Treatment portals cover at least the true pelvis with 1.5- to 2.0-cm margin beyond the pelvic rim. Superiorly, the field extends to either L4–5 or L5–S1 to cover the pelvic lymph nodes up to the common iliacs (some choose to cover the common iliacs in more advanced disease, which may extend the superior border to as high as L3) and extends distally to the introitus to include the entire vagina. Lateral fields, if used, should extend anteriorly to adequately include the external iliac nodes, anterior to the pubic symphysis, and at least to the junction of S2–3 posteriorly. At-risk inguinal nodes should be covered and attention should be given to field arrangement or the addition of supplemental electron fields to assure that the inguinal nodes receive sufficient dose.

In patients with tumors involving the middle and lower vagina with clinically negative groins, the bilateral inguinofemoral lymph node regions should be treated electively to 45 to 50 Gy. Planning CT is recommended to determine adequately the depth of the inguinofemoral nodes. A number of techniques have been used to treat the areas at risk without overtreating the femoral necks. Some of the most commonly used techniques include the use of unequal loading (2:1, AP/PA), a combination of low- and high-energy photons (4 to 6 MV, AP, and 15 to 18 MV, PA), or equally weighted beams with a transmission block in the central AP field, utilizing small AP photon or electron beams to deliver a daily boost to the inguinofemoral nodes, or, more recently, the use of IMRT. When using IMRT, it is advisable that the radiation oncologist and radiation team have experience and recognize the importance of adequate target delineation, as well as a quality assurance program that takes into account target shrinkage and interfractional/intrafractional motion.

For patients with positive pelvic nodes or for those patients with advanced disease not amenable to interstitial implant, additional boost to the areas of gross disease, as defined by CT scan, should be given using conformal therapy to deliver a total dose between 65 and 70 Gy, when feasible, with high-energy photons. Boost to the areas of gross nodal disease, as defined by CT scan, should be given using small fields (similar to the parametrial boost with midline shielding) to deliver a total dose between 60 and 65 Gy with high-energy photons. In patients with clinically palpable inguinal nodes, additional doses of 15 to 20 Gy (calculated at a depth determined by CT scan) are necessary with reduced portals. This can generally achieved by using low-energy photons and/or electron beam (12 to 18 MeV), or IMRT techniques. Although the role of IMRT for treatment of vaginal cancer remains undefined, its benefit in reducing GI, GU, and bone marrow toxicity while providing excellent local tumor control has been well documented in other gynecologic sites. M.D. Anderson reported on the use of IMRT in 13 patients with very advanced vaginal cancer patients or with extensive rectovaginal septum involvement that precluded brachytherapy. At 18-month median follow-up, there were no pelvic recurrences, although 2 patients did develop fistulas after treatment. Recently, Stanford University published their experience with the use of IMRT in 10 patients with vaginal SCC showing excellent locoregional control with no grade 3 or 4 toxicities.

Overall treatment time (7 to 9 weeks) has been found to be a significant treatment factor predicting tumor control, although this has not been universally recognized.

Low-Dose Rate Intracavitary Brachytherapy

VAIN and small T1 lesions with less than a 0.5-cm depth can be adequately treated with ICB alone. LDR-ICB is performed using vaginal cylinders loaded with cesium-137 (^{137}Cs) radioactive sources. Ninety-five percent of vaginal lymphatic channels are located within a 3-mm depth from the vaginal surface, confirming the adequacy of prescribing the dose to a depth of 5 mm for superficially invasive lesions.

It is recommended that the largest possible diameter that can be comfortably accommodated by the patient should be used to improve the ratio of mucosa-to-tumor dose and eliminate vaginal rugations. In general, the vulva is sutured closed for the duration of the implant in order to secure the position of the applicators.

In patients with upper vagina lesions with less than a 0.5-cm depth of invasion, vaginal colpostats alone (after hysterectomy) or in combination with intrauterine tandem, loaded with ^{137}Cs sources similar to that used in treatment of cervical cancer, can be used to treat the proximal vagina to a minimum dose of 65 to 70 Gy, estimated to 0.5-cm depth, including the contribution of EBRT if given. When indicated, the remainder of the vagina can be treated by performing a subsequent implant using vaginal cylinders (generally 50 to 60 Gy prescribed to the vaginal surface).

High-Dose Rate Intracavitary Brachytherapy

The International Commission of Radiation Units defines HDR brachytherapy as exceeding 12 Gy/h. HDR-ICB is typically performed with a 10 Ci single iridium-192 (^{192}Ir) source (microSelectron HDR, Nucletron). The applicators are similar to those described for LDR. Generally, the number of insertions ranges from 1 to 6 (median, 3), with the dose per fraction ranging from 300 to 800 cGy (median, 700 cGy). Complications analyses from retrospective data show no significant differences between the HDR and the LDR. The choice of vaginal cylinder mirrors the LDR technique in that the cylinder chosen should be the largest comfortable for the patient. Dose target remains the same (EQD2), but the prescription dose may be at the surface or 5 mm below the mucosal surface. Since the cylinder is in the vagina for only a short time (15 to 45 minutes), it is usually held in place by an immobilization board, rather than a vaginal stitch.

Interstitial Brachytherapy

ITB is an important component in the treatment of more advanced primary vaginal carcinomas, typically in combination with EBRT and/or ICB. As a general rule, temporary implants are more commonly used in the curative treatment of larger gynecologic malignancies, whereas permanent implants are usually performed for smaller volume disease. When performing an interstitial procedure, freehand implants or template systems designed to assist in preplanning and to guide and secure the position of the needles in the target volume can be employed. These templates generally consist of a perineal template, vaginal obturator, and 17-gauge hollow guides of various lengths that can be afterloaded with ^{192}Ir sources. The vaginal obturator is centrally drilled so that it can allow the placement of a tandem to be loaded with ^{137}Cs sources or to accommodate the HDR ^{192}Ir. This makes it possible to combine an interstitial and intracavitary application simultaneously. The major advantage of these systems is greater control of the placement of the sources relative to tumor volume and critical structures owing to the fixed geometry provided by the template. In order to improve the accuracy of target localization and needle placement as well as to improve avoidance of normal structures, several investigators have explored performing ITB under transrectal ultrasound, CT, MRI-planned implants with endorectal coil, laparotomy, and laparoscopic guidance.

Tewari and associates described results in 71 patients who underwent ITB with (61 patients) or without (10 patients) EBRT. Each implant delivered a total tumor dose reaching 80 Gy integrated with EBRT. Local control was achieved in 53 patients (75%). By stage, 5-year DFS rates included stage I, 100%; stage IIA, 60%; stage IIB, 61%; stage III, 30%; and stage IV, 0%. Significant complications occurred in 9 patients (13%) and included necrosis ($n = 4$), fistulas ($n = 4$), and small bowel obstruction ($n = 1$).

Role of Chemotherapy and Radiation

The control rate in the pelvis for stage III and IV patients is relatively low, and about 70% to 80% of the patients have persistent disease or recurrent disease in the pelvis in spite of high doses of EBRT and brachytherapy. Failure in distant sites does occur in about 25% to 30% of the patients with locally advanced tumors, which is much less than pelvic recurrences. Therefore, there is a need for better approaches to the management of advanced disease such as the use of concomitant chemoradiotherapy. Agents such as 5-FU, mitomycin, and cisplatin have shown promise when combined with RT, with complete response rates as high as 60% to 85%, but long-term results of such therapy have been variable, in part owing to the advanced stage of the patients included in these small studies. Extrapolating from published data on locally advanced cervical cancer demonstrating an advantage in locoregional control, overall survival, and DFS for patients receiving cisplatin-based chemotherapy concurrently with RT as well as data on locoregionally advanced vulvar cancer, consideration should be given to a similar approach in patients with advanced vaginal cancer.

PATTERNS OF FAILURE IN SQUAMOUS CELL CARCINOMA

At least 85% of patients who recur will have a component of locoregional failure, and the vast majority of these recurrences will be confined to the pelvis and vagina. The rate of locoregional recurrence in stage I is approximately 10% to 20% versus 30% to 40% in stage II. The pelvic control rate for patients with stage III and stage IV is relatively low, and about 50% to 70% of the patients have recurrences or persistence in spite of well-designed RT. The median time to recurrence is 6 to 12 months. Tumor recurrence is associated with a dismal prognosis, with only a few long-term survivors after salvage therapy. Failure in distant sites alone or associated with locoregional failure does occur in about 25% to 40% of patients with locally advanced tumors.

TREATMENT COMPLICATIONS

KEY POINTS

- At least 85% of patients who recur will have a component of locoregional failure, with the vast majority of these recurrences being confined to the pelvis and vagina.
- The median time to recurrence is 6 to 12 months.
- Tumor recurrence is associated with a dismal prognosis.
- Acute radiation toxicity usually resolves within 2 to 3 months after completion of therapy.

The anatomic location of the vagina places the lower gastrointestinal and genitourinary tracts at greatest risk for complications after surgery or RT.

Acute toxicity from vaginal irradiation includes edema, erythema, moist desquamation, and confluent mucositis with or without ulceration, and the severity of the acute effects varies in intensity and duration depending upon patient age, hormonal status, tumor size, stage, RT dose, and personal hygiene. These effects usually resolve within 2 to 3 months after the completion of therapy. Chemotherapy concurrently with RT enhances the acute mucosal response to both EBRT and brachytherapy. The effects of chemotherapy on the incidence of late complications, if any, are unclear.

Late effects include the development of vaginal atrophy, fibrosis, and stenosis. Telangiectasias are commonly seen in the vagina. Care should be taken in treating these if symptomatic as they can precipitate vaginal necrosis. Vaginal narrowing or shortening, paravaginal fibrosis, loss of elasticity, and reduced lubrication often result in dyspareunia and sexual dysfunction. More severe complications include necrosis with ulceration that can progress to fistula formation (rectovaginal, vesicovaginal, and urethrovaginal). Most series report major complication rates (>Gr 2) of 16% to 17% at 10 years.

The RT tolerance limit of the surface of the proximal vagina is 140 Gy. The distal vaginal tolerance is lower and should be limited to surface doses of less than 90 Gy. In addition, the posterior wall of the vagina is more prone to radiation injury than the anterior and lateral walls, and the dose should be kept below 80 Gy in order to minimize the risk of rectovaginal fistula.

CLEAR CELL CARCINOMA OF THE VAGINA

Stage I CCA of the vagina is adequately managed with surgery, with one series of 142 cases noting an 8% risk of recurrence after radical surgery ($n = 117$) and an 87% survival. As the majority of CCAs occur in the upper third of the vault, the largest series addressing the surgical approach to these lesions have advocated radical hysterectomy, pelvic and para-aortic lymphadenectomy, and sufficient colpectomy to achieve negative margins. Wharton et al. advocate intracavitary or transvaginal irradiation for the treatment of small tumors because this may yield excellent tumor control with a functional vagina and preservation of ovarian function. A combination of wide local excision and extraperitoneal node dissection followed by brachytherapy is an acceptable alternative for patients desirous of fertility preservation.

Most patients with stage II vaginal CCA should be treated with combination EBRT and brachytherapy; however, small, easily resectable lesions in the upper fornix might undergo resection, allowing better preservation of coital and ovarian function.

NONEPITHELIAL TUMORS OF THE VAGINA

> **KEY POINT**
> - As distant disease is the predominant pattern of failure in patients with vaginal melanoma, quality of life should be optimized by offering management with wide excision followed by RT and avoiding disfiguring radical surgery.

Melanoma of the Vagina

Vaginal melanoma is an exceedingly rare entity, and with its propensity to develop distant metastases and its lack of a recognized precursor lesion, it has presented therapeutic challenges with generally disappointing results irrespective of treatment modality. Because vaginal melanoma was deemed a relatively radioresistant tumor, radical surgery had been the treatment of choice in operable patients. However, most series report 5-year survival rates of 5% to 30% regardless of radicality of surgery. As distant disease is the predominant pattern of failure in these patients, quality of life should be optimized by wide excision followed by RT to affect local control, while obviating the need for disfiguring radical surgery.

Recent retrospective data also suggest that vaginal melanoma is reasonably radioresponsive and possibly radiocurable. Volumes and doses of irradiation are similar to those used for epithelial tumors, ranging from 50 Gy for subclinical disease to 75 Gy for gross tumors. Several series have now shown that prolonged local control can be obtained with RT as an adjunct to more limited surgery, or even with RT alone, primarily in patients with lesions ≤3 cm in diameter. The use of systemic chemotherapy and/or immunotherapy has been very disappointing in the limited published data. Due to an extremely high risk of local recurrence of distant metastasis, the prognosis of vaginal melanoma continues to be very poor regardless of treatment delivered.

Sarcomas of the Vagina

Sarcomas represent 3% of vaginal primaries with leiomyosarcoma representing 50% to 65% of vaginal sarcomas, with the majority arising from the posterior vaginal wall. Histopathologic grade appears to be the most important predictor of outcome. Radical surgical resection, such as posterior pelvic exenteration, offers the best chance for cure for vaginal leiomyosarcomas. Sarcomas are relatively resistant to chemotherapy, and the most common site of failure is the pelvis. In 50% of patients with recurrence, it is the only site of failure. Five-year survival rates are generally better in patients with leiomyosarcoma than in patients with carcinosarcoma.

Adjuvant RT seems to be indicated in patients with high-grade tumors and locally recurrent low-grade sarcomas.

Embryonal RMS of the vagina, the most common pediatric vaginal tumor, is appropriately managed through the use of multimodality therapy. A series of reports from the Intergroup Rhabdomyosarcoma Study Group have reported survival rates in excess of 85% utilizing VAC chemotherapy and wide excision with or without adjuvant RT, sparing the great majority of patients from exenterative surgery. However, due to the high rates of local recurrence in patients who did not receive adjuvant RT in the IRS III and IV trials, the recent Children's Oncology Group ARST0331 study amended their protocol to require adjuvant RT at week 13 for all patients with vaginal primaries. This study is closed to accrual and currently completing follow-up assessments.

SALVAGE THERAPY

This group represents a heterogeneous population, and careful workup to establish the extent of disease is crucial. Local recurrences should be confirmed by biopsy. In most cases, only patients with small-volume local recurrences and no metastatic disease are curable.

Generally, patients with isolated pelvic or regional recurrences after definitive surgery who have not received prior RT are managed with EBRT, often in conjunction with brachytherapy. Concurrent cisplatin-based chemotherapy may also be recommended, and extrapolation from the available data for locally advanced cervical and vulvar cancer suggests that a combined modality approach with chemoradiation may improve the locoregional control and survival in patients with isolated pelvic recurrences. Salvage options for patients with central recurrence after definitive or adjuvant RT are limited to radical surgery, usually exenterative, or, in selected patients with small volume disease, reirradiation using interstitial radiation implants or highly conformal 3D EBRT. In patients with small, well-defined vulvovaginal or pelvic recurrences, reirradiation using primarily interstitial techniques has been attempted with control rates between 50% and 75% and grade 3 or higher complication rates between 7% and 15%. Recently, stereotactic body irradiation using high-dose, localized therapy has been reported with acceptable palliative outcomes and toxicity; however, studies are few, small, and retrospective.

PALLIATIVE THERAPY

Radiation Therapy

At the present time, there is no curative option for patients who present with stage IVB disease. Many of these patients suffer from severe pelvic pain or bleeding. Palliative radiation with either ICB (for vaginal bleeding) or EBRT can result in good tumor regression and excellent palliation of symptoms. The RTOG published on a palliative schedule that is well tolerated with good symptomatic results. The treatment is 370 cGy BID for two days. Three courses are delivered, with a field reduction on the third. Combination with taxol chemotherapy has been reported as well.

Chemotherapy in Advanced and Recurrent Vaginal Cancer

Treatment of recurrent or metastatic disease is confined to a handful of phase II clinical trials and anecdotal reports. In general, regimens that are active in cervical cancer are usually active in vaginal cancer. Regimens including cisplatin, mitoxantrone, 5-FU, mitomycin C, bleomycin, vincristine, and MVAC (methotrexate, vinblastine, doxorubicin, and cisplatin) have been reported with varying success.

SUGGESTED READINGS

Beriwal S, Demanes DJ, Erickson B, et al. American Brachytherapy Society consensus guidelines for interstitial brachytherapy for vaginal cancer. *Brachytherapy.* 2012;11:68–75.

Blanchard P, Monnier L, Dumas L, et al. Low-dose-rate definitive brachytherapy for high-grade vaginal intraepithelial neoplasia. *Oncologist.* 2011;16:182–188.

Carrascosa LA, Yashar CM, Paris KJ, et al. Palliation of pelvic and head and neck cancer with paclitaxel and a novel radiotherapy regimen. *J Palliat Med.* 2007;10:877–881.

Chaudhuri S, Das D, Chowdhury S, et al. Primary malignant melanoma of the vagina: A case report and review of literature. *South Asian J Cancer.* 2013;2:4.

Chyle V, Zagars GK, Wheeler JA, et al. Definitive radiotherapy for carcinoma of the vagina. *Int J Radiat Oncol Biol Phys.* 1996;35:891–905.

Creasman WT, Phillips JL, Menck HR. The National Cancer Data Base report on cancer of the vagina. *Cancer.* 1998;83:1033–1040.

Daling JR, Madeleine MM, Schwartz SM, et al. A population-based study of squamous cell vaginal cancer: HPV and cofactors. *Gynecol Oncol.* 2002;84(2):263.

Frank SJ, Jhingran A, Levenback C, et al. Definitive radiation therapy for squamous cell carcinoma of the vagina. *Int J Radiat Oncol Biol Phys.* 2005;62:138–147.

Hiniker SM, Roux A, Murphy JD, et al. Primary squamous cell carcinoma of the vagina: Prognostic factors, treatment patterns, and outcomes. *Gynecol Oncol.* 2013;131(2):380–385.

Iavazzo C, Pitsouni E, Athanasiou S, et al. Imiquimod for treatment of vulvar and vaginal intraepithelial neoplasia. *Int J Gynecol Obstet.* 2008;101:3–10.

Kirkbride P, Fyles A, Rawlings GA, et al. Carcinoma of the vagina-experience at the Princess Margaret Hospital (1974–1989). *Gynecol Oncol.* 1995;56:435–443.

Kucera H, Vavra N. Radiation management of primary carcinoma of the vagina: Clinical and histopathological variables associated with survival. *Gynecol Oncol.* 1991;40:12–16.

Kunos CA, Debernardo E, Radivoyevitch T, et al. Hematological toxicity after robotic stereotactic body radiosurgery for treatment of metastatic gynecologic malignancies. *Int J Radiat Oncol Biol Phys.* 2012;84:e35–e41.

Kunos CA, Fabien J, Zhang Y, et al. Gynecologic cancer. In: Simon S. Lo, Bin S. Teh, Jiade J. Lu, et al., eds. *Stereotactic Body Radiation Therapy.* Berlin, Germany: Springer; 2012:211–225.

Magné N, Pacaut C, Auberdiac P, et al. Sarcoma of the vulva, vagina and ovary. *Best Pract Res Clin Obstet Gynaecol.* 2011;25(6):797–801.

Murakami N, Kasamatsu T, Sumi M, et al. Radiation therapy for primary vaginal carcinoma. *J Radiat Res.* 2013;54:931–937.

Perez CA, Grigsby PW, Garipagaoglu M, et al. Factors affecting long-term outcome of irradiation in carcinoma of the vagina. *Int J Radiat Oncol Biol Phys.* 1999;44:37–45.

Spanos W Jr, Guse C, Perez C, et al. Phase II study of multiple daily fractionations in the palliation of advanced pelvic malignancies: Preliminary report of RTOG 8502. *Int J Radiat Oncol Biol Phys.* 1989;17:659–661.

Vera R, Eifel PJ, Jhingran A, et al. Intensity-modulated radiation therapy (IMRT) in the treatment of carcinoma of the vagina. *Int J Radiat Oncol Biol Phys.* 2007;69:S396.

Wee WW, Chia YN, Yam PK. Diagnosis and treatment of vaginal intraepithelial neoplasia. *Int J Gynecol Obstet.* 2012;117:15–17.

Wharton JT, Routledge FN, Gallager HS, et al. Treatment of clear cell adenocarcinoma in young females. *Obstet Gynecol.* 1975;45:365–368.

Xia L, Han D, Yang W, et al. Primary malignant melanoma of the vagina: A retrospective clinicopathologic study of 44 cases. *Int J Gynecol Cancer.* 2014;24:149–155.

The Uterine Cervix

EPIDEMIOLOGY

Worldwide, cervical cancer is the fourth most common cancer (after breast and colorectal) in women and is the leading cause of death of women from cancer in developing countries. Approximately one half million new cases occur each year, with the majority of cases occurring in developing countries lacking access to routine Papanicolaou (Pap) smear screening. Cervical carcinoma is the 14th most common malignant tumor in women in the United States. In 2013, an estimated 12,340 women will be diagnosed with invasive cervical cancer in the United States, and an estimated 4,030 women will die from the disease. While the incidence and mortality of this disease in North America have declined during the last half-century, black and Hispanic women continue to be disproportionately affected, especially in the southern United States.

RISK FACTORS AND ETIOLOGY

KEY POINTS

- Cervical cancer is a sexually transmitted disease associated with chronic infection by oncogenic types of human papillomavirus (HPV).
- Tobacco smoking may be a cofactor for the development of high-grade cervical dysplasia in women who have chronic HPV infections.
- HPV 16 and 18 account for approximately 70% of cervical cancers.

Cervical cancer is a sexually transmitted disease associated with chronic infection by oncogenic types of HPV. Therefore, risk factors for cervical cancer are the same as those for sexually transmitted disease, including early age at onset of sexual activity, multiple pregnancies, long duration of oral contraceptive use, other sexually transmitted infections including chlamydia and herpes simplex virus, immunosuppressed states such as renal transplant, and multiple sexual partners. Tobacco smoking is also a risk factor for cervical cancer and may be a cofactor for development of high-grade cervical dysplasia in women who have chronic HPV infections.

Human Papillomavirus

HPV is a double-stranded DNA virus, with more than 30 recognized oncogenic and more than 70 nononcogenic strains of HPV being described to date. In the United States, HPV 16 and 18 account for approximately 70% of cervix cancers. High-risk HPV genotypes code for three early proteins (E5, E6, and E7) with cellular growth–stimulating and transforming properties. The E6 protein binds to p53, results in chromosomal instability, activates telomerase, inhibits apoptosis, and results in cellular immortalization. The E7 protein binds to retinoblastoma protein (Rb), inactivating the Rb-related pocket proteins, activates cyclins E and A, inhibits cyclin-dependent kinase inhibitors, and also results in cellular immortalization. HPV E6 and E7 lead to dysplasia and malignant transformation of cervical epithelium. High-risk HPV types are identified in a high percentage of patients with adenocarcinoma of the cervix and small cell carcinoma of the cervix in addition to the more common squamous carcinoma of the cervix.

Cellular and humoral immune responses are likely to be involved in the resolution of HPV infection, and deficiencies, such as caused by human immunodeficiency virus (HIV) infection, may result in more rapid progression to dysplasia and carcinoma.

Almost 50% of women will be infected with the HPV within 4 years after the onset of sexual activity, with prevalence peaking between 25 to 35 years of age. Despite a high prevalence of HPV, only 5% to 15% will develop cervical dysplasia.

Concurrent Infection with HPV and Human Immunodeficiency Virus

HIV is a sexually transmitted virus that results in a decline in circulating CD4+ cells over time. Concurrent infection with HIV and HPV may result in more rapid progression from chronic HPV infection to dysplasia and cancer, and HIV+ patients with concurrent HPV infection must be followed closely and aggressively treated for squamous intraepithelial lesions. Although it has been long believed that antiretroviral therapy does not affect HPV-related disease in HIV-infected patients, recent data from the Canadian Women's HIV Study show that HIV+ patients on antiretroviral therapy experience higher likelihood of regression of cervical SIL.

ANATOMY

The cervix is an extension of the lower uterine segment of the uterus. The cervix varies in length, averaging 3 to 4 cm. Centrally in the vaginal portion is the external cervical os, which connects to the endocervical canal, the internal cervical os, and the endometrial canal.

The cervix is lined by squamous and columnar cells. The transition from columnar cells to squamous cells occurs in the region of the cervical os known as the transformation zone. Most cervical dysplasias and invasive cancers arise from this area. The endocervix contains mostly mucinous glandular epithelium.

The uterus has five ligamentous attachments: the round, broad, utero-ovarian, cardinal, and uterosacral ligaments. Within the leaves of the broad ligament are extraperitoneal connective tissues, known as the parametrium. The blood supply of the uterus is mainly through the uterine artery, originating from the anterior division of the hypogastric artery. The lymphatics of the cervix drain into the paracervical and parametrial lymph nodes and to the internal, external, and common iliac chains. The obturator lymph nodes are the most medial portion of the external iliac nodal region. Other lymphatic drainage routes include the inferior and superior gluteal lymph nodes and the superior rectal, presacral, and para-aortic lymph nodes. The innervations of the cervix are from the sacral roots (S2–4).

NATURAL HISTORY

KEY POINTS

■ An interval of epithelial dysplastic changes, typically in the transformation zone, known as cervical intraepithelial neoplasia (CIN), precedes the development of invasive cancer.

■ The reported rate of progression of carcinoma *in situ* (CIS) to invasive cancer ranges from 12% to 22%.

■ The pattern of lymphatic metastases is predictable and orderly as the rate of paraaortic lymph node metastasis is very rare if the pelvic nodes are uninvolved.

■ The most common sites of hematogenous spread include the lung, mediastinum, bone, and liver.

■ Most recurrences occur in the first 24 months, with a median of 17 months.

Preinvasive Disease

Cervical cancer is preceded by an interval of epithelial dysplastic changes, typically in the transformation zone, known as, which may progress to invasive cancer. Low-grade dysplasia (CIN 1) is confined to the basal one third of the epithelium, and most low-grade lesions will regress to normal in about 24 months. Full thickness involvement is known as CIN 3 or CIS. Overall, the reported rate of progression of CIS to invasive cancer ranges from 12% to 22%.

Patterns of Spread

Cervical cancer can spread through direct extension to the endocervix, lower uterine segment, parametrium, vagina and, less often, to the bladder and/or rectum. It can also spread through the lymphatics to the parametrial, obturator, and internal, external, and common iliac lymph nodes. The pattern of spread is usually predictable and orderly as the rate of para-aortic lymph node metastasis is very rare if the pelvic nodes were spared. The overall risk of pelvic lymph node metastasis in stage IB is about 17%. The risk of paraaortic nodal metastasis is higher with advanced stage, with rates of 16% and 25% for stages II and III, respectively. The most common sites of hematogenous spread include the lung, mediastinum, bone, and liver. Most recurrences occur in the first 24 months with a median of 17 months.

CLINICAL PRESENTATION AND DIAGNOSTIC EVALUATION

KEY POINTS

■ The two primary means of obtaining and diagnosing cervical dysplasia are the conventional Papanicolaou smear and the liquid-based thin-layer preparation.

■ The combination of negative cytology and HPV testing carries a high negative predictive value of over 95% regarding the development of CIN 3 or invasive cancer.

■ HPV testing is more sensitive in detecting high-grade disease compared to conventional smears, but it has a lower specificity rate.

■ Indications for colposcopy include an abnormal-appearing cervix, persistent postcoital bleeding or discharge, persistent CIN 1, 2, or 3 on cytology, *in utero* exposure to diethylstilbestrol (DES), and atypical squamous cells of uncertain significance (ASCUS) smears with positive high-risk HPV testing.

Preclinical Invasive Disease

Screening and Cytology

The two primary means of obtaining and diagnosing cervical dysplasia are the conventional Pap smear and the liquid-based thin-layer preparation. Although the data are conflicting, it appears that liquid-based cytology may be superior to conventional cytology, increasing detection rates of low- and high-grade abnormalities. The American Cancer Society (ACS) updated their cervical cancer screening guidelines in 2012. The current recommendation is to start cytologic screening at age 21. For women aged 21 to 29 years, screening should be performed every 3 years with conventional or liquid-based Pap tests. From ages 30 to 65, combination HPV and cytology screening (cotesting) every 5 years or cytology screening alone every 3 years is recommended. ACS recommends stopping at age 65 if there have been three consecutive negative cytology tests or two consecutive negative HPV and Pap tests in the past 10 years, with the most recent screening occurring within 5 years.

According to the ACS, women with HIV infection, immunosuppression, or in utero DES exposure will require more frequency screening. ACOG recommends annual screening for women who have been treated in the past for CIN 2, CIN 3, or cervical cancer. ACOG recommends screening twice in the 1st year for women who are immunocompromised and annually thereafter.

HPV Testing

The combination of negative cytology and HPV testing carries a high negative predictive value of over 95% regarding the development of CIN 3 or invasive cancer, providing great reassurance for low-risk women and lengthening the interval of screening in that population to 3 years.

HPV testing is much more sensitive in detecting high-grade disease compared to conventional smears but with a lower specificity rate. Screening women younger than 30 years may lead to unnecessary testing as many HPV infections are transient, and most women will not develop dysplasia with HPV infection. In low-grade squamous intraepithelial lesion, more than 85% of cases test positive for HPV. Therefore, HPV testing is not encouraged. HPV testing appears to be useful in triage of ASCUS smears, possibly reducing colposcopic referrals by almost 50%.

Colposcopy

Colposcopy examines the lower genital tract including the vulva, vagina, and epithelium of the cervix and opening of the endocervix. The use of acetic acid and Lugol solution assists in highlighting abnormal changes that could signify high-grade disease such as aceto-white plaques and vascular abnormalities (punctations, mosaicism, and abnormal branching). Indications for colposcopy include an abnormal appearing cervix; persistent postcoital bleeding or discharge; persistent CIN 1, 2, or 3 on cytology; *in utero* exposure to diethylstilbestrol; and ASCUS smears with positive high-risk HPV testing. Adequate colposcopic examination mandates full visualization of the entire transformation zone endocervical curettage (ECC) and concordance on biopsy with Pap smear results.

Conization Biopsy

Cervical conization refers to the surgical removal of the squamocolumnar junction. This may be done in the operating suite through a classical cold knife conization technique or as an outpatient using thermal cautery with loop excision. Indications for conization include inadequate colposcopy; positive ECC; persistent CIN 1 (usually >1 year); CIN 2, 3; or CIS; and discrepancy between cytologic, colposcopic, or pathologic findings.

Clinical Disease

Symptoms and Complaints

The most common presentations of invasive cervical cancer are abnormal vaginal bleeding, postcoital bleeding, and vaginal discharge. As the tumor enlarges, it can cause local symptoms such as pelvic pain and difficulty with urination or defecation. As the disease metastasizes to regional lymph nodes, back pain, leg swelling (especially unilateral), and neuropathic pain may occur. Local extension can cause urinary or rectal symptoms or pain.

Physical Findings

The most common finding on physical examination is an abnormal lesion on the cervix, at times necrotic and friable. Possible extension onto the vaginal wall should be assessed. Determination of parametrial, sidewall, and uterosacral ligament involvement must be done through a rectovaginal examination. Other areas of concern are the superficial groin and femoral lymph nodes and the supraclavicular region.

Staging

KEY POINTS

- Cervical cancer is clinically staged by physical examination and limited radiographic evaluation.
- Positron emission tomography (PET) has emerged as a superior method of imaging nodal disease in cervical cancer.
- Surgical findings and radiographically guided biopsies of suspected lesions cannot be used to change or modify clinical FIGO staging.
- The diagnosis of microinvasive disease (MID) must be made on a conization or hysterectomy specimen.

Laboratory Studies

A complete peripheral blood count is indicated to evaluate for anemia, which might warrant correction. Serum chemistries with attention to serum creatinine are essential to evaluate for renal failure or assess renal function in patients who will receive cisplatin-based chemoradiotherapy. Additional tests should include liver functions and urinalysis.

Radiographic Studies

Cervical cancer is clinically staged by physical examination and limited radiographic evaluation. Computed tomography (CT) and magnetic resonance imaging (MRI) are used extensively to delineate disease extent and improve treatment planning but do not change the assigned Fédération Internationale de Gynécologie et d'Obstetrique (FIGO) staging. American Joint Commission on Cancer has a less used but similar staging system but does take radiologic findings into account. Several studies and a meta-analysis have shown an increased sensitivity for MRI as compared with CT for the evaluation of tumor size, uterine body involvement, and extent of disease.

Modern imaging techniques, such as CT and MRI, have low sensitivities for detecting disease in the paraaortic nodes less than 1 cm. PET has emerged as a superior method of imaging nodal disease in cervical cancer. The reported sensitivity is about 85% to 90% and the specificity about 95% to 100%.

FIGO and American Joint Committee Commission on Cancer Staging

The staging system most commonly used for cervical cancer is based on the 2009 FIGO staging system and is shown in Table 7.1. Stage IA1 is defined as stromal invasion to less than or equal to 3 mm in depth and no wider than 7 mm; stage IA2 is defined as stromal invasion of 3 to 5 mm with width of no greater than 7 mm. In addition to size criteria, the Society of Gynecologic Oncologists (SGO) also considers negative lymphovascular space invasion (LVSI) and margin status as criteria for MID. The horizontal spread must be 7 mm or less to be considered MID according to FIGO, but SGO does not include lateral spread in defining MID. The diagnosis of MID must be made on a conization or hysterectomy specimen. Punch biopsies are not adequate. Stage IB is divided into IB1, which includes all lesions greater than IA2 and no more than 4 cm in greatest dimension, and stage IB2, a lesion limited to the cervix measuring greater than 4 cm.

Table 7.1	FIGO Staging of Carcinoma of the Uterine Cervix (Updated 2009)

Stage I: The carcinoma is strictly confined to the cervix (extension to the corpus would be disregarded).

    IA: Invasive carcinoma that can be diagnosed only by microscopy, with deepest invasion ≤5 mm and largest extension ≤7 mm.

        IA1: Measured stromal invasion of ≤3.0 mm in depth and extension of ≤7.0 mm.

        IA2: Measured stromal invasion of >3.0 mm and not >5.0 mm with an extension of not more than 7.0 mm.

    IB: Clinically visible lesions limited to the cervix uteri or preclinical cancers greater than stage IA.[a]

        IB1: Clinically visible lesion ≤4.0 cm in greatest dimension.

        IB2: Clinically visible lesion >4.0 cm in greatest dimension.

Stage II: Cervical carcinoma invades beyond the uterus, but not to the pelvic wall or to the lower third of the vagina.

    IIA: Without parametrial invasion.

        IIA1: Clinically visible lesion ≤4.0 cm in greatest dimension.

        IIA2: Clinically visible lesion >4 cm in greatest dimension.

    IIB: With obvious parametrial invasion.

Stage III: The tumor extends to the pelvic wall and/or involves lower third of the vagina and/or causes hydronephrosis or nonfunctioning kidney.[b]

    IIIA: Tumor involves lower third of the vagina, with no extension to the pelvic wall.

    IIIB: Extension to the pelvic wall and/or hydronephrosis or nonfunctioning kidney.

Stage IV: The carcinoma has extended beyond the true pelvis or has involved (biopsy proven) the mucosa of the bladder or rectum. A bullous edema, as such, does not permit a case to be allotted to Stage IV.

    IVA: Spread of the growth to adjacent organs.

    IVB: Spread to distant organs.

[a]All macroscopically visible lesions—even with superficial invasion—are allotted to stage IB carcinomas. Invasion is limited to a measured stromal invasion with a maximal depth of 5.00 mm and a horizontal extension of no >7.00 mm. Depth of invasion should not be >5.00 mm taken from the base of the epithelium of the original tissue—superficial or glandular. The depth of invasion should always be reported in millimeter, even in those cases with "early (minimal) stromal invasion" (~1 mm).

[b]On rectal examination, there is no cancer-free space between the tumor and the pelvic wall. All cases with hydronephrosis or nonfunctioning kidney are included, unless they are known to be due to another cause.

Source: From Pecorelli S. Revised FIGO staging for carcinoma of the vulva, cervix, and endometrium. *Int J Gynaecol Obstet.* 2009;105:103–104.

Surgical findings and radiographically guided biopsies of suspected lesions cannot be used to change or modify clinical FIGO staging. Stage IVA requires biopsy confirmation of bladder or rectal mucosal involvement. Stage IIIB indicates pelvic sidewall involvement or demonstration of a nonfunctioning kidney or hydronephrosis.

A TNM (Tumor, Node, Metastasis) staging system is proposed by American Joint Committee Commission on Cancer (AJCC) and is mainly used in documenting findings on surgical and pathologic evaluations as the pathologic stage of the disease. If there is ambiguity regarding the correct stage when two qualified professionals evaluate the patient, the lower stage is assigned.

Pretreatment Nodal Staging

The presence of paraaortic lymph node metastases is known to have a significant impact on progression-free and overall survival. Pretreatment knowledge of paraaortic spread could potentially direct treatment in a manner that could improve outcomes. Given the limitations of imaging in reliably detecting paraaortic micrometastases, surgical staging has been used. However, the role of surgical staging for locally advanced cervical cancer remains unclear.

PATHOLOGY

KEY POINTS

- Squamous CIS is a precursor lesion of invasive squamous carcinoma.
- Untreated squamous CIS results in invasive carcinoma in about one third of cases over a period of 10 years.
- Adenocarcinoma accounts for 20% to 25% of cervical carcinomas and is associated with HPV (usually type 18, but sometimes type 16).
- Adenosquamous carcinomas appear to be either histologically more aggressive or diagnosed at a later stage than adenocarcinomas of the uterine cervix.

Squamous Cell Carcinoma

Preinvasive Disease

Squamous CIS is a precursor lesion of invasive squamous carcinoma, and it is characterized by full-thickness atypia of the cervical epithelium. Endocervical glands may also be involved. The normal maturation of squamous epithelium is absent. There is no breach of the underlying basement membrane.

Microinvasive Carcinoma

Microinvasive squamous carcinoma is associated with squamous intraepithelial neoplasia, and it is characterized by small nests of cells that have escaped the basement membrane of the surface or glandular epithelium. Microinvasive carcinoma often displays cells that are larger, with more abundant eosinophilic cytoplasm than cells in the adjacent dysplasia.

A diagnosis of microinvasive squamous carcinoma of the cervix requires a loop electrosurgical excisional procedure or conization biopsy that encompasses the entire lesion and has negative margins (Fig. 7.1).

Invasive Squamous Cell Carcinoma

Invasive cervical carcinoma arises from high-grade dysplasia, which may be detected up to 10 years before invasive carcinoma develops. Untreated squamous CIS results in invasive carcinoma in about one third of cases over

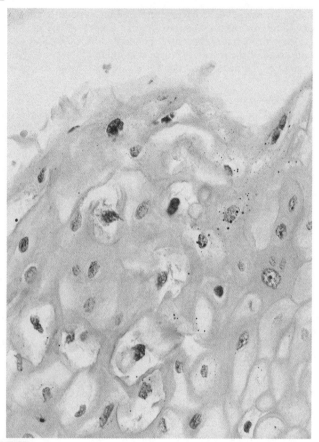

FIGURE 7.1 HPV changes. This squamous epithelium displays cells with large halos surrounding atypical nuclei ("koilocytotic atypia").

a period of 10 years. Invasive carcinoma occurs most often after the age of 40 years, although it may be seen in young women. It is associated with HPV infection in more than 99% of cases. These tumors may consist of firm, indurated masses, or they may be ulcerated or polypoid. Microscopic examination reveals irregular, haphazardly infiltrating nests of cells with eosinophilic cytoplasm and enlarged, atypical, hyperchromatic nuclei.

Lymphatic and vascular space invasion may be present, especially in more deeply invasive tumors. Invasive squamous carcinomas are also graded, although treatment protocols do not depend on grade, and the histologic grade may not correlate with prognosis. Lesions are graded 1 to 3 (well, moderately, and poorly differentiated). Grade 2 (moderately differentiated) tumors represent the majority of invasive squamous carcinomas of the uterine cervix and are usually nonkeratinizing squamous carcinomas with nuclear pleomorphism, numerous mitoses, and an infiltrative pattern. Grade 3 (poorly differentiated) tumors either have smaller cells without neuroendocrine differentiation or are pleomorphic with anaplastic nuclei and sometimes a tendency to form spindle cells that must be distinguished from sarcoma by positive cytokeratin stains.

Adenocarcinoma

While the incidence of squamous carcinoma of the cervix has decreased in the past decades owing to cytologic screening, the number of cases of cervical adenocarcinoma has increased. Adenocarcinoma accounts for 20% to 25% of cervical carcinomas.

Adenocarcinoma *in situ* (AIS) is a precursor of invasive adenocarcinoma. It is found adjacent to many invasive adenocarcinomas, often accompanied by squamous dysplasia. Both AIS and invasive adenocarcinoma of the cervix are associated with HPV (usually type 18, but sometimes type 16).

AIS is characterized by preservation of the overall endocervical gland architecture. However, endocervical glands and surface epithelium are replaced to varying degrees by cells displaying atypia. Most adenocarcinomas *in situ* occur near the transformation zone, and skip lesions are unusual.

Other Epithelial Tumors

Adenosquamous carcinoma is a tumor composed of admixed malignant glandular and squamous elements. A recent multi-institutional study found that adenosquamous carcinomas are more commonly associated with higher tumor grade ($p < 0.001$) and vascular invasion ($p = 0.002$) than are adenocarcinomas. Adenosquamous carcinomas appear to be either histologically more aggressive or diagnosed at a later stage than adenocarcinomas of the uterine cervix.

Small Cell Carcinoma

Most neuroendocrine tumors seen in the uterine cervix represent small cell carcinomas. Even a small component of small cell carcinoma in a tumor of mixed type is associated with adverse outcome. These tumors are morphologically identical to those seen in small cell carcinoma of the lung. They are aneuploid tumors that show a strong association with type 18 HPV. Immunohistochemical stains for neuroendocrine markers, such as chromogranin and synaptophysin, may be helpful in the diagnosis. CD56 (neural cell adhesion molecule) is a sensitive marker for the diagnosis of small cell cancer in the cervix.

Mixed Epithelial, Mesenchymal Tumors, and Other Malignant Tumors

Uncommon malignant tumors of the cervix include sarcomas, malignant mixed müllerian tumors, endometrial stromal sarcomas, melanomas, granulocytic sarcomas, primitive neuroectodermal tumors, desmoplastic small round cell tumors, and primary germ cell tumors. Primary extranodal lymphomas of the uterine cervix are usually diffuse B-cell neoplasms.

PROGNOSTIC FACTORS

KEY POINTS

- Size of the primary tumor, depth of stromal invasion, lymphovascular invasion, and parametrial involvement have been correlated with disease-free survival in patients undergoing radical hysterectomy (RH).
- While FIGO stage is prognostically significant in predicting outcome, lymph node involvement is, in most studies, the most significant negative prognostic factor.

Tumor Size, Volume, and Margin Status

Size of the primary tumor, depth of stromal invasion, and parametrial involvement have been correlated with disease-free survival in patients undergoing RH. Lymphovascular space invasion and depth of cervical stromal invasion have also been associated with significantly poorer prognosis.

Size has also been correlated with increased pelvic failure rates in patients treated definitively with radiation. In patients with stage IB cervical cancer treated surgically, with or without RT, positive margin status conveyed a hazard ratio of 3.92 compared to negative margins. Also, margin status (distance in millimeter in patients with close margins) was significantly associated with an increased recurrence rate. In this series, postoperative RT eliminated local recurrences in patients with close margins and halved the recurrence rate in patients with positive margins.

Stage

The FIGO stage is universally accepted for its prognostic significance. Paraaortic node metastasis confers a much greater risk than measures of tumor volume, however, and emphasizes the fact that FIGO staging does not take into account important prognostic information such as nodal status.

Nodal Status

Lymph node involvement is, in most studies, the most significant negative prognostic factor. Reports emphasize higher 5-year survival rates (90% or higher) among surgically treated patients with no evidence of metastasis in the regional nodes, compared to patients with positive pelvic (50% to 60%) or paraaortic nodes (20% to 45%).

Lymphovascular Space Invasion

LVSI proved to be a significant prognostic factor in a surgical–pathologic study of 542 patients completed by the Gynecologic Oncology Group (GOG). Disease-free survivals were 77% and 89%, respectively, in patients with and without LVSI. Furthermore, LVSI was shown to correlate with pelvic adenopathy and with time to recurrence.

Hypoxia and Anemia

The presence of both hypoxia and anemia has been independently correlated in multiple studies with adverse outcomes in patients with cervical cancer. The data regarding anemia's impact are largely retrospective, while hypoxia has been studied through direct tumor measurements in patients treated definitively with surgery as well as with radiation therapy. Studies have not confirmed the hypothesis of a direct correlation between anemia and tumor hypoxia, and the relationship between these two prognostic factors is complex. Several authors have suggested that a lower hemoglobin level could also be a marker for more aggressive disease as opposed to a physiologic variable that could be manipulated for therapeutic benefit.

Histopathology

Conflicting data exist regarding the prognostic significance of adenocarcinoma as compared with squamous cell carcinoma, with some studies suggesting similar survival rates for comparable stages and others suggesting inferior survival in the adenocarcinoma subgroup. There is evidence that adenosquamous carcinoma is either a histologically more aggressive tumor than cervical adenocarcinoma or is diagnosed later in the disease course.

Higher tumor grade and vascular invasion are statistically more common in adenosquamous carcinoma than adenocarcinoma of the cervix. The presence of small cell neuroendocrine carcinoma in any amount, even when associated with other types of neoplasm, is an independent prognostic factor associated with aggressive tumor behavior.

GENERAL MANAGEMENT AND RESULTS OF TREATMENT

KEY POINTS

- A quadrivalent vaccine targeting HPV types 16, 18, 6, and 11 is now recommended for all women of ages 9 to 26.
- As up to 30% of CIN and invasive cancers are caused by strains not in the vaccine, women who receive the vaccine are recommended to be followed according to guidelines already set for cytologic smears.
- Severe dysplasia/CIN and CIS are adequately managed with local therapies such as conization, laser ablation, cryotherapy, or a simple hysterectomy.
- Stage IA1 carcinoma is usually treated with conization or hysterectomy.
- Stage IA2 squamous cell carcinoma is a modified (type II) radical hysterectomy (MRH) and pelvic lymphadenectomy, although curative-intent RT is an equivalent option.
- Radical surgery and definitive chemoradiation have similar good outcomes for stage IB to IIA nonbulky tumors.
- Bulky IB2, IIB, IIIB, and IVA tumors are treated with curative-intent chemoradiation.

PREVENTION: HPV VACCINATION

Currently, there are two FDA-approved HPV vaccines that have been shown in randomized clinical trials to be highly effective in protecting against high-risk HPV infections. Both Gardasil (quadrivalent vaccine) and Cervarix (bivalent vaccine) protect against HPV types 16 and 18, the cause of 70% of cervical cancers and 50% of precancerous cervical lesions. Gardasil also protects against HPV 6 and 11, which are responsible for approximately 90% of genital warts. In addition to cervical cancer prevention, Gardasil is also approved for prevention of anal, vaginal, and vulvar cancers in women, as well as the prevention of anal and penile cancers in men. The American College of Obstetricians and Gynecologists recommends the quadrivalent or bivalent HPV vaccine for all women aged 9 to 26 years. As up to 30% of CIN and invasive cancers are caused by strains not in the vaccine, all women who receive the vaccine should follow standard screening recommendations. The HPV vaccine is given at 0, 2, and 6 months. The HPV vaccine is not effective in those with active HPV infection and abnormal cytology.

Severe Dysplasia and Carcinoma *In Situ*

Patients with severe dysplasia/CIN and CIS have essentially no risk of lymphatic involvement and are often treated with local therapies such as conization, laser ablation, cryotherapy, or a simple hysterectomy. These various techniques have comparable efficacy. Patients with HIV infection, high HPV viral load, positive margins, older age, and residual high-risk infection following conservative management have a higher recurrence rate. Reported rates of recurrent CIS and invasive cancer following therapeutic conization are low (<5%).

Factors associated with persistent disease or invasive cancer following cold knife conization include residual CIN 3, positive ectocervical and endocervical margins, multiquadrant disease, age greater than 50, and positive endocervical curettings. Patients with positive ECC after conization or positive endocervical margins on a cone specimen for CIS should have repeat conization prior to hysterectomy to avoid inappropriate treatment for invasive disease.

Since patients with CIS have virtually no risk of pelvic adenopathy, it is also appropriate to treat with only intracavitary RT. Tumor control rates of 100% have been reported. Grigsby and Perez successfully treated 21 such patients with a single intracavitary implant, delivering a mean point A dose of 46.12 Gy; no treatment sequelae were observed.

Stage IA

The concept of "microinvasion" (equating to FIGO stage IA) should define tumors that penetrate the basement membrane but have little or no risk of nodal involvement or dissemination. All macroscopically visible lesions are considered stage IB tumors.

Stage IA1 carcinoma is usually treated with conization or extrafascial hysterectomy. The control rate approaches 100%. Absence of LVSI plays a key role in opting for the conservative management of patients with MID as its presence may herald a higher incidence of lymphatic involvement as well as tumor recurrence.

Patients with FIGO IA2 disease with LVSI are not candidates for conservative surgical approaches in most circumstances. The recommended treatment for stage IA2 squamous cell carcinoma is a modified (type II) RH and pelvic lymphadenectomy, although curative-intent RT is an equivalent option. The average pelvic lymphatic metastasis rate from reported data is 5% to 13%. In patients who are medically inoperable, intracavitary RT may be used, with several series documenting excellent outcomes and low complication rates.

Adenocarcinoma Early Disease

The incidence of cervical adenocarcinoma has increased in the past 40 years. Almost all AIS lesions are associated with HPV, with 18 being the predominant type. The management of AIS is controversial. The term "microinvasion" may be inaccurate in describing glandular lesions as an accurate measurement of depth of invasion in glands may be difficult. The overall rate of residual disease in hysterectomy specimens after conization with negative margins is 25% and with positive margin is around 50%. Given the critical role of margin status post-conization, a cold knife technique may be preferred in patients with AIS. The recommended surveillance after conization for AIS includes cytology and ECC every 4 months. The most successful conservative management protocols require negative margins and no LVSI, and careful counseling and follow-up are warranted.

Stages IB to IIA (Nonbulky)

Stage IB is divided into IB1 (lesions < 4 cm) and IB2 (lesions confined to cervix > 4 cm). IB1 lesions and selected IIA lesions without extensive vaginal involvement can be treated with either RH and PLD (followed by tailored chemoradiation as indicated by surgical findings) or primary chemoradiation. Surgery is the preferred option in younger women as ovarian function and vaginal length, and thus sexual function, can generally be maintained. Transposition of the ovaries to the abdominal wall or the gutters away from the field of RT may prevent radiation-induced ovarian failure. Retention of ovarian function following ovarian transposition and postoperative radiation has been reported to range from 53% to 71%. The rate of ovarian metastasis is very low, about 0.9%, and thus, salpingo-oophorectomy is not part of RH.

Radical surgery and definitive chemoradiation have similar good outcomes. Typically, 5-year survival for stage IB patients is 85% to 90% and 65% to 75% for stage IIA. In a prospective study of RH ± RT (patients with parametrial involvement, deep stromal invasion, and/or positive nodes received postoperative RT) versus RT alone, no difference was seen in disease-related outcome. In the RH arm, 54% (62 out of 114) and 84% (40 out of 55) of stages IB1 and IB2 received postoperative RT, respectively. Severe morbidity was seen in 28% in the surgical arm (mostly combined surgery and RT) compared to 12% in the RT arm.

Stage IB patients who undergo radical surgery and are found to have poor prognostic pathologic features should receive adjuvant RT to decrease their risk for local recurrence. This high-risk group of patients is defined by the presence of two more of the following risk factors: lymphovascular space involvement, >1/3 stromal invasion, tumor size >4 cm. In a prospective study of adjuvant RT versus observation in this group of high-risk stage IB patients after surgery, adjuvant RT decreased the rate of local recurrence by 46% and progression-free survival by 42% at 10-year median follow-up for patients still alive at last contact.

Fertility-Sparing Surgery/Radical Vaginal and Abdominal Trachelectomy

Almost 30% of women diagnosed with cervical cancer will be less than 40 years of age and 40% will have early stage I disease. Preservation of fertility can be a major consideration in treatment if an acceptable oncologic outcome can be obtained. Recently, there have been major advances in fertility-sparing surgery (FSS) in women with stage IA2 to IB1 cervical cancers with the introduction of a procedure that involves transvaginal resection of cervical and paracervical tissues (vaginal radical trachelectomy) and proximal vaginal, placement of a permanent cerclage at the cervicouterine junction, and a laparoscopic pelvic lymphadenectomy.

The overall recurrence rate in the literature is about 4%, comparing favorably with standard treatment. Appropriate lesions include FIGO stage IA1 without extensive LVSI and IA2 or IB1 lesions less than 2 cm with limited endocervical involvement. A review reported that of patients electing FSS, 43% attempt conception, 70% conceive, 49% deliver at term, and 15% have cervical stenosis causing infertility.

Bulky IB Carcinoma of the Cervix

Bulky endocervical tumors and the so-called barrel-shaped cervix cancers have a higher incidence of central recurrence, pelvic and paraaortic lymph node metastasis, and distant dissemination. Historically, adjuvant extrafascial hysterectomy following preoperative RT was an accepted treatment approach. The GOG performed a randomized trial in which 256 eligible patients with carcinomas of the cervix ≥4 cm were treated with external beam and intracavitary irradiation, or with a slightly lower dose of intracavitary irradiation and the same external beam pelvic irradiation followed by an extrafascial hysterectomy. The 3-year disease-free survival and overall survival rates were 79% and 83%, respectively, and were virtually identical in the irradiation-alone and the combined irradiation and surgery groups. The incidence of progression was somewhat higher in the irradiation-alone group (46%) compared to the combined therapy group (37%) ($p = 0.07$). However, it appears that surgery does not contribute to increased survival compared to RT alone in patients with "bulky" stage IB disease. Furthermore, combined modality therapy was associated with a higher incidence of any reported adverse effects compared to RT alone (63% vs. 56%).

Stages IIB, IIIB, and IVA

Most patients in the United States with stage IIB disease are treated with curative-intent chemoradiation. With RT alone, the 5-year survival rate has historically been 60% to 65%, and the pelvic failure rate 18% to 39%. Similarly, most patients with stage III and IVA tumors are best treated with concurrent chemoradiation. Based on multiple randomized clinical trials, concurrent chemotherapy with irradiation is considered the standard of care. Although the studies used a variety of agents, the de facto standard has become once weekly cisplatin at a dose of

40 mg/m^2 for six cycles. Other chemotherapy agents used successfully include 5-FU, mitomycin, carboplatin, paclitaxel, and epirubicin. Considering all eligible patients with stage IIB to IVA carcinomas enrolled in GOG-85, a 55% survival rate with platinum-based chemotherapy with RT was demonstrated after a median follow-up of 8.7 years. In this same group of patients, GOG-120 found a 66% survival rate with platinum-based chemoradiation. More recently, an international phase III randomized trial investigated whether the addition of concurrent and two additional cycles of adjuvant gemcitabine to cisplatin-based irradiation could further enhance clinical outcomes in stage IIB to IVA disease. At 3-year follow-up, progression-free and overall survival was higher in the gemcitabine arm compared to the standard regimen of cisplatin-based chemoradiation. This study, however, has been criticized for its statistical design and the paucity of late toxicity follow-up data.

The value of adjuvant chemotherapy following cisplatin-based chemoradiation in locally advanced cervical cancer patients is currently being explored in the OUTBACK study. This prospective, randomized, phase III trial endorsed by the GOG and RTOG randomizes patient to adjuvant carboplatin and paclitaxel or no additional therapy following primary cisplatin-based chemoradiation. The primary outcome to be addressed in this trial is improvement in overall survival.

External Irradiation Alone

Rarely, brachytherapy procedures cannot be performed because of medical reasons or unusual anatomic configuration of the pelvis or the tumor (e.g., extensive lesion and inability to identify the cervical canal, presence of a fistula). These patients may be treated with higher doses of external irradiation alone, although the results are inferior to those obtained with combined external beam and intracavitary irradiation.

UNUSUAL CLINICAL SITUATIONS

Invasive Carcinoma Treated by Simple Hysterectomy

Although uncommon, simple hysterectomy for an unrecognized invasive cervical cancer can occur in patients operated on for what is felt to be CIS, "microinvasive" disease, incorrectly diagnosed endometrial carcinoma, or for "benign" indications. If only microinvasive carcinoma is found, with no evidence of LVSI, no additional therapy is necessary. However, in patients with more advanced disease, simple extrafascial abdominal hysterectomy is not curative because the paravaginal/paracervical soft tissue, vaginal cuff, and pelvic lymph nodes are not removed.

While technically difficult, an adequate radical operation after previous simple hysterectomy may be appropriate for selected patients. Another approach favored by some is the use of adjuvant pelvic RT in patients with invasive disease of severity greater than microinvasive.

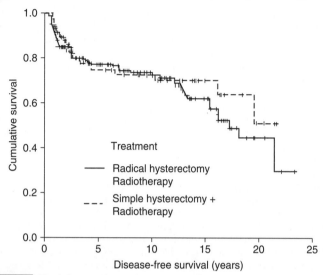

FIGURE 7.2 The influence of type of treatment on disease-free survival in patients undergoing RH with and without RT and those who had simple hysterectomy followed by adjuvant RT. (Kaplan-Meier analysis, p = not significant.) *Source:* From Munstedt K, Johnson P, von Georgi R, et al. Consequences of inadvertent, suboptimal primary surgery in carcinoma of the uterine cervix. *Gynecol Oncol.* 2004;94:515–520.

In an exhaustive review of the literature comparing series of patients having reoperation with radical parametrectomy and LND versus those having postoperative RT, the weighted average 5-year survivals favored RT (68.7% vs. 49.2%).

If the postoperative RT approach is chosen, postoperative irradiation should be administered immediately after recovery from operation, as prognosis is much worse if therapy is delayed. The potential contribution of concurrent platinum-based chemotherapy must be considered, particularly in view of the randomized study of patients treated after RH with high-risk features (Fig. 7.2).

Small Cell Carcinoma of the Cervix

Small cell carcinomas account for less than 3% of cervical neoplasms and are not often confined to the cervix and surrounding tissues at diagnosis. Lymph node involvement is present in over 50%, and vascular invasion is frequently present. One small retrospective study suggested no patient with greater than stage IB1 survived, and even for stage IB1 patients, the survival was much worse than would be expected in more common histologies. Given the propensity to distant metastasis, the use of combination chemotherapy has been widely accepted in these patients. Prophylactic cranial RT has also been given following this chemoradiation in the absence of progression.

SURGERY

> ### KEY POINTS
> - Class I extrafascial hysterectomy is the most common hysterectomy performed for a variety of gynecologic disorders.
> - Class II or MRH involves resection of the parametrial tissue medial to the ureter and a 1- to 2-cm vaginal margin.
> - Class III or radical abdominal hysterectomy involves resection of parametrial tissue to the pelvic sidewall along with a 2- to 3-cm vaginal margin.

A generally accepted classification of types of hysterectomy is given in Table 7.2 and described below.

Class I Extrafascial Hysterectomy

This is the most common hysterectomy performed for a variety of gynecologic disorders. It consists of removing the uterus and cervix with very little removal of vaginal mucosa. This hysterectomy is adequate for the treatment of stage IA1 and advocated by some for stage IA2. This procedure can be accomplished abdominally, vaginally, or laparoscopically.

Class II or Modified Radical Hysterectomy

MRH involves dissection of the uterine artery at its junction with the ureter. The parametrial tissue is resected medial to the ureter. The ureterosacral ligaments are isolated, and the proximal portions medial to the ureter are resected. A 1- to 2-cm vaginal margin is resected along with the cervix. A pelvic lymphadenectomy is typically performed along with MRH. Type II MRH is reserved for microscopic or smaller tumors depending on the surgeon's experience and preference.

Class III or Radical Abdominal Hysterectomy

The RH differs from the MRH in the amount of dissection and resection. The ureters are dissected to their insertion into the bladder trigone. The cardinal ligaments are resected to the pelvic sidewall. The ureterosacral ligaments may be either dissected to their attachment or in select cases resected midway to their attachment. Resection of 2 to 3 cm of proximal vagina is usual, but the operation can be tailored according to tumor size and patient anatomy.

Class IV or Extended Radical Hysterectomy

There is little indication for extended radical hysterectomy (ERH) with availability of modern RT and chemosensitization for locally advanced tumors. ERH involves complete dissection of the ureter off the vesicouterine ligament, sacrifice of the superior vesical artery, and resection of three fourths of the vagina. The risk of bladder dysfunction and fistula formation is greatly increased compared to type I to III hysterectomies.

Table 7.2 Types of Abdominal Hysterectomy

Type of Surgery	Intrafascial	Extrafascial Type 1	Modified Radical Type II	Radical Type III
Cervical fascia	Partially removed	Completely removed	↑	↑
Vaginal cuff removal	None	Small rim removed	Proximal 1–2 cm removed	Upper one third to one half removed
Bladder	Partially mobilized	↑	↑	Mobilized
Rectum	Not mobilized	R-V septum partially mobilized	↑	Mobilized
Ureters	Not mobilized	↑	Unroofed in ureteral tunnel	Completely dissected to bladder entry
Cardinal ligaments	Resected medial to ureters	↑	Resected at level of ureter	Resected at pelvic sidewall
Uterosacral ligaments	Resected at level of cervix	↑	Partially resected	Resected at postpelvic insertion
Uterus	Removed	↑	↑	↑
Cervix	Partially removed	Completely removed	↑	↑

Note: Type IV, extended RH (partial removal of bladder or ureter), in addition to type III.
Source: From Stehman FB, Perez CA, Kurman RJ, et al. Chapter 31—Uterine cervix. In: Hoskins WJ, Perez CA, Young RC, eds. *Principles and Practice of Gynecologic Oncology*, 3rd ed. Philadelphia, PA: Lippincott Williams & Wilkins; 2000:864.

Class V Hysterectomy

A rarely performed operation, a type V hysterectomy, involves resection of the distal ureter or bladder with reimplantation of ureter if needed.

Pelvic Exenteration

Total pelvic exenteration (TPE) is mainly used for select stage IVA patients or with limited central recurrences and no metastatic disease following treatment with primary RT or combined surgery and RT. It involves *en bloc* removal of the bladder, uterus, rectum, vagina and, at times, vulva, depending on the exact site and extent of recurrence. The procedure can be tailored to remove only the anterior or posterior structures including the bladder (anterior exenteration) or rectum (posterior exenteration). Reported 5-year survivals are approximately 40%, ranging from 18% to 70% in the literature.

Sidewall extension, metastatic disease, and, usually, hydronephrosis are possible contraindications to the procedure. Perioperative complications can include bleeding, infection, cardiac and pulmonary complications, gastrointestinal and urinary leaks, fistulas, bowel obstruction, and reconstruction flap failure. Sexual dysfunction and psychosocial effects are often longer-term sequelae that can be permanent. The mortality rate from TPE is about 5%, even with careful patient selection.

RADIATION THERAPY

KEY POINTS

- Radiation portals are designed to encompass gross disease and regional areas at risk for microscopic spread.
- Extended field radiation therapy (EFRT) can be used either prophylactically or therapeutically to treat the lymph nodes located in the paraaortic chain.
- Results from RTOG 90–01 show that pelvic RT combined with platinum-based chemotherapy is superior to adjuvant EFRT (without chemotherapy) in patients with locally advanced disease and negative paraaortic nodes.
- Chemotherapy can feasibly be added to EFRT in patients with gross metastases to the paraaortic nodes, although at the expense of an increased acute toxicity.
- Brachytherapy allows for the delivery of high doses of radiation safely to the tumor and has been a major factor in the ability of RT to cure cervical cancer.
- Standard doses to the whole pelvis with external beam radiation therapy (EBRT) are 45 to 50.4 Gy, and are combined with low-dose-rate (LDR), pulse-dose-rate, or high-dose-rate (HDR) brachytherapy.
- LDR brachytherapy is delivered over one or two treatments to a point A dose of 40 to 55 Gy, resulting in a total point A dose of 85 to 90 Gy (EBRT + LDR brachytherapy) depending on tumor stage. HDR brachytherapy is usually delivered over four to six treatments to the same LDR-equivalent point A dose.
- Newer techniques such as intensity-modulated radiation therapy (IMRT) and image guided brachytherapy may improve side effects and allow simultaneous dose intensification.

External Irradiation

Standard Fields (Non-Intensity-Modulated Radiation Therapy)

Treatment of invasive carcinoma of the uterine cervix requires delivery of adequate doses of irradiation to the pelvic lymph nodes. The superior border of the pelvic portal should be at the L4–5 interspace to include the external iliac and hypogastric lymph nodes. Some have recommended extension of the superior border to the confluence of the common iliac artery and veins. This has not been tested in a trial but should be considered, especially in those patients with positive pelvic nodes. This increase in the superior border will expose more normal tissue to irradiation. A 2-cm margin on the AP:PA fields lateral to the bony pelvis is adequate. If there is no vaginal extension, the lower margin of the portal is at the midportion to inferior border of the obturator foramen or 3 to 4 cm below any visible or palpable disease, whichever is lower. When there is vaginal involvement, the field should extend distally beyond the tumor a minimum of 3 to 4 cm, although some contend that the entire length of vagina should be treated down to the introitus. It is important to identify the distal extension of the tumor in some manner at the time of initial simulation, for example, by inserting a small rod with a radiopaque marker in the vagina, or by placement of fiducial markers. Often, vaginal extension will not be clearly defined by CT scan but may be better appreciated on MRI. In patients with involvement of the distal third of the vagina (stage IIIA), portals should cover the inguinal lymph nodes because of the increased probability of metastases. The lateral portal anterior margin is placed 1 cm anterior to the pubic symphysis to include the anterior extent of the external iliac nodes. The posterior margin usually covers at least 50% of the rectum in stage IB tumors, and extends to cover the entire sacrum in patients with more advanced tumors (Fig. 7.3B). Routinely placing the posterior border at S3

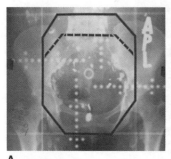 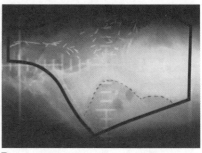

A **B**

FIGURE 7.3 **A:** Anteroposterior simulation film of the pelvis illustrating portals used for external irradiation. The 15 × 15 cm portals at source-skin distance are used for stage IB (*broken line*), and 18 × 15 cm portals are used for more advanced disease (*solid line*). This allows better coverage of the common iliac lymph nodes. The distal margin is usually placed at the bottom of the obturator foramina. **B:** Lateral simulation film of the pelvis illustrating portals used for external irradiation. *Source:* From Stehman FB, Perez CA, Kurman RJ, et al. Uterine cervix. In: Hoskins WJ, Perez CA, Young RC, et al., eds. *Principles and Practice of Gynecologic Oncology*, 3rd ed. Philadelphia, PA: Lippincott-Raven; 2000:867.

interspace (to cover the uterosacral ligament and presacral nodes) may result in inadequate coverage of the planning target volume. Ideally, three-dimensional (3-D) imaging with CT, MRI, or both will be used to ensure adequate coverage. Contouring of the structures at risk with blocks based on these contours forms the mainstay of current therapy—3-D conformal.

Intensity-Modulated External Radiation Therapy

Intensity-modulated radiation therapy (IMRT) refers to the delivery of radiation beams with varying intensity patterns that create a dose distribution, which covers the target with the prescribed dose while limiting doses to normal surrounding structures. Treatment planning is based on 3-D imaging utilizing CT, most commonly. MRI and PET images can be fused with planning CT scans to more accurately delineate the treatment volume (Fig. 7.4).

Published benefits of IMRT include the ability to preferentially limit the dose of radiation to normal tissues, safely deliver higher tumor doses, and enable treatment and retreatment of tumors that are not otherwise treatable. For example, in patients with bulky, unresectable lymph nodes, IMRT can be utilized to boost dose to the involved nodes. A small, single-institution, prospective Chinese study by Du et al. compared treatment of paraaortic node metastasis with IMRT versus conventional paraaortic field irradiation. The investigators found significantly higher rates of tumor response and overall survival at 2 and 3 years, accompanied by lower hematologic and gastrointestinal toxicity rates, in patients treated with IMRT. The mean dose delivered to the target volume was 59 Gy with IMRT versus 49 Gy with conventional paraaortic field irradiation. Despite the higher dose, IMRT provided better critical organ sparing than the conventional RT technique. To date, the weight of opinion does not support the ability of IMRT techniques to replace intracavitary brachytherapy for the treatment of cervical cancer.

A concern and possible pitfall from the implementation of IMRT for gynecologic cancers include the problem of organ and tissue motion. Other concerns include an increase in the incidence of secondary radiation-induced malignancies, limitations of imaging in accurately defining pelvic disease, increased dose heterogeneity, and problems with quality assurance. Although there are institutional reports on the dosimetric and clinical benefits of IMRT, it should only be undertaken in a facility with experience and robust quality assurance, preferably in a clinical trial setting, until more prospective data and long-term follow-up are available. Currently, there is an international, multi-institution, phase II/III study (INTERTECC) evaluating the role of IMRT with concurrent cisplatin for stage I–IVA cervical cancer. Toxicity and locoregional tumor control are the main outcomes being assessed in this study. In addition, there is an ongoing randomized trial at Tata Memorial in Mumbai, India, on Stage IIB cervical carcinoma.

Extended Field Radiation Therapy

EFRT can be used either prophylactically or therapeutically to treat the lymph nodes located in the paraaortic chain. The paraaortic chain is surrounded by organs of limited radiation tolerance, that is, the spinal cord, kidneys, and small intestine; thus, there are concerns regarding its use related to increased acute and late toxicities. Conventional techniques for

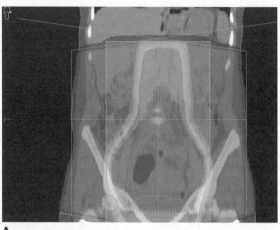

A

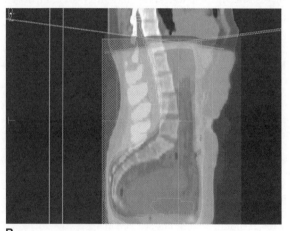

B

FIGURE 7.4 This figure shows dose distribution from extended field RT given with a four-field isocentric technique with all fields treated in continuity. The AP-PA fields **(A)** are weighted 70:30 in relation to the lateral fields **(B)**, limiting the dose to the kidneys, as shown in the DVH in Figure 7.5. This patient had a large pelvic mass, compromising the ability to spare the rectum and bladder.

treatment include the use of opposed anterior and posterior fields and a four-field technique (AP:PA and opposed laterals). Careful determination of the kidney location with an intravenous pyelogram or CT scan and knowledge and respect of normal tissue tolerance limits (kidneys, small bowel, and spinal cord) are critical when designing fields and beam weighting. A dose–volume histogram (DVH) of such a treatment is shown in Figure 7.5.

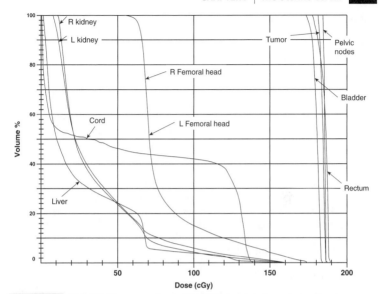

FIGURE 7.5 This DVH from an extended field RT plan plots the volume of various organs or structures versus the dose received. It shows excellent coverage of tumor and nodal regions while the normal structures, for example, the kidneys, spinal cord, etc., receive limited dose. This provides quantitative measures of dose distribution for use in evaluating and comparing treatment plans.

Elective Paraaortic Lymph Node Irradiation

Occult involvement of the paraaortic lymph nodes is a potential cause of treatment failure in carcinoma of the cervix. Adjuvant or EFRT is a logical treatment strategy that seeks to avoid the risks and treatment delays associated with surgical staging. Retrospective and prospective data suggest that EFRT can be delivered safely and with reasonable efficacy in high-risk patients. In a prospective RTOG trial that randomized 367 patients (stage IIB or stages IB to IIA, 4 cm) to pelvic RT versus EFRT, elective EFRT translated into overall survival of 67% at 5 years, and 55% at 10 years compared with 55% and 44%, respectively, for those treated to the pelvis only ($p = 0.02$). Locoregional failures were similar at 10 years for both arms (pelvic only, 35%; EFRT, 31%). When the first disease failure patterns were examined, more patients failed distantly when treated only with pelvic RT compared to those receiving EFRT ($p = 0.053$). The EFRT arm was associated with more grade 4 and 5 complications, particularly in patients with prior abdominal surgery (11% vs. 2%).

Results from RTOG 90–01 show that pelvic RT combined with platinum-based chemotherapy is superior to adjuvant EFRT (without chemotherapy) in patients with locally advanced disease. EFRT combined with chemotherapy could offer opportunities for improved outcomes in patients at high risk of metastatic paraaortic disease.

Possible indications for consideration of EFRT include positive PET scans in the paraaortic region; high pelvic lymph nodes involved, for example, common iliac; gross nodal metastases in the pelvis; bilateral positive pelvic lymph nodes; adenocarcinoma histology with any number of positive pelvic lymph nodes; and squamous cell histology with four positive pelvic lymph nodes.

Therapeutic Paraaortic Lymph Node Irradiation
Data from the GOG suggest that patients with stage IB, II, III, and IVA cervical cancers will have spread to the paraaortic lymph nodes in 5%, 16%, 25%, and 13%, respectively. Tumor involvement in paraaortic lymph nodes is quite uncommon in the absence of pelvic lymph node metastasis. The degree to which RT demonstrates curative potential in this group of patients is quite variable and is mostly related to selection factors in the patient population so treated.

Therapeutic EFRT in patients with paraaortic metastases appears to be efficacious, resulting in long-term survivals of 25% to 50%. Chemotherapy can feasibly be added to EFRT in these patients, although at the expense of increased acute toxicity. While the optimum chemotherapy agents and schedule remain to be determined, weekly cisplatin is a reasonable suggestion based on current knowledge.

Brachytherapy

Brachytherapy refers to the placement of radioactive sources at a short distance from the intended target. Brachytherapy allows the delivery of high doses of radiation safely and has been a major factor in the ability of RT to cure cervical cancer. For details on brachytherapy, please refer to Chapter 2.

Doses of Irradiation

Invasive carcinoma of the cervix is treated with a combination of whole pelvis and intracavitary therapy. Standard doses to the whole pelvis with external irradiation are 45 to 50.4 Gy, delivered by four-field box or IMRT technique. This is usually combined with one or two LDR intracavitary insertions for approximately 40 to 55 Gy to point A, depending on tumor stage (volume). Usual doses to point A from both the external irradiation to the whole pelvis and the LDR intracavitary brachytherapy range from 70 Gy for small (1 cm) stage IB tumors to 90-Gy for stage IIB or IIIB tumors. In some patients, an additional parametrial dose is administered in patients with IIB, III, or IVA tumors (considering the dose delivered to the side wall by the brachytherapy). The recommended HDR brachytherapy prescription in GOG cervical cancer protocols is 5 fractions of 6 Gy (to point A) in addition to EBRT. Another commonly used HDR schedule is 4 fractions of 7 Gy.

Overall Treatment Time

Several studies have demonstrated lower pelvic tumor control and survival rates after definitive RT in invasive carcinoma of the uterine cervix when the overall treatment time is prolonged. Combining the published results, one can suggest that pelvic control will suffer at an approximate rate of 1% per day that treatment extends beyond 52 days. This impact will be potentially seen in all stages of localized disease, and survival will be negatively affected.

CHEMOTHERAPY

Chemotherapy is increasingly utilized in the management of cervical cancer, both in primary management and for recurrent and metastatic disease. Conventional agents that are able to induce a response rate of at least 20% in measurable disease include cisplatin, paclitaxel, topotecan, ifosfamide, doxorubicin, epirubicin, and vinorelbine. Doublets that combine these agents with cisplatin result in a doubling of response rate and improved progression-free survival but little or no improvement in overall survival when compared to cisplatin as a single agent. Three- and four-drug chemotherapy regimens further increase the response rate without improvement in overall survival at the expense of increased toxicity.

COMBINED MODALITY TREATMENT

Adjuvant Hysterectomy after Radiation Therapy

The main impetus for adjuvant hysterectomy postradiation therapy (AHPRT) is to decrease the incidence of pelvic recurrence; however, its use remains controversial because overall survival appears to be unaffected. A randomized trial to address this question was performed by the GOG in 256 patients with cervix cancers more than 4 cm in size who were randomized to curative doses of pelvic RT with brachytherapy versus preoperative doses of RT and brachytherapy plus AHPRT. The relapse rate was significantly lower in the AHPRT arm versus RT alone (27% vs. 14%). The incidence of progression was somewhat higher in the RT-alone group at 46% versus 37% ($p = 0.07$) in the AHPRT group. However, no overall survival advantage was seen, and the toxicities were similar in both groups.

Adjuvant Postoperative Pelvic RT

KEY POINTS

- Two groups of patients with early-stage cervical cancer warrant treatment with postoperative radiation: those with intermediate risk features (presence of two out of three risk factors of large tumor size, lymphovascular invasion, and deep stromal invasion) and those with high-risk features (positive nodes, margins, or parametria).
- A phase III GOG trial in women with intermediate risk cervical cancer treated with RH ± RT showed a 46% reduction in the risk of recurrence in the RT arm compared to the observation arm ($p = 0.007$) and a reduction in the risk of progression or death ($p = 0.009$).
- A phase III intergroup trial in high-risk women treated with RH and postoperative radiation ± chemotherapy showed a significant improvement in 3-year survival with concurrent cisplatin/5-fluorouracil and irradiation followed by adjuvant chemotherapy compared with pelvic irradiation alone (87% vs. 77%, respectively).
- An ongoing randomized cooperative group trial is presently investigating the benefit of adjuvant carboplatin and taxol chemotherapy following postoperative chemoradiation in women with early-stage high-risk cervical cancer.

The most common failure pattern following radical surgery for cervical carcinoma is pelvic relapse. Based on an extensive GOG clinicopathologic study, recommendations were made to separate patients into intermediate- and high-risk groups. Intermediate-risk criteria relate to tumor size, depth of stromal invasion, and LVSI. High-risk criteria include positive pelvic nodes, close or positive margins, and parametrial extension. Retrospective and prospective data suggest that adjuvant pelvic RT significantly improves pelvic control rates and disease-free survivals in patients with risk factors for recurrence who have completed radical surgery. The role of chemotherapy, particularly in high-risk patients, has also become established.

Intermediate Risk, Node Negative

The GOG conducted a Phase III trial comparing RH alone with RH and postoperative pelvic RT in patients with node-negative stage IB cervical carcinomas, with prognostic features correlated with an intermediate risk of recurrence (GOG-92). Eligibility criteria for this study are given in Table 7.3. There were 277 patients randomized after RH: 137 to pelvic RT and 140 to no further therapy. RT consisted of 46 Gy to a whole pelvic field. No brachytherapy was used. After a median follow-up of 5 years for living patients, recurrence was observed in 28% of the patients in the control group and in 15% of the radiated patients. There was a statistically significant reduction in the risk of recurrence (relative risk = 0.53, $p = 0.008$) in the irradiated group. Severe or life-threatening adverse effects were observed in 7% of the radiated patients, versus 2.1% of the controls. After additional follow-up and data maturation, a final report from GOG-92 showed a 46% reduction in the risk of recurrence in the RT arm compared to the observation arm ($p = 0.007$) and a reduction in the risk of progression or death ($p = 0.009$). Particularly striking was the impact of postoperative RT in patients with adenocarcinoma or adenosquamous histologies; among this subset, only 8.8% recurred in the RT arm versus 44% in the observation arm. There was a strong trend toward improved survival in the RT arm, but this did not reach statistical significance ($p = 0.074$).

Management of patients with stage IB2 tumors is somewhat controversial in that some favor initial surgery followed by adjuvant RT, while others recommend curative-intent chemoradiation to avoid the use of two local modalities.

Table 7.3	**GOG-92 Eligibility Criteria**	
Capillary Lymphatic Space Involvement	Stromal Invasion	Tumor Size
Positive	Deep 1/3	Any
Positive	Middle 1/3	≥2 cm
Positive	Superficial 1/3	≥5 cm
Negative	Deep or middle 1/3	≥4 cm

Node-Positive/High-Risk Patients

Metastatic disease in the pelvic lymph nodes is a poor prognostic sign. An intergroup study was conducted by the Southwest Oncology Group (SWOG), GOG, and RTOG in women with FIGO stages IA2, IB, or IIA carcinoma of the cervix and found to have metastatic disease in the pelvic lymph nodes, positive parametrial involvement, or positive surgical margins at time of primary RH, and total pelvic lymphadenectomy with confirmed negative paraaortic lymph nodes. One hundred twenty-seven patients were randomized between pelvic EBRT with 5-FU infusion and cisplatin, and 116 were treated with pelvic external beam irradiation alone. The median follow-up for survivors was 43 months. Three-year survival was significantly improved with concurrent cisplatin/5-fluorouracil and irradiation followed by adjuvant chemotherapy compared with pelvic irradiation alone (87% vs. 77%, respectively). Chemotherapy appeared to reduce both pelvic and extrapelvic recurrences.

Close or Positive Margins/Parametrial Involvement

Eighty-five percent of patients accrued on the SWOG/GOG/RTOG Intergroup study were eligible based on pelvic node involvement. Only 5% of patients accrued to this intergroup study had positive margins. Nevertheless, patients with positive or close margins and/or parametrial involvement are considered to be at high risk and, based on this randomized trial, should be considered for adjuvant chemoradiation.

Radiation Therapy Dose and Technique

Vaginal intracavitary RT alone can be appropriate for patients with CIS with minimally invasive carcinoma at the vaginal margin of resection as the only risk factor. Outpatient HDR brachytherapy is commonly employed because it prevents the prolonged immobilization required for LDR brachytherapy. The usual dose per fraction prescribed at 0.5 cm depth is 7 Gy; 3-weekly fractions are typically given. The upper 3 to 5 cm of the vagina should be targeted.

When external RT is used, patients generally should not receive more than 45 Gy to the whole pelvis. Doses up to 50.4 Gy are acceptable when treating smaller fields that exclude more small bowel. Brachytherapy or small-field external beam boosts can be given, within tolerance, to increase dose to the central pelvis.

The use of IMRT with chemotherapy has been reported to maintain excellent pelvic control rates, with better acute tolerance and fewer chronic toxicities compared to conventional four-field box RT.

Chemotherapy in Combinations for Localized Carcinoma of the Cervix Neoadjuvant Chemotherapy Followed by Radiotherapy

Randomized trials of neoadjuvant chemotherapy (NACT) followed by radiation versus radiation alone in patients with locally advanced cervical cancer (mainly stages III and IV) have been disappointing, in terms of both complete response rates and increase in survival. A meta-analysis of 18 randomized clinical trials of neoadjuvant chemotherapy, including 2074 patients, compared NACT followed by RT to RT alone and demonstrated no advantage of neoadjuvant chemotherapy with regard to progression-free survival, locoregional disease-free survival, metastasis-free survival, or overall survival. NACT followed by RT for patients with locally advanced cervical cancer should not be performed based on existing data.

Neoadjuvant Chemotherapy Followed by Surgery

Numerous nonrandomized studies reported in the 1990s suggested that NACT followed by surgery might be an attractive approach, and some but not all of the randomized trials show a trend in favor of this combined approach. A meta-analysis of five randomized clinical trials and 872 patients who received NACT followed by surgery ± RT was compared to RT alone. There was a significant improvement in progression-free survival, locoregional disease-free survival, metastasis-free survival, and overall survival for those who were resectable following NACT. Nevertheless, based on the available data, NACT remains investigational.

Adjuvant Chemotherapy

Several nonrandomized studies suggest a beneficial effect of adjuvant chemotherapy given after radical surgery in patients at high risk for recurrence. Two randomized trials with a very limited number of patients have tried to evaluate the effect of adjuvant chemotherapy in patients with high-risk cervical cancer after RH. The results of both studies were inconclusive. An ongoing randomized cooperative group trial is presently investigating the benefit of adjuvant carboplatin and taxol chemotherapy following postoperative chemoradiation in women with early-stage high-risk cervical cancer.

TREATMENT OF RECURRENT CARCINOMA OF THE CERVIX

The main cause of death among women with cervical cancer is uncontrolled disease in the pelvis. However, a subset of patients with recurrent disease confined to the pelvis following definitive therapy, whether that therapy is surgery or RT, is potentially curable.

When curative-intent salvage treatment is contemplated, the local recurrence should be biopsy proven, and the patient should be evaluated for regional and distant metastases by physical examination and imaging. PET scanning may be the most accurate test in terms of assessing metastasis prior to embarking on local salvage therapy. Generally, patients with pelvic or regional recurrences after definitive surgery alone are managed with RT or chemoradiation, often with brachytherapy. Salvage options for patients with central recurrence after definitive or adjuvant RT are limited to radical, usually exenterative, surgery, and in selected patients, reirradiation using interstitial radiation implants or highly conformal EBRT or IMRT. Chemotherapy-responsive patients can obtain meaningful palliation in many cases (Table 7.4).

In addition to cytotoxic therapies, targeted agents against molecular signaling pathways have also been studied in the setting of recurrent

Table 7.4	Randomized Studies of Cisplatin-Based Combinations versus Single-Agent Cisplatin in Patients with Cervical Cancer				
Arms of Studies and Study Drug	No. of Patients	CR, n (%)	PR, n (%)	CR + PR, n (%)	Median Survival (months)
MMC/VCR/BLM/CDDP	54	4 (7)	8 (15)	12 (22)	6.9
vs.					
MMC/CDDP	51	2 (4)	11 (21)	13 (25)	7
vs.					
CDDP	9	1 (11)	2 (22)	3 (33)	17
DVA/BLM/MMC/CDDP	143	11 (8)	33 (23)	44 (31)[a]	10
vs.					
CDDP	144	8 (6)	20 (14)	28 (19)[a]	9.4
DBD/CDDP	153 (147)[b]	14 (9)	17 (12)	31 (21)	7.3
vs.					
IFOSF/CDDP	155 (151)[b]	19 (12.5)	28 (18.5)	47 (31)[c]	8.3
vs.					
CDDP	146 (140)[b]	9 (6.5)	16 (11.5)	25 (18)P[c]	8
BLM/IFOSF/CDDP	50 (46)[b]	12 (26)	12 (26)	24 (52)[d]	8
vs.					
CDDP	56 (51)[b]	5 (10)	10 (20)	15 (29)[d]	6

[a]$p = 0.03$.
[b]Numbers evaluable for response.
[c]$p = 0.004$.
[d]$p < 0.01$.
CR, complete response; PR, partial response; MMC, mitomycin C; VCR, vincristine; BLM, bleomycin; CDDP, cisplatin (dose in all studies and in all arms 50 mg/m^2); DVA, vindesine; DBD, dibromodulcitol; IFOSF, ifosfamide.

cervical disease. Bevacizumab is a recombinant antibody against the vascular endothelial growth factor, a known driver of tumor progression. The GOG 227C phase III trial examined the role of single-agent bevacizumab in the treatment of persistent or recurrent squamous cell carcinoma of the cervix. In the 46 patients who were enrolled, 11 survived progression free for at least 6 months and 5 experienced partial responses. The median progression-free survival and overall survival were 3.4 and 7.3 months, respectively. Overall, bevacizumab was well tolerated; there was no incidence of grade 4 or higher hematologic toxicity. Given these encouraging results in comparison with historical GOG trials in this patient population, a further phase III study may be warranted.

COMPLICATIONS AND SEQUELAE OF TREATMENT

KEY POINTS

- Complications following RH include ureteral injuries, vesicovaginal or ureterovaginal fistulas (1% to 2% of cases), bladder atony (5%), lymphocyst formation (1.6%), and lymphedema (3.6%).
- Grade 2 or higher late sequelae of pelvic RT occur in 5% to 15% of cases and may include chronic proctosigmoiditis, rectal stricture, rectal ulcer, bowel obstruction, malabsorption syndrome, chronic cystitis, bladder contracture, urethral stricture, incontinence, vaginal stenosis/fibrosis, dyspareunia, vault necrosis, and rectovaginal or vesicovaginal fistulae.
- Concurrent chemoradiation results in additional acute hematologic toxicity although most phase III studies show no significant increase in late toxicity.

Surgery Related

The most common complications with conization include infection, bleeding, damage to surrounding structures (bladder, rectum, and vagina), and cervical incompetence with predisposition to preterm labor in future pregnancies. RH and lymphadenectomy may result in additional and somewhat unique complications. Urologic complications, such as ureteral injuries and vesicovaginal or ureterovaginal fistulas, are reported in 1% to 2% of cases; this rate may increase in patients requiring postoperative RT. The majority of vesicovaginal fistulas will heal spontaneously with continuous bladder drainage for 6 to 8 weeks and treatment of any underlying infection. Conservative management of ureterovaginal fistulas can include ureteral stenting and drainage of the urinary system via percutaneous nephrostomy, which may lead to healing of the fistula. Surgical repair of fistulas may be required for those that do not resolve with conservative management. Fistulas that occur following pelvic RT are less likely to heal with conservative management and may require earlier surgical treatment. As surgical repair after RT has a lower success rate, urinary diversion may be required as definitive treatment.

Lymphocyst formation is about 1.6%, and the lymphedema rate is about 3.6% following pelvic LND. Located over the sacral promontory, the hypogastric plexus contains sympathetic fibers that fuse with parasympathetic fibers located in the parametrium and allows for bladder contraction and compliance. Surgical disruption of this plexus results in bladder atony and dysfunction in about 5% of patients, possibly requiring continuous or intermittent drainage for a few weeks.

Rectal function can also be impacted by RH. In a study utilizing a questionnaire to evaluate rectal function after RH in 48 patients, 18% had constipation, 33% required chronic straining, and 60% required laxative or manual assistance with defecation. The incidence of chronic constipation was more than 20%.

Radiation Therapy Related

Acute effects during external pelvic RT most typically include diarrhea and bladder irritation. These are usually self-limited and can be managed effectively with conservative measures. Most late gastrointestinal and urologic complications occur within the first 3 years after RT, with an overall fistula rate of about 2%. Factors that may increase the rate of fistula are combined treatment (surgery and RT), smoking, thin habitus, inflammatory bowel diseases, and diabetes and other vasculopathies.

Commonly reported late sequelae of pelvic RT by site are as follows:

1. Rectosigmoid complications: chronic proctosigmoiditis, rectal stricture, and rectal ulcer
2. Small intestine complications: obstruction and malabsorption syndrome
3. Genitourinary (GU) complications: chronic cystitis, bladder contracture, urethral stricture, and incontinence
4. Vaginal complications: vaginal stenosis/fibrosis, dyspareunia, vault necrosis, and rectovaginal or vesicovaginal fistulae

There is approximately a 5% rate of major late sequelae in patients with stage I cervical carcinoma treated with RT and a rate of approximately 10% in patients with stage II to IVA diseases. Grade 2 complications are seen in 10% to 15% of patients with all stages treated with RT alone. Risk is related to a number of factors, mainly dose and volume treated. A greater incidence of pelvic complications has been consistently observed in patients treated with higher doses to the whole pelvis (above 40 to 50 Gy). Injury to the gastrointestinal tract is the most frequent late complication of RT for cervical cancer.

Combined Modality Related

Irradiation Followed by Surgery

One larger retrospective series of patients with stage IB cervical carcinoma treated with RT reported an incidence of major complications at 3 and 5 years of 7.7% and 9.3%, respectively; the actuarial risk of major complications was 14.4% at 20 years. The rate of fistula formation was doubled in those who underwent adjuvant hysterectomy (5.3% vs. 2.6%). In a GOG study, 256 patients with stage IB carcinomas of the cervix—4 cm confined to cervix—were treated either with external RT and intracavitary irradiation or with external RT and a lower dose of intracavitary irradiation followed by an extrafascial hysterectomy. The toxicities were similar in both groups, with grade 3 and 4 toxicities of about 10% in each arm.

Surgery Followed by Irradiation

Radical surgery commonly results in intestinal adhesions to denuded surfaces in the pelvis. When postoperative RT is given, complications are more likely. The GOG demonstrated a significant increase in grade 2 late complications among patients undergoing pre-RT surgical staging, particularly with a transperitoneal approach compared with a retroperitoneal approach.

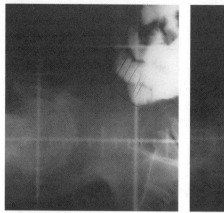
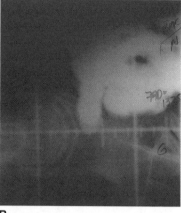

A   B

FIGURE 7.6 **A, B**: Lateral radiographs with and without bladder distention in a patient with contrast in the small intestine.

Pretreatment laparotomy also increased the rate of fistula formation (5.2% vs. 2.9%) as well as small bowel obstruction (14.5% vs. 3.7%). An extra-peritoneal approach to lymph node staging lessens these complications.

In a randomized study of postoperative RT versus no further treatment (NFT) after RH, grade 3 to 4 GU toxicities were noted in 3.1% versus 1.4% in the RT as compared to the NFT arm, respectively. Similarly, grade 3 and 4 GI toxicities were 3.1% versus 0.8%, respectively. Overall, grade 3 and 4 toxicities were 6% in the RT group versus 2.1% in the NFT arm.

Methods to decrease the volume of small bowel irradiated will further lessen enteric morbidity. Figures 7.6 and 7.7 show the effect of treating

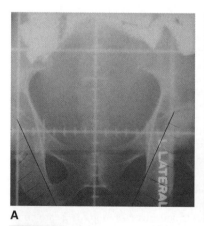
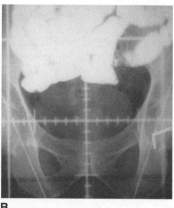

A   B

FIGURE 7.7 **A, B**: Anterior–posterior radiographs with and without bladder distention in a patient with contrast in the small intestine.

patients in the prone position with a full bladder as a means of limiting the volume of small bowel irradiated. Similarly, IMRT techniques can also be used to limit doses to normal tissues.

Concurrent Chemoradiation

Concurrent chemoradiation results in additional acute hematologic toxicity. A major concern has been the possible need to delay treatment, thus potentially compromising outcomes. Typical RT fields radiate some pelvic bone marrow, and the use of IMRT to limit hematologic toxicity in some patients is currently being investigated. Although some early series suggested that concurrent chemotherapy increased late complications in patients receiving curative-intent RT, most studies suggest no significant impact.

Thromboembolic Complications

Thromboembolic complications were reported in a series of 281 consecutive patients who underwent radical surgery for cervical and uterine malignancies. Postoperative thromboembolic complications occurred in 7.8% of patients despite regular use of low dose heparin and antiembolism stockings during the postoperative hospitalization. A second series noted a 16.7% incidence of thromboembolic complications in 48 patients who received chemoradiation therapy without surgery. Brachytherapy alone is associated with a very low rate of thromboembolic complications: 0.3% in one series.

Erythropoietin has been utilized to maintain normal hemoglobin levels during chemoradiation. Reports of increased incidence of thromboembolic complications have been noted in patients who receive erythropoietin during RT. The routine use of erythropoietin to maintain normal hemoglobin levels during chemoradiation should be discouraged.

SUGGESTED READINGS

Blitz S, Baxter J, Raboud J, et al. Evaluation of HIV and highly active antiretroviral therapy on the natural history of human papillomavirus infection and cervical cytopathologic findings in HIV-positive and high-risk HIV-negative women. *J Infect Dis.* 2013;208:454–462.

Bohlius J, Langensiepen S, Schwarzer G, et al. Recombinant human erythropoietin and overall survival in cancer patients: Results of a comprehensive meta-analysis. *J Natl Cancer Inst.* 2005;97:489–498.

Center for Disease Control. *Cervical Cancer Rates by Races and Ethnicity.* http://www.cdc.gov/cancer/cervical/statistics/race.htm

Delgado G, Bundy B, Zaino R, et al. Prospective surgical-pathological study of disease-free interval in patients with stage IB squamous cell carcinoma of the cervix: A Gynecologic Oncology Group study. *Gynecol Oncol.* 1990;38:352–357.

Du XL, Sheng XG, Jiang T, et al. Intensity-modulated radiation therapy versus para-aortic field radiotherapy to treat para-aortic lymph node metastasis in cervical cancer: Prospective study. *Croat Med J.* 2010;51:229–236.

Dueñas-González A, Zarbá JJ, Patel F, et al. Phase III, open-label, randomized study comparing concurrent gemcitabine plus cisplatin and radiation followed by adjuvant gemcitabine and cisplatin versus concurrent cisplatin and radiation in patients with stage IIB to IVA carcinoma of the cervix. *J Clin Oncol.* 2011;29:1678–1685.

Eifel PJ, Morris M, Wharton JT, et al. The influence of tumor size and morphology on the outcome of patients with FIGO stage IB squamous cell carcinoma of the uterine cervix. *Int J Radiat Oncol Biol Phys.* 1994;29:9.

Garland SM, Hernandez-Avila M, Wheeler CM, et al. Quadrivalent vaccine against human papillomavirus to prevent anogenital diseases. *N Engl J Med.* 2007;356:1928–1943.

Haie-Meder C, Potter R, Van Limbergen E, et al. Recommendation from Gynecological (GYN) GEC ESTRO Working Group. Concepts and terms in 3D image-based treatment planning in cervix cancer brachytherapy with emphasis on MRI assessment of GTV and CTV. *Radiother Oncol.* 2005;74:235–245.

Keys HM, Bundy BN, Stehman FB, et al. Radiation therapy with and without extrafascial hysterectomy for bulky stage IB cervical carcinoma: A randomized trial of the Gynecologic Oncology Group. *Gynecol Oncol.* 2003;89:343–353.

Landoni F, Maneo A, Colombo A, et al. Randomised study of radical surgery versus radiotherapy for stage IB-IIA cervical cancer. *Lancet.* 1997;350:535–540.

Leblanc E, Narducci F, Frumovitz M, et al. Therapeutic value of pretherapeutic extraperitoneal laparoscopic staging of locally advanced cervical carcinoma. *Gynecol Oncol.* 2007;105:304–311.

Monk BJ, Sill MW, Burger RA, et al. Phase II trial of bevacizumab in the treatment of persistent or recurrent squamous cell carcinoma of the cervix: A gynecologic oncology group study. *J Clin Oncol.* 2009;27:1069–1074.

Morris M, Eifel PJ, Lu J, et al. Pelvic radiation with concurrent chemotherapy compared with pelvic and paraaortic radiation for high-risk cervical cancer. *N Engl J Med.* 1999;340:1137–1143.

National Cancer Institute. *Cancer Advances in Focus: Cervical Cancer.* http://www.cancer.gov/cancertopics/factsheet/cancer-advances-in-focus/cervical

Peters WA III, Liu PY, Barrett RJ, et al. Concurrent chemotherapy and pelvic radiation therapy compared with pelvic radiation therapy alone as adjuvant therapy after radical surgery in high-risk early-stage cancer of the cervix. *J Clin Oncol.* 2000;18:1606–1613.

Rose PG, Bundy BN, Watkins EB, et al. Concurrent cisplatin-based radiotherapy and chemotherapy for locally advanced cervical cancer. *N Engl J Med.* 1999;340:1144–1153.

Rotman M, Pajak TF, Choi K, et al. Prophylactic extended-field irradiation of para-aortic lymph nodes in stages IIB and bulky IB and IIA cervical carcinoma. *JAMA* 1995;274:387.

Rotman M, Sedlis A, Piedmonte MR, et al. A phase III randomized trial of postoperative pelvic irradiation in stage IB cervical carcinoma with poor prognostic features: Follow-up of a Gynecologic Oncology Group study. *Int J Radiat Oncol Biol Phys.* 2006;65:169–176.

Siegel R, Naishadham D, Jemal A. Cancer statistics, 2013. *CA Cancer J Clin.* 2013;63:11.

Stehman FB, Bundy BN, DiSaia PH, et al. Carcinoma of the cervix treated with irradiation therapy. I. A multi-variate analysis of prognostic variables in the Gynecologic Oncology Group. *Cancer.* 1991;67:2776.

Tierney J; the Neoadjuvant Chemotherapy for Cervical Cancer Meta-analysis Collaboration. Neoadjuvant chemotherapy for locally advanced cervical cancer: A systematic review and meta-analysis of individual patient data from 21 randomized trials. *Eur J Cancer.* 2003;39:2470–2486.

8 The Corpus: Epithelial Tumors

In the United States, endometrial cancer is the most prevalent of all gynecologic malignancies. It is estimated that 49,560 new cases of endometrial cancer will be diagnosed in 2013, and this disease will account for an estimated 8,190 deaths. Factors influencing its rising incidence include prolonged life expectancy, earlier diagnosis, and obesity. Currently, endometrial adenocarcinoma is the fourth most common cancer in females, behind breast, colorectal, and lung cancers. It is the seventh leading cause of death from malignancy in women. The lifetime risk of endometrial cancer is 2.6% among American women, with a 0.5% lifetime mortality risk.

In 75% of all cases, the tumor is confined to the uterine corpus at the time of diagnosis, and survival rates of 75% or more are expected. In the past 50 years, the treatment of this cancer has evolved from a regimen of preoperative radiation therapy followed by hysterectomy 6 weeks later, to individualized management consisting of surgical treatment with or without additional therapy depending on whether various risk factors are identified. Currently, endometrial cancer is surgically staged using the 2009 International Federation of Gynecology and Obstetrics (FIGO) staging system (Table 8.1).

EPIDEMIOLOGY AND RISK FACTORS

KEY POINTS

- Type I cancers are estrogen related, and type II cancers are not.
- Type II cancers represent the more aggressive phenotypes.
- There is a high risk of an invasive cancer in the presence of biopsy-proven complex atypical hyperplasia (CAH).

Two broad histologic categories of endometrial cancer have been described (Table 8.2), termed type I and II carcinomas. They appear to have different patterns of molecular alterations that underlie their pathogenesis and clinical outcomes.

Type I endometrial cancers are associated with unopposed estrogen exposure and are often preceded by premalignant disease. They are usually early stage at diagnosis, are low-grade tumors (predominantly of endometrioid histology), and carry a favorable prognosis. Obesity and family history remain two of the strongest risk factors for endometrial cancer. Hereditary cancers are most clearly linked to Lynch syndrome (hereditary nonpolyposis colorectal cancer [HNPCC]), an autosomal dominant cancer susceptibility syndrome. Diabetes and hypertension, once thought to be risk factors for endometrial cancer, are probably surrogates for obesity; as a result, they

Table 8.1	FIGO Staging of Carcinoma of the Endometrium (Updated 2009)
Stage 1	Tumor Confined to the Corpus Uteri
IA[a]	No or less than half the myometrial invasion
IB[a]	Invasion equal to or more than half of the myometrium
Stage II[a]	Tumor invades cervical stroma but does not extend beyond the uterus[b]
Stage III[a]	Local and/or regional spread of the tumor
IIIA[a]	Tumor invades the serosa of the corpus uteri and/or adnexae[c]
IIIB[a]	Vaginal and/or parametrial involvement[c]
IIIC[a]	Metastases to pelvic and/or paraaortic lymph nodes[c]
IIIC1[a]	Positive pelvic nodes
IIIC2[a]	Positive paraaortic lymph nodes with or without positive pelvic lymph nodes
Stage IV[a]	Tumor invades bladder and/or bowel mucosa, and/or distant metastases
IVA[a]	Tumor invasion of bladder and/or bowel mucosa
IVB[a]	Distant metastases, including intra-abdominal metastases and/or inguinal lymph nodes

[a]G1, G2, or G3.
[b]Endocervical glandular involvement only should be considered as stage I and no longer as stage II.
[c]Positive cytology has to be reported separately without changing the stage.
Source: From Pecorelli S. Revised FIGO staging for carcinoma of the vulva, cervix, and endometrium. *Int J Gynaecol Obstet.* 2009;105:103–104, with permission.

Table 8.2	Comparison between Type I and Type II Endometrial Cancers	
	Type I	Type II
CLINICAL FEATURES		
Risk factors	Unopposed estrogen	Age
Race	White > black	White = black
Differentiation	Well differentiated	Poorly differentiated
Histology	Endometrioid	Nonendometrioid
Stage	I/II	III/IV
Prognosis	Favorable	Not favorable
MOLECULAR FEATURES		
Ploidy	Diploid	Aneuploid
K-ras overexpression	Yes	Yes
Her-2/neu overexpression	No	Yes
P53 overexpression	No	Yes
PTEN mutations	Yes	No
MSI	Yes	No

probably should not be considered as important independent risk factors. Finally, tamoxifen (a common agent for the treatment of breast cancer) is a risk factor for the development of type I endometrial carcinoma, though the benefits of treatment (for breast cancer) far outweigh the risk of disease.

In contrast, type II endometrial cancers represent estrogen-independent tumors and are associated with a more aggressive clinical course. Unlike type I tumors, there is no readily observed premalignant phase. Both clear cell and serous carcinoma and perhaps grade 3 tumors comprise these histologic phenotypes. Some experts also classify uterine carcinosarcomas as a representative of type II histology (Table 8.2).

The molecular defects associated with endometrial cancers are stratified between type I and type II cancers. Type I cancers frequently have *PTEN*, *KRAS*, and *PIK3CA* mutations, and this is also varied by race, whereas type II cancers are more likely to have *TP53* mutations. Among women belonging to families with the autosomal dominant HNPCC syndrome, the most common extracolonic malignancy is endometrial carcinoma with a lifetime risk of 40% to 60%.

PATHOLOGY OF PREINVASIVE DISEASE

The current classification of endometrial hyperplasia accepted by both the International Society of Gynecologic Pathologists (ISGP) and the World Health Organization (WHO) is based on the schema of Kurman et al., which divides hyperplasia on the basis of architectural features into simple or complex and on the basis of cytologic features into typical or atypical. The resulting classification relies on a combination of architectural and cytologic criteria. It comprises four categories as follows: simple hyperplasia (SH), complex hyperplasia (CH), simple atypical hyperplasia (SAH), and CAH. Endometrial hyperplasia appears to arise as a result of unopposed and prolonged estrogen stimulation. Therefore, some hyperplasias may regress if the estrogenic stimulus is removed.

The probability of progression to adenocarcinoma is related to the degree of architectural or cytologic atypia. While progression occurs rarely for patients with SH or CH (incidence is 1% and 3%, respectively), progression from atypical hyperplasia is much higher: 8% and 29% for patients with SAH or CAH, respectively (Table 8.3). However, coexistent

Table 8.3	Classification of Endometrial Hyperplasia
Types of Hyperplasia Progressing to Cancer	%
Simple (cystic without atypia)	1
Complex (adenomatous without atypia)	3
Atypical	
Simple (cystic with atypia)	8
Complex (adenomatous with atypia)	29

adenocarcinoma may be present in up to 40% of hysterectomies performed to treat CAH.

Mutter et al. have proposed an alternative classification of hyperplasia based on a combination of morphologic, molecular, and morphometric information. This includes the use of a new term, endometrial intraepithelial neoplasia (EIN), as the histopathologic presentation of a monoclonal endometrial preinvasive glandular proliferation that is considered the immediate pathologic precursor of endometrioid endometrial adenocarcinoma. Almost 40% of women with an EIN diagnosis will be diagnosed with endometrial carcinoma within 1 year, and for those who do not develop cancer within 12 months, there is a 45-fold increased risk of future endometrial cancer. Correspondingly, absence of an EIN lesion in an initial representative biopsy, including those with only benign hyperplasia, confers very high (99%) negative predictive value for concomitant or future adenocarcinoma.

In contrast, endometrial intraepithelial carcinoma (EIC) has recently been recognized as a histologically distinctive lesion that is proposed to represent a form of intraepithelial tumor. It appears to be the likely precursor to serous carcinoma of the endometrium.

PATHOLOGY OF ENDOMETRIAL CANCER

Uterine tumors are classified based on the ISGP and WHO classification system, which is a relatively simple classification scheme and accommodates the vast majority of endometrial carcinoma. It has been shown to accurately distinguish prognostic classes of endometrial neoplasms.

The differentiation of a carcinoma is expressed as its grade. Grade 1 lesions are well differentiated and are generally associated with a good prognosis. Both architectural criteria and nuclear grade are used to determine grade. The architectural grade is determined based upon the amount of the tumor growth in solid sheets (Table 8.4). The FIGO rules for grading

Table 8.4	Histologic Grade and Depth of Invasion			
	Grade, No. of Patients (%)			
Depth	G1 (%)	G2 (%)	G3 (%)	Total (% of Total)
Endometrium only	44 (24)	31 (11)	11 (7)	86 (14)
Superficial	96 (53)	131 (45)	54 (35)	281 (45)
Middle	22 (12)	69 (24)	24 (16)	115 (19)
Deep	18 (10)	57 (20)	64 (42)	139 (22)
Total	180 (100)	288 (100)	153 (100)	621 (100)

Source: Reprinted from Creasman WT, Morrow CP, Bundy BN, et al. Surgical pathologic spread patterns of endometrial cancer: A Gynecologic Oncology Group study. *Cancer.* 1987;60:2035–2041, with permission.

state that notable nuclear atypia, inappropriate for architectural grade, raises the grade of a grade 1 or grade 2 tumor by 1. Though FIGO did not define notable nuclear atypia, it has been interpreted to include tumors with a majority of cells having nuclei of grade 3, which portends a significantly worse behavior and justifies upgrading by one grade. Some cell types (i.e., serous and clear cell) are not easily architecturally graded because their growth patterns are architecturally limited, and in these cases the nuclear grading is more universally applicable. In instances where two distinctive cell types are identified within a single tumor (mixed carcinomas), classification is based on the component that constitutes at least 10% of the tumor.

Molecular Alterations in the Pathogenesis and Progression of Endometrial Adenocarcinoma

Deletions or mutations of the *PTEN* gene and microsatellite instability (MSI) due to hypermethylation of the promoter for the mismatch repair gene, *hMLH1*, are both relatively common and early events in the development of a significant proportion of endometrioid adenocarcinomas. In contrast, these molecular alterations do not appear critical in the pathogenesis of serous or clear cell carcinoma. There are relatively few data to inform the importance of MSI as a prognostic factor in endometrial cancer, although defects in mismatch repair systems may alter responsiveness to chemotherapy or radiation.

Mutations in the p53 gene are found with high frequency not only in invasive serous carcinoma but also in EIC, the noninvasive precursor of serous carcinoma, suggesting that a different pathway is followed in the development of this second type of endometrial adenocarcinoma. These mutations appear to be an early event in the development of serous carcinoma, but a late event in endometrioid carcinomas for which it serves as an indicator of poor prognosis. In addition to the very frequent overexpression of p53 protein in serous carcinoma, it has also been related to high FIGO stage, clear cell histology, higher histologic grade, and increasing depth of myometrial invasion.

The *KRAS, CTNNB1* (β-catenin), *PIK3CA*, and *FGFR2* genes are also commonly mutated in endometrial cancer.

Cell Types

Endometrioid

Endometrioid adenocarcinoma is the most common form of carcinoma of the endometrium, comprising 75% to 80% of the cases. It varies from well differentiated to undifferentiated. Characteristically, the glands of endometrioid adenocarcinoma are formed of tall columnar cells that share a common apical border. With decreasing differentiation, there is a preponderance of solid growth rather than gland formation.

Foci of squamous differentiation are found in about 25% of endometrial adenocarcinomas. In a Gynecologic Oncology Group (GOG) study of early-stage disease, it was noted that these tumors with squamous regions behave in a fashion similar to endometrioid carcinomas without squamous differentiation. Historically, the tumors were sometimes separated into adenoacanthoma or adenosquamous carcinoma based on whether the squamous component appeared histologically benign or malignant; however, the terms are confusing, are not prognostically relevant, and have been abandoned. Pure squamous carcinoma of the endometrium is extremely rare, representing less than 1% of endometrial carcinoma, and with only about 60 reported cases.

Serous

Serous carcinoma of the endometrium closely resembles serous carcinoma of the ovary and fallopian tube because its papillary growth and cellular features are similar. It is usually found in an advanced stage in older women, when comprehensive surgical staging is performed. Serous carcinoma represents about 10% of endometrial carcinomas. The tumors often deeply invade the myometrium, and unlike typical endometrioid adenocarcinoma, there is a propensity for peritoneal spread.

Unfortunately, advanced-stage disease or recurrence is common even when serous carcinomas are apparently only minimally invasive or even confined to the endometrium in polyps. Since the metastatic disease is often identified only microscopically, about 60% of patients are upstaged following complete surgical staging. A recent report by Wheeler et al. stressed the prognostic importance of meticulous surgical–pathologic staging. They and others found that serous carcinoma truly confined to the uterus had an overall excellent prognosis, while those with extrauterine disease, even if only microscopic in size, almost always suffered recurrence and death from tumor.

There has been considerable confusion about the definition and significance of papillary carcinoma of the endometrium. A variety of cell types of endometrial adenocarcinoma with differing biologic behavior, including serous, clear cell, mucinous, and villoglandular carcinoma, may grow in a papillary fashion. Thus, the adjective papillary does not represent a cell type but rather an architectural pattern and should no longer be used in describing serous carcinomas.

Other Cell Types

Clear cell adenocarcinoma of the endometrium represents approximately 4% of all uterine tumors. It is generally recognized and defined on the basis of the distinctive clearing of the cytoplasm of neoplastic cells. These are biologically aggressive neoplasms with 5-year survival of approximately 40% regardless of stage. These results are attributed to a high propensity for extrauterine spread and frequent recurrence. In fact, occult extrauterine metastasis is present in 40% of patients with disease clinically confined to the uterus.

Mucinous adenocarcinoma is rare in the endometrium, representing approximately 1% of endometrial adenocarcinomas. Mucinous carcinoma of the endometrium has the same prognosis as common endometrial carcinoma. If an endometrial carcinoma manifests two or more different cell types, each representing at least 10% or more of the tumor, the term mixed cell type is appropriate.

Malignancies in other organs may metastasize to the endometrium. The most common extragenital sites are the breast, stomach, colon, pancreas, and kidney, although any disseminated tumor could involve the endometrium. The ovaries are the most likely genital sources of metastasis.

Cancers of an identical cell type may be discovered in the ovary and endometrium simultaneously. Usually, the primary site is assigned to the area having the largest tumor mass and most advanced stage. In certain situations, primary malignancies in the endometrium and ovary may coexist. This "field effect" of the "extended müllerian system" may occur in 15% to 20% of endometrioid carcinomas of the ovary. In a review of a GOG study of 74 patients with simultaneously detected endometrial and ovarian carcinoma with disease grossly limited to the pelvis, only 16% of women suffered a recurrence of disease, with a median follow-up of 80 months. This group of patients was atypical, with 86% having endometrioid histology in both sites. Recurrence was statistically related to the presence of microscopic metastases or high histologic grade.

CANCER PREVENTION AND SCREENING FOR ENDOMETRIAL CANCER

KEY POINTS
- All women should be encouraged to promptly report abnormal vaginal bleeding.
- Women taking tamoxifen (usually as breast cancer prevention or treatment) do not require endometrial screening in the absence of symptoms.

Many cases of endometrial cancer develop by way of a precursor lesion. Estrogen-related cancers frequently develop secondary to atypical endometrial hyperplasia. Serous tumors also may develop EIC through a precursor lesion. Prompt recognition of precursor lesions with institution of proper treatment will prevent cancers and their sequelae. Many endometrial cancers may be preventable, particularly those that are estrogen related.

Because 95% of endometrial carcinomas occur in women 40 years and older and because endometrial hyperplasia, the precursor state, tends to be a premenopausal and perimenopausal condition, it is appropriate to evaluate individuals past their fourth decade of life if there is abnormal bleeding. Similarly, a higher degree of suspicion should be held for younger patients with high-risk characteristics including significant obesity, polycystic ovarian syndrome/chronic anovulation, or tamoxifen exposure.

Evaluation can be by endometrial biopsy or by dilatation and curettage (D&C) if the biopsy is unsuccessful or the results are unclear. Patients with complex and atypical hyperplasia may be treated by hysterectomy or by periodic use of progestins, depending on age and reproductive desires. Hysterectomy is the preferred treatment in the patient with complex atypical endometrial hyperplasia. This approach not only cures the usual presenting symptoms of abnormal bleeding but confers prophylaxis against the almost 30% risk of later developing endometrial carcinoma. Since coexistent invasive endometrial cancer may be present in up to 40% of women with CAH, frozen section and surgical staging should be available at the time of hysterectomy.

Those with CAH treated with progestins should have a D&C performed before treatment to rule out the occasional occult carcinoma not detected by biopsy. A progestin should be administered at least 10 to 14 days each month, and endometrial biopsies should be performed at 3- to 4-month intervals to assess treatment results. Women with a uterus should never be prescribed estrogen-only preparations of hormone replacement therapy because unopposed estrogen greatly increases their risk of endometrial cancer. The addition of progestins to the regimens of patients treated with exogenous estrogen may prevent endometrial hyperplasia and subsequent cancer and may protect against the development of carcinoma.

Women taking tamoxifen and have their uterus intact should be informed of the increased risk of endometrial cancer. Education regarding the onset of vaginal bleeding is important, and patients should be advised to report symptoms early. All women on tamoxifen who present with abnormal vaginal bleeding should be investigated promptly. However, screening of asymptomatic women on tamoxifen therapy with ultrasound or endometrial biopsies is not recommended.

Considering the available knowledge about the disease and available tests, it seems unlikely that screening would be generally advised in the near future. This has also been the view in statements from official organizations like the International Union Against Cancer and the American Cancer Society (ACS). The ACS does recommend annual endometrial biopsies starting at age 35 for women known to have or be at risk for HNPCC. Obese patients should be counseled that a healthy diet and regular exercise could reduce their risk of endometrial cancer (in addition to other known benefits).

DIAGNOSTIC EVALUATION

KEY POINTS
- All postmenopausal bleeding should be evaluated.

Endometrioid adenocarcinoma is likely to present with disease confined to the uterus, while serous and clear cell tumors are more likely to have extrauterine spread and preoperative CA-125 and/or imaging is warranted.

Approximately 90% of patients will present with abnormal vaginal discharge, of which 80% will report abnormal bleeding (usually postmenopausal) and 10% show leukorrhea. Other signs and symptoms of more advanced disease include pelvic pressure and other symptoms indicative of uterine enlargement or extrauterine tumor spread (abdominal bloating, pain, shortness of breath).

The standard method of assessing uterine bleeding is formal fractional D&C. Outpatient procedures, such as endometrial biopsy or aspiration curettage coupled with endocervical sampling, may be indicated if the clinical suspicion is sufficiently high. However, sampling techniques may not provide sufficient diagnostic information, in which case the fractional

D&C is mandatory. Results of endometrial biopsies correlate well with endometrial curettings.

After the diagnosis of endometrial carcinoma has been histologically confirmed, the patient should undergo a thorough clinical evaluation consisting of a physical examination and careful medical history, complete blood count, liver and renal function tests, and chest x-ray. Further imaging can be guided by the risk of extrauterine spread. In general, women with well-differentiated endometrioid tumors do not need to undergo an extensive metastatic workup. However, patients with high-grade tumors should undergo further evaluation. This may include intravenous including intravenous pyelogram, cystoscopy, and proctoscopy if there is suspicion for extrauterine disease; body imaging by computed tomography (CT) with or without 18F-fluorodeoxyglucose–positron emission tomography (PET); or magnetic resonance imaging (MRI) of the pelvis (particularly indicated if cervical involvement is suspected). In addition, a CA-125 may be useful; if elevated, it becomes a way to evaluate progress during treatment and, subsequently, during surveillance.

Preoperative assessments of lymph node involvement have been proposed by some authors as useful techniques to assess for metastasis. However, only a few pretreatment imaging tests have been described. Both CT and MRI are extensively used to assess nodal spread of disease in patients with malignant tumors, including endometrial cancer. Both techniques have based the detection of pathologic nodes on measurements of node size: a short-axis diameter greater than 10 mm is the most accepted criterion for the diagnosis of suspicious nodal involvement. Unfortunately, these morphologic imaging techniques have low sensitivity ranging from about 20% to 65% with specificity between 73% and 99%.

PET/CT recently has been evaluated for endometrial cancer. Signorelli et al. performed a retrospective study to determine the diagnostic accuracy of 18F-FDG PET/CT in detecting nodal metastases in patients with high-risk endometrial cancer; pelvic node metastases were found at histopathologic analysis in 9 of the 37 patients (24.3%). Patient-based sensitivity, specificity, positive predictive value, negative predictive value, and accuracy were 77.8%, 100.0%, 100.0%, 93.1%, and 94.4%, respectively. Nodal lesion site–based sensitivity, specificity, positive predictive value, negative predictive value, and accuracy were 66.7%, 99.4%, 90.9%, 97.2%, and 96.8%, respectively. From these data, it appears that 18F-FDG PET/CT is accurate in pelvic node staging workup of high-risk endometrial cancer, allowing the best planning of primary surgical treatment in this subset of patients. The GOG is conducting an ongoing prospective assessment of PET/CT in patients with endometrial and cervical cancer (GOG 233).

PATHOLOGIC FACTORS OF PROGNOSTIC SIGNIFICANCE

The importance of uterine and extrauterine risk factors is determined by how they affect the probability of retroperitoneal lymph node involvement and subsequent survival.

FIGO Stage

The prognostic utility of surgicopathologic stage has been confirmed in multiple studies of large numbers of patients, using both univariate and multivariate analyses. FIGO stage is often the single strongest predictor of outcome for women with endometrial adenocarcinoma in studies using multivariate analyses. Although the FIGO clinical staging system of 1971 was generally useful, retrospective comparison of the two methods demonstrated the clear superiority of surgicopathologic staging over clinical staging in predicting outcome (Tables 8.4 and 8.5).

Histologic Cell Types

The histologic classification of endometrial adenocarcinoma is important because it has consistently been recognized as an important predictor of biologic behavior and probability of survival. Endometrioid adenocarcinoma accounts for the majority of tumors in the corpus and, fortunately, usually has a relatively good prognosis.

Adenocarcinoma with squamous differentiation is similar to typical endometrioid adenocarcinoma with respect to the distribution by age and frequency of nodal metastasis but is associated with a slightly increased probability of survival. Villoglandular carcinomas have a biologic behavior similar to that of endometrioid adenocarcinoma. Serous carcinoma is an aggressive tumor, with overall survival (OS) rates varying from 40% to 60% at 5 years. Clear cell carcinoma is also a highly aggressive tumor, with 5-year survival rates of 30% to 75%.

Grade

The degree of histologic differentiation has long been considered one of the most sensitive indicators of tumor spread. The GOG and other studies have confirmed that as grade becomes less differentiated, there is a greater tendency for deep myometrial invasion (Table 8.4) and, subsequently, higher rates of pelvic and paraaortic lymph node involvement (Tables 8.5 and 8.6). In fact, 50% of grade 3 lesions have greater than one

Table 8.5	Grade, Depth of Invasion, and Pelvic Node Metastasis		
	Grade		
Depth of Invasion	G1 ($N = 180$)	G2 ($N = 288$)	G3 ($N = 153$)
Endometrium only ($N = 86$)	0 (0%)	1 (3%)	0 (0%)
Inner ($N = 281$)	3 (3%)	7 (5%)	5 (9%)
Middle ($N = 115$)	0 (0%)	6 (9%)	1 (4%)
Deep ($N = 139$)	2 (11%)	11 (19%)	22 (34%)

Source: From Creasman WT, Morrow CP, Bundy BN, et al. Surgical pathologic spread patterns of endometrial cancer: A Gynecologic Oncology Group study. *Cancer.* 1987;60:2039–2041, with permission.

Table 8.6	Grade, Depth of Invasion, and Aortic Node Metastasis		
	Grade		
Depth of Invasion	G1 ($N = 180$)	G2 ($N = 288$)	G3 ($N = 153$)
Endometrium only ($N = 86$)	0 (0%)	1 (3%)	0 (0%)
Inner ($N = 281$)	1 (1%)	5 (4%)	2 (4%)
Middle ($N = 115$)	1 (5%)	0 (0%)	0 (0%)
Deep ($N = 139$)	1 (6%)	8 (14%)	15 (23%)

Source: From Creasman WT, Morrow CP, Bundy BN, et al. Surgical pathologic spread patterns of endometrial cancer: A Gynecologic Oncology Group study. *Cancer.* 1987;60:2039–2041, with permission.

half myometrial invasion, with pelvic and paraaortic lymph node involvement approaching 30% and 20%, respectively. Survival has also been consistently related to histologic grade, and in a GOG study of more than 600 women with clinical stage I or occult stage II endometrioid adenocarcinoma, the 5-year relative survival was as follows: grade 1—94%; grade 2—84%; grade 3—72%.

Myometrial Invasion

The depth of myometrial invasion should be recorded in all pathology reports, preferably in both millimeters and in the percentage of total myometrial thickness. Extension of tumor into adenomyosis is not regarded as invasion. Deep myometrial invasion is one of the more important factors correlated with a diminished probability of survival and is associated with a higher probability of extrauterine tumor spread, treatment failure, and recurrence. In a GOG study of over 400 women with clinical stage I and occult stage II endometrioid adenocarcinoma, the 5-year relative survival was 94% when tumor was confined to the endometrium, 91% when tumor involved the inner third of the myometrium, 84% when the tumor extended into the middle third, and 59% when the tumor invaded into the outer third of the myometrium. Although the depth of invasion is often inversely related to the degree of differentiation, myometrial invasion is an independent predictor of outcome for women with early-stage endometrial carcinoma.

Vascular Space Invasion

Several studies have suggested that lymphatic vascular space invasion (LVSI) is a strong predictor of recurrence and death and is independent of depth of myometrial invasion or histologic differentiation. Zaino et al. found that vascular invasion was a statistically significant indicator of death from tumor in early clinical stage but not in early surgical stage endometrial adenocarcinoma. This suggests that lymphatic invasion helps to identify patients likely to have spread to lymph nodes or distant sites, but that its importance is diminished for those in whom thorough sampling of nodes has failed to identify metastasis. Vascular space invasion or capillary-like space involvement with tumor exists in approximately 15% of uteri containing adenocarcinoma. Nodal metastases are more common when capillary invasion is identified. Capillary invasion is identified in 35% to 95% of serous carcinomas of the endometrium, where it has generally been associated with an elevated risk of tumor recurrence or death from disease.

Adnexal Involvement

Six percent of clinical stage I and occult stage II patients have spread of tumor to the adnexa. Of these, 32% have pelvic node metastases, compared with 8% pelvic node positivity if adnexal involvement is not present. Twenty percent have positive paraaortic node metastases, which is four times greater than if adnexal metastases are not present. Gross intraperitoneal spread without adnexal metastases correlates highly with the involvement of pelvic and paraaortic lymph nodes.

Peritoneal Cytology

About 12% to 15% of patients who undergo surgical staging have positive peritoneal cytology. Of these, 25% have metastases to pelvic lymph nodes, and 19% have metastases to paraaortic lymph nodes. In addition, 35% of patients with extrauterine disease (adnexal, nodal, or intraperitoneal spread) have positive cytologic washings. However, 4% to 6% of patients with positive washings have no evidence of extrauterine disease. Published opinions are mixed about the significance of this finding. Several small series show no outcome differences. However, two large series show peritoneal cytology to be, by itself, a poor prognostic factor. Nonetheless, in 2009 FIGO removed peritoneal washings as a formal component of endometrial cancer staging and suggests that positive cytology should be reported separately but does not affect stage. *p cytology in endometrial Ca*

Pelvic and Paraaortic Lymph Nodes

In the 1987 GOG study of 621 clinical stage I and occult stage II patients, 70 (11%) had metastases to pelvic or paraaortic lymph nodes. Of this number, 22 patients had metastases to both the pelvic and paraaortic regions and 12 had metastases to the paraaortic nodes only. The highest rate of paraaortic node metastases (32%) occurred if pelvic nodes were involved. The frequency of pelvic and paraaortic nodal metastases with respect to depth of invasion and grade is shown in Tables 8.5 and 8.6.

DETERMINING THE SURGICAL PROCEDURE

KEY POINTS
- Surgical staging is a critical component for the proper diagnosis and management of all endometrial carcinomas.
- FIGO stage is the most powerful predictor of prognosis.
- Surgical staging is feasible by laparoscopy.

Contemporary management for most patients with endometrial cancer remains surgical. Although the tradition has been to do this abdominally, laparoscopic management has increasingly been integrated into the forefront of surgical staging. Surgery for endometrial cancer includes, at the minimum, an initial surgical exploration with collection of peritoneal fluid for cytologic evaluation (intraperitoneal cell washings), thorough inspection of the abdominal and pelvic cavities with biopsy or excision of any extrauterine lesions suspicious for tumor, and total extrafascial hysterectomy with bilateral salpingo-oophorectomy (BSO). The uterus should be observed for tumor breakthrough of the serosal surface. The distal ends of the fallopian tubes are clipped or ligated to prevent possible tumor spill during uterine manipulation. To complete the surgical staging of endometrial cancer, the removal of bilateral pelvic and paraaortic lymph nodes is also required. While the current FIGO staging system removed the status of cytology as a stage-defining criterion, it remains an important piece of information, especially in women with high-risk histologies (e.g., serous carcinoma) with very early-stage disease.

In cases with gross omental or intraperitoneal disease spread, cytoreductive surgery is usually performed, especially if the surgeon believes a complete or optimal cytoreduction is possible. This may require total omentectomy, radical peritoneal stripping, and, occasionally, bowel resection.

In cases complicated by medical comorbidity, advanced age, or obesity, or when nodal dissection cannot or will not be performed, total vaginal hysterectomy with or without laparoscopic assistance may be utilized. Following surgical assessment, patients may be classified based on pathologic features as to their risk of recurrence, and those deemed to be at sufficient risk may be offered adjuvant therapies. An algorithm for surgical approach can be found in Figure 8.1.

Nonsurgical Management

Patients with significant medical comorbidities who are not acceptable candidates for surgery (e.g., markedly advanced age, diminished performance status, or severe cardiac/pulmonary disease) may be managed by alternative means. Importantly, obesity in and of itself should not preclude surgical management. Patients who are obese but otherwise surgical candidates may undergo an abdominal panniculectomy to enhance surgical exposure to facilitate hysterectomy and nodal dissection. Primary radiation therapy without surgery has been used and is discussed later in this chapter.

Approximately 5% of women with endometrial cancer are diagnosed under the age of 40. For some of these patients, the standard treatment of hysterectomy is unacceptable due to desires to maintain fertility. Ideally, eligibility for nonoperative management should be limited to patients without myometrial invasion. Pelvic MRI may be useful to better assess for myometrial involvement. In patients who are offered nonsurgical treatment, progestational therapy, delivered orally or intrauterinely, has been successful in reversing malignant changes in up to 76% of cases. Increasingly, there has been a consideration for progestin-based intrauterine devices, although the data are limited. In a 2012 systematic review of the literature, 74% of

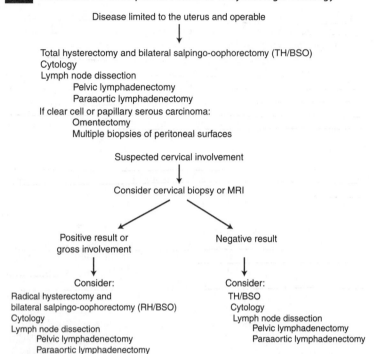

FIGURE 8.1 Surgical management of early-stage endometrial cancer (stages I and II). Patients with stage I and II endometrial cancers are treated with total hysterectomy (TH), BSO, peritoneal cytology, and pelvic and paraaortic lymphadenectomy. Many advocate lymphadenectomy when feasible for all patients with early-stage endometrial cancer regardless of grade or depth of myometrial invasion. *Source*: From Markman M, ed. *Atlas of Cancer*, 2nd ed. Philadelphia, PA: Current Medical Group; 2008.

atypical endometrial hyperplasia and 72% of grade 1 endometrial cancer patients achieved a pathologic complete response (CR) for 6 months or longer with oral progestins. The range of CRs was 50% to 95% for atypical endometrial hyperplasia and 50% to 100% for grade 1 cancer. The mean time required to achieve the CR was 6 months. Of the 22 patients reported with grade 1 cancer treated with progesterone-releasing intrauterine device, 68% achieved a CR. Because response may be temporary or incomplete, periodic sampling of the endometrium is advised.

Surgical Recommendations

The contemporary management of endometrial cancer continues to evolve, and the indications for lymph node dissection remain controversial. For most patients, however, comprehensive staging most accurately assigns stage and associated prognosis. Staging also allows for a more tailored approach to the use of adjuvant therapies. Patients who *a priori* are deemed not to be candidates for staging should be considered for vaginal or laparoscopic-assisted vaginal hysterectomies. Laparoscopic techniques have been shown to result in comparable surgery to open procedures. For patients with resectable intraperitoneal disease, cytoreductive surgery may improve outcomes.

Nodal Dissection

The value of surgical staging is a source of controversy and has been the subject of increased scrutiny and debate over the last several years. Proponents of routine surgical staging suggest that the ability to identify otherwise unrecognized disease spread to the nodes changes the postoperative therapies that are given and is the most accurate way to assess risk. Most controversial is the assertion that surgical staging has a therapeutic benefit independent of the node status (positive or negative for metastatic disease). Fundamentally, surgeons must determine for themselves whether or not surgical staging has sufficient value to offer it to all patients or only to those selected based on risk factors identified preoperatively and intraoperatively. The principal risks attributable to nodal dissections include increased operative time, potential for blood loss associated with vascular injury, genitofemoral nerve injury with resulting numbness and paresthesias over medial thighs, lymphocyst formation, and lymphedema. In general, the risks associated with nodal dissections are low and acceptable. The principal advantage of comprehensive staging is that the physician and patient are provided with the greatest amount of information. In the contemporary management of endometrial cancer, this information results in less use of radiation and substitution of vaginal cuff brachytherapy for pelvic radiation.

The importance, extent, and technique of nodal dissection are hotly debated. Questions relate to which patients should be offered and could benefit from surgical staging (all, some, or none), and what is the optimal surgical procedure to be performed (biopsy of enlarged/visible nodes, lymphadenectomy). Controversy also exists between those surgeons who perform only pelvic dissections and those who advocate pelvic and para-aortic nodal dissection.

Arguments against Routine Nodal Dissection

Most patients with endometrial cancer will present with low-risk features. In the entire GOG 33 study population of 621 patients, 75% had grade 1 to 2 tumors, and 59% had inner one third or less myometrial invasion. Only 9% of patients had positive lymph nodes. The Post Operative Radiation Therapy in Endometrial Cancer (PORTEC) trial evaluated patients with stage IC, grade 1; stages IB and IC, grade 2; or stage IB, grade 3 who underwent hysterectomy without lymph node dissection and compared observation to postoperative pelvic radiation. This patient population managed without nodal dissection and had favorable outcomes with or without radiation therapy (5-year survival rates of 85% observation, 81% with pelvic radiation).

Two randomized trials comparing hysterectomy with or without lymphadenectomy have been reported. A Study in the Treatment of Endometrial

Cancer (ASTEC) randomized patients with endometrial cancer treated with hysterectomy to pelvic lymphadenectomy or not. Following surgery, patients with stage I and IIA diseases were then randomized again to observation or pelvic radiation therapy if they had grade 3, serous, or clear cell histology; more than 50% myometrial invasion; or endocervical glandular invasion (stage IIA). Treatment centers were also permitted to use vaginal cuff brachytherapy regardless of pelvic radiation assignment. The results show no evidence of benefit in terms of overall or recurrence-free survival for pelvic lymphadenectomy in women with early endometrial cancer.

A similar study was performed by Italian investigators (CONSORT trial). In this trial, 514 patients were assigned to hysterectomy with or without pelvic lymphadenectomy. Patients were required to have myometrial invasion, and patients with grade 1 tumors and less than 50% invasion were excluded. In the no-LND group, 22% of patients had nodal dissections due to clinical suspicion with 14% of these cases, or 3% of the entire no-LND arm, having node-positive disease. In the LND group, the median number of nodes removed was 26. Paraaortic dissection could be performed at the surgeon's discretion and was done in 26% of cases. In the LND group, 13% were found to have positive nodes. Postoperative therapy was not protocol prescribed, but the use of radiation therapy was more common in the no-LND group (25% vs. 17%). The 5-year disease-free survival (DFS) was 81% in both groups, and 5-year survival was 90% in the no-LND group versus 86% in the LND group (hazard ratio [HR] 1.2, $p = 0.5$). The authors concluded that pelvic lymphadenectomy could not be recommended as a routine procedure for therapeutic purposes.

Arguments for Selective Nodal Dissection

Increasingly, some form of nodal assessment has been integrated into the upfront management of endometrial cancer, and nodal assessment has been incorporated into the staging of endometrial cancer since 1988. Surgical staging is the most accurate way to determine the extent of disease spread. Palpation of pelvic lymph nodes is not sufficiently accurate.

Based on pathologic information available at the time of surgery, the risk for nodal metastasis may be estimated. Physicians who selectively perform nodal dissections frequently do so based on the presence of uterine risk factors, which suggest the potential for nodal disease. In the surgical–pathologic study GOG 33, pelvic and paraaortic nodal diseases were more frequent with increasing grade (% pelvic nodal metastases: 3% grade I, 9% grade II, 18% grade 3), depth of invasion (1% endometrium only, 5% inner 1/3, 6% middle 1/3, 25% outer 1/3 myometrial invasion), and LVSI (27% with LVSI, 7% without LVSI). Pelvic and paraaortic nodal metastases were also more common with cervical involvement, when peritoneal cytology was positive, and when extranodal (adnexal, intraperitoneal sites) disease was found.

In 2000, the Mayo group described a model that could classify a group with a low risk of nodal disease spread and high DFS based on frozen section evaluation of the uterus. Mariani et al. determined that patients with grade 1 or 2 histology, myometrial invasion less than 50%, and tumor size less than 2 cm were at a low risk for lymph node involvement. In this large series of 381 patients with grade 1 or 2 endometrioid endometrial cancer and less than 50% myometrial invasion, no patients with tumor size less than 2 cm had lymph node involvement. Of the patients with tumors greater than 2 cm, 8 of 107 (7%) had lymph node involvement. Overall, grade 1 and 2 tumors had 4% (5/126) and 7% (4/61) lymph node involvement, respectively. Given these findings, the authors recommended consideration of lymph node sparing surgeries in patients with grade 1 or 2 tumors of endometrioid histology, tumor size less than 2 cm, and myometrial invasion less than 50%. These findings have further been validated in subsequent retrospective studies.

Arguments for Routine Nodal Dissection

Many gynecologic oncologists have moved toward performing uniform comprehensive surgical staging for nearly all patients with endometrial cancer. The rationale for uniform staging includes the lack of a patient population for whom nodal disease is so low that nodes should be omitted, the inaccuracy of preoperative or intraoperative assessments predicting the risk for nodal disease, the potential for therapeutic benefit in node-positive and node-negative patients, and the lack of significant morbidity associated with the procedure. Postoperative adjuvant decisions are best made with the most complete information. If nodal assessment is the predominant factor by which to categorize patients into risk groups, routine nodal dissection is the best method by which to determine which few patients will require adjuvant therapy.

Laparoscopic Management

Laparoscopic management of endometrial cancer has increasingly been integrated into standard practice. Laparoscopic techniques are utilized in the initial treatment of endometrial cancer (laparoscopic-assisted vaginal hysterectomy, total laparoscopic hysterectomy), to stage patients with laparoscopic pelvic and paraaortic nodal dissection, and to restage patients following incomplete surgical staging.

The largest and most comprehensive data set to date comes from the large prospective randomized trial conducted by the GOG (LAP2 trial). The study was designed to compare laparoscopic hysterectomy with comprehensive surgical staging to the traditional laparotomy technique (using a 2:1 randomization favoring the laparoscopic arm) to determine the complete staging rates, safety, short-term surgical outcomes, and long-term cancer recurrence and survival. The study enrolled 920 patients to the open arm and 1,696 to laparoscopy. The rate of conversion from laparoscopy to open procedure was 26% and was most frequently related to poor visibility (15%), extrauterine cancer spread (4%), and bleeding (3%). The conversion rate increased with an increasing patient obesity, with laparoscopic success rate being 90% with a BMI < 20, 65% with BMI = 35, and 34% with BMI = 50. Median number of removed nodes was similar between each technique, as were the frequencies of patients found to have positive lymph nodes. Complication rates (combined rates of vascular, urinary, bowel, nerve, or other complications) for those who had an open procedure were 7.6%, compared to 9.5% of patients randomized to laparoscopy.

Of the 1,242 patients randomized to laparoscopy who had the procedure successfully completed laparoscopically, the complication rates were 4.9%. Comparing patients who underwent open surgery versus successful completion of laparoscopy, operative time was longer (median, 70 minutes) but hospital time was shorter (2 vs. 4 days) with laparoscopy. Postoperative arrhythmia, pneumonia, ileus, antibiotic use, and any complication greater than grade 2 were lower in the laparoscopic group. The authors concluded that laparoscopic surgical staging is an acceptable and possibly a better option, particularly when the surgery can be successfully completed laparoscopically. In a subsequent evaluation of recurrence and survival data from the GOG LAP2 trial published in 2012, 3-year recurrence rates were 11.4% with laparoscopy versus 10.2% with open surgery, and 5-year survival was 90% in each arm.

Laparoscopic surgery has demonstrated an important role in the management of endometrial cancer. The demonstration of comparable surgical end points (similar numbers of nodes removed, similar frequency of positive nodes) along with shortened hospital stay and quicker recovery compared to open procedures suggests that appropriate patients should be counseled regarding this option.

Robotic surgery may represent the next step forward in minimally invasive surgery. Since FDA approval for hysterectomy and myomectomy procedures in 2005, there has been an increasing utilization of robotic surgery within gynecologic oncology practice. A number of retrospective series have described robotic experience or compared outcomes to laparoscopy and/or open procedures. Proposed robotic surgery advantages include improved visualization with 3D optics, "wristlike" motion of instruments that allow for greater dexterity, reduction in tremor, an easier learning curve for adoption compared to straight–stick laparoscopy, and more comfortable ergonomics. Published data suggest comparable outcomes with respect to blood loss, nodal counts, and operative time compared to laparoscopy, with several series suggesting lower postoperative complications compared to open surgery. Robotic surgery may offer unique opportunities for obese patients.

ROLE OF ADJUVANT THERAPY

KEY POINTS

- Women with a very low risk of endometrial cancer do not require any postoperative treatment. In these patients, the risks of therapy outweigh the minimal benefits associated with treatment.
- Adjuvant radiation for early-stage disease can reduce local recurrence with no appreciable effect on OS.
- Intravaginal radiation therapy is probably sufficient for comprehensively staged patients with early-stage disease.
- Chemotherapy is preferable to whole abdominal radiation in advanced-stage disease.
- Combination therapy is currently being studied in advanced-stage disease.

A postoperative treatment plan should take into account the prognostic factors determined by the surgical–pathologic staging. Patients can be classified into three categories: those who show a high rate of cure without postoperative therapy, those who yield a low rate of cure without postoperative therapy, and those who demonstrate a reduced rate of surgical cure and may benefit from additional therapy. The postoperative treatment plan should also consider the available postoperative treatment methods and their morbidities. Chemotherapy as adjuvant treatment for patients with stage III and IV endometrial carcinomas is recently supported by data from GOG 122 and is discussed separately. Adjuvant radiation therapy is continually evolving, and currently, intravaginal brachytherapy and external beam whole-pelvic therapy with or without an extended field are commonly employed (Table 8.9).

ADJUVANT RADIATION THERAPY

Radiation therapy plays a significant role in the management of endometrial cancer. It is often used as an adjuvant treatment after surgery or as definitive treatment for patients who are medically inoperable, or with local recurrence. In the past, most patients were treated with preoperative intracavitary brachytherapy with or without external beam radiotherapy followed by hysterectomy. This approach is not without merit, especially in patients with gross cervical involvement. However, most patients nowadays undergo surgery first; then, depending on the prognostic features obtained from the pathology review, the need for radiotherapy is determined.

It should be noted that patients with very low risk (grade 1 or II, disease limited to the endometrium, not demonstrating a high-risk histology) should not receive adjuvant radiation therapy. A 2012 Cochrane meta-analysis showed that adjuvant pelvic radiation therapy in these patients resulted in a 2.5-fold higher risk of death compared to observation alone (relative risk 2.64, 95% CI: 1.05 to 6.66). Although brachytherapy may be a more reasonable approach to adjuvant treatment, it is also associated with side effects, including genitourinary symptoms (e.g., incontinence) that raise significant doubts about the benefit–risk relationship.

Early-Stage Disease

Most of the data on adjuvant radiation in endometrial cancer pertain to patients with early-stage (I and II) disease. The role of radiation in this group of patients, however, has been undergoing significant scrutiny in the last 10 years. The questions to be resolved are elucidating the benefits of radiation, clarifying which patients will be best served by this additional therapy, and determining the most appropriate radiation strategy.

Two prospective randomized trials compared surgery alone to surgery and postoperative external beam radiation. The first trial was conducted by the GOG (GOG 99). In this trial, 390 patients with stage IB and IIB endometrial cancers who underwent a total abdominal hysterectomy and BSO and pelvic/paraaortic lymph nodes sampling were randomized to observation (*n* = 202) or postoperative pelvic radiation (*n* = 190). With a median follow-up of 69 months, the 4-year survival rate was 92% in the irradiation arm, compared with 86% in the observation arm ($p = 0.6$). The 2-year estimated progression-free survival (PFS) rate was 97% versus 88% in favor of the irradiation arm ($p = 0.007$), with the greatest decrease seen in vaginal/pelvic recurrences. The second trial was the PORTEC study, in which 714 patients with stage IB grades 2 and 3, and stage IC grades 1 and 2 were randomized after total abdominal hysterectomy and BSO and no lymph node sampling to observation ($n = 360$) or pelvic radiation ($n = 354$). With a median follow-up of 52 months, the 5-year vaginal/pelvic recurrence rate was 4% in the radiation arm compared to 14% in the observation arm ($p < 0.001$). The corresponding 5-year survival rates were 81% and 85%, respectively ($p = 0.37$).

Despite the fact that adjuvant radiation significantly improved local–regional control, most of the debate focuses on the lack of improvement in OS. Because of relatively high incidence of other comorbidities, the chance of dying from an intercurrent illness is as high if not higher than dying from endometrial cancer. In addition, many of the patients who develop local recurrence after surgery alone are often salvaged with subsequent radiation. Even in patients who die from endometrial cancer, the most common cause is distant rather than local relapse.

An update with a median follow-up of 13.3 years has been published recently. The actuarial 15-year locoregional recurrence was statistically different at 6% versus 15% for those with adjuvant irradiation compared to observation with no statistical difference in OS or failure-free survival, distant metastases, or secondary cancers. Most recurrences in the observation arm were vaginal (11% of the 15%).

In a follow-up study including 427 patients with higher-risk disease (age >60 years plus grade 1 to 2 and outer 50% invasion, or grade 3 with inner 50% invasion, or stage IIA [1988 FIGO] disease), the PORTEC 2 study compared pelvic radiation therapy to vaginal brachytherapy. None of the patients underwent nodal assessment, and 5-year PFS (78% to 83%) and survival (80% to 85%) suggested that in this population vaginal brachytherapy was equivalent to pelvic radiation.

Type of Radiation

There are two types of radiation (intravaginal brachytherapy and external beam radiation) that could be used either alone or in combination for early-stage endometrial cancer. A significant reduction in local recurrence rates has been seen with the addition of pelvic radiation to intravaginal brachytherapy (1.9% vs. 6.9%, $p < 0.01$). With regard to OS, there was no significant difference between the two treatments, but in the subset of patients with grade 3 disease and deep myometrial penetration, there was a survival advantage (cause-specific survival) of 18% versus 7% in favor of the pelvic radiation arm.

With the increase in surgical lymph node staging, the use of postoperative intravaginal brachytherapy alone regained its appeal. The rationale was that full surgical lymph node staging could potentially eliminate the need for pelvic radiation while vaginal brachytherapy could still address the risk of vaginal cuff recurrence. Several reports in the past 5 years showed a very low rate of recurrence either in the vagina or in the pelvis with such an approach.

From the above discussion, it is clear that the options available for patients with early-stage endometrioid endometrial cancer are numerous. Perhaps, it is better to consider different options based on following factors: stage and grade, whether surgical lymph nodes staging was done, and the risk of nodal versus vaginal recurrence. The therapeutic ratio of adjuvant external beam radiation is very likely to benefit from the advances in intensity-modulated radiation therapy by providing the most conformal dose distribution to the tumor volume while sparing the surrounding normal structures.

Surgically Staged Patients
A reasonable alternative to observation in patients who had surgical lymph node staging is intravaginal brachytherapy alone. Horowitz et al. reported on 81 patients with stage IB grade 3-IC who were treated with surgery including lymph node dissection followed by high-dose rate intravaginal brachytherapy. Of the 81 patients, only 2 (2.4%) had vaginal recurrence and only 1 (1%) had pelvic recurrence.

No Surgical Lymph Node Staging
In those patients with stage IB grade 3-IC without surgical lymph node staging, intravaginal brachytherapy alone does not seem to be adequate. Pelvic radiation alone is sufficient without the addition of intravaginal radiation. In patients without comprehensive surgical staging, completion lymphadenectomy is also a reasonable consideration in an attempt to minimize the delivery of unnecessary whole pelvic radiation. The results of the GOG 249 and PORTEC 3 trials may help us segregate these patients into low risk, who may be appropriate for observation or cuff brachytherapy alone, or high risk, who may need more aggressive therapy, including a combination of irradiation and chemotherapy.

Advanced-Stage Disease

For patients with more advanced disease (stage III and cytoreduced stage IVA disease), the standard of care has evolved from radiation therapy to the increased use of platinum-based chemotherapy. However, in light of the benefits of local control with radiation therapy, combined modality is often administered. The GOG is currently conducting clinical trials evaluating this.

Chemotherapy
The data to support chemotherapy come from the GOG 122 trial, which included 396 patients with stage III and optimally debulked stage IV disease who were randomly assigned to treatment with whole-abdomen radiation ($n = 202$) or to doxorubicin–cisplatin (AP) chemotherapy ($n = 194$). With a median follow-up of 74 months, there was significant improvement in both PFS (50% vs. 38%; $p = 0.007$) as well as OS (55% vs. 42%; $p = 0.004$), respectively, in favor of chemotherapy.

However, a separate study showed that radiation therapy was at least equivalent to chemotherapy. In this study, which included stage I patients, patients were randomly assigned to radiation therapy or doxorubicin–cisplatin–cyclophosphamide (TAP). With a median follow-up of 95.5 months, the 5-year DFS was 63% in both arms ($p = 0.44$), and the 5-year OS rate was 69% in the radiation arm compared to 66% in the chemotherapy arm ($p = 0.77$).

As the follow-up study to GOG 122, GOG 184 evaluated the combination of irradiation and chemotherapy in 552 women with stage III and IV diseases. Of note, after 66 patients were enrolled, those with upper abdominal disease were excluded from the study. Treatment consisted of tumor volume directed irradiation (51% received 5,040 cGy pelvis irradiation alone, and 49% received 4,320 to 4,350 cGy of extended field for positive paraaortic disease or undissected paraaortics) followed by randomly assigned treatment with AP or TAP. TAP did not improve the risk of recurrence compared to AP, nor did it improve the recurrence-free survival, and it was associated with a worse toxicity profile. The OS data are pending.

On the basis of these data, AP was the preferred adjuvant chemotherapy regimen. However, on the basis of GOG 209, carboplatin and paclitaxel are now the more routinely administered regimen. In this trial, almost 1,300 women with recurrent or advanced endometrial cancer (including stage III disease) were randomly assigned to TAP or carboplatin plus paclitaxel. As presented at the 2012 Society of Gynecologic Oncologists Annual Meeting, women who were treated with carboplatin and paclitaxel had a similar overall response rate to those treated with TAP (51% in both arms). In addition, survival results were no different (PFS, 13 months in each arm; OS 37 vs. 40 months, respectively). However, carboplatin and paclitaxel were significantly more tolerable.

Postoperative Surveillance

> ### KEY POINTS
> - Routine physical examination in combination with prompt reporting of symptoms is probably the best method for detecting recurrent disease.
> - Pap smears detect only a small fraction of recurrent disease.

The frequency and extent of follow-up visits and surveillance tests for patients with a history of gynecologic cancer have traditionally been based on arbitrary guidelines that have been established and perpetuated at various institutions throughout the United States. Since the majority of patients with endometrial cancer will do well, and there is no clear evidence that early detection of disease recurrence will improve outcome, it has become necessary to reevaluate the practice of routine intensive surveillance in women with a history of endometrial cancer.

Physicians should educate patients regarding the signs and symptoms of recurrent disease and act promptly to evaluate symptomatic patients with diagnostic tests targeted toward the symptoms. Obtaining Pap smears routinely at each follow-up visit does not appear to be beneficial. Elevated levels of the tumor-associated antigen CA-125 have been documented in patients with advanced/recurrent endometrial cancer; however, the value of surveillance CA-125 levels is limited and best reserved for patients with an elevated value at initial diagnosis. Based on the knowledge that the majority of recurrences occur within the first 3 years after surgery, it is recommended that patients undergo semiannual pelvic examinations for 3 years, then annually thereafter. There is no evidence in the literature that routine chest x-rays improve survival, and Pap smears do not improve the outcome of patients with isolated vaginal recurrences. Low-risk women may be able to be followed less frequently to allow more detailed investigation of the high-risk women.

SPECIAL SITUATIONS

Serous and Clear Cell Histologies

Serous cancer and, to a lesser extent, clear cell cancer tend to spread in a fashion similar to ovarian cancer with a high propensity for upper abdominal relapse. Therefore, whole abdomen radiation and chemotherapy have both been studied in this group of patients. Patients with early-stage disease who are surgically staged can be treated with intravaginal radiation given with carboplatin/taxol chemotherapy while those with advanced stage are given tumor-directed radiation and/or chemotherapy.

Definitive Radiation for Inoperable Disease

Patients with medically inoperable stage I to II uterine cancers are usually treated in a fashion similar to those with cervical cancer by using intracavitary applicators with or without pelvic radiation. For patients with clinical stage I grade 1 or 2 and no evidence of myometrial invasion or lymph node metastasis on MRI, intracavitary brachytherapy alone is sufficient. More recently, high-dose-rate brachytherapy is also being employed.

COMPLICATIONS OF RADIATION

Pelvic Radiation

In the PORTEC randomized trial, the overall (grades 1 to 4) rate of late complications was 26% in the RT group compared to 4% in the observation group ($p < 0.0001$). Most of the late complications in the RT group, however, were grades 1 and 2 (22%) and only 3% were grades 3 and 4. It is also important to note that many patients in this trial were treated with AP/PA fields where the overall rate of complications was 30% compared to 21% for those treated with 4-field box ($p = 0.06$).

Whole-Abdomen Radiation

The toxicity is more pronounced than pelvic radiation but not as high as expected. In GOG 94, grade 4 gastrointestinal toxicity was seen in 6 patients (3.8%). Severe liver toxicity was seen in 3 out of 158 evaluable patients (2%), with 2/3 recovering without sequelae. There were no grade 3 and 4 genitourinary toxicities.

Intravaginal Brachytherapy

The main advantage of this treatment is its ability to deliver a relatively high dose of radiation to the vagina while limiting the dose to the surrounding normal structures such as bowels and bladder. This advantage is manifested with the low rate of severe late toxicity seen with this treatment technique ranging from 0% to 1%. But such a low rate of severe complications cannot be taken for granted because special attention needs to be paid to the depth of prescription, dose per fraction, the length of vagina treated, and the diameter of the cylinder used.

TREATMENT OF RECURRENT DISEASE

KEY POINTS
- Radiation therapy is useful for local recurrences in patients who have not been irradiated previously.
- Surgery is an excellent option for isolated disease that can be completely resected.
- Hormonal therapy is often active in patients with well-differentiated tumors.
- Multiagent chemotherapy is more active than single agents, and the optimal combination is under active investigation.

Patients with recurrent endometrial cancer must be fully evaluated for sites of recurrent disease. Depending on the site of the recurrence and prior therapy, patients may be treated for palliation or for cure. Treatment may consist of irradiation, surgery, endocrine therapy, or cytotoxic chemotherapy. These agents may be used singly or in combination. It is uncommon for patients with recurrent disease to be cured unless the recurrence is only in the vaginal cuff or central pelvis.

For women with an isolated vaginal recurrence who have not received prior radiotherapy, salvage radiotherapy is an excellent choice for treatment. As demonstrated in PORTEC 1, 87% of women with an isolated recurrence treated by radiotherapy had a CR. Vaginal recurrences within a previously irradiated field carry a worse prognosis. In PORTEC 1, the 3-year OS rate in this patient population was 43%, much lower than the 65% reported for radiotherapy-naive patient with isolated vaginal recurrences. Despite the lower rate of response to radiotherapy and higher risk of side effects, this option should not be completely excluded from the list of treatment options but likely needs to be administered at a specialized center capable of tailoring the approach to minimize toxicity to normal, surrounding tissues.

SYSTEMIC THERAPIES

Endocrine Therapy

Hormonal agents have been found to be valuable, particularly in the patient with recurrent disease, and reviews of their use have been extensively published. Response rates to a variety of endocrine agents including progestins, antiestrogens, and aromatase inhibitors are presented in Table 8.7. The overall response to progestins is approximately 25%. A higher dose of progestin does not appear to increase the response rate. Tamoxifen has been investigated in patients with recurrent disease in several studies. Results have varied, but in general, response rates have been modest in untreated patients. The possibility of alternating tamoxifen

Table 8.7	Response to Endocrine Therapy		
Hormonal Agent	Average Dose	Response Rate (%)	Range (%)
Hydroxyprogesterone caproate (Delalutin)	1–3 g IM q wk	29	9–34
Medroxyprogesterone acetate (Provera)	200–1,000 mg IM q wk or po qd	22	14–53
Megestrol acetate (Megace)	40–800 mg po qd	20	11–56
Tamoxifen (Nolvadex)	20–40 mg po qd	10	0–53
Goserelin acetate	3.6 mg SC q mo	11	NA
Anastrozole (SERM)	1 mg po qd	9	NA
Arzoxifene (SERM)	20 mg po qd	31	NA

NA, not applicable; SERM, selective estrogen receptor modulator.

with megestrol acetate in order to exploit the recruitment of progesterone receptors by tamoxifen has also been tested with some success by the GOG.

Cytotoxic Chemotherapy

Both single-agent and combination regimens are capable of inducing objective responses, yet the median time to treatment failure is on average 3 to 6 months and the OS of patients with metastatic endometrial cancer is generally less than 12 months. The role of chemotherapy in the recurrent disease setting remains palliative, and minimizing side effects is of equal importance when selecting a regimen.

Single-Agent Trials

A wide variety of single agents have been tested. Despite the number of drugs evaluated, the most commonly used single agents today based on response rates of at least 20% include cisplatin, carboplatin, doxorubicin, epirubicin, ifosfamide, docetaxel, paclitaxel, and topotecan. Frequent variability in response rate has been noted for the same agent and is probably related to several factors, including prior treatment, performance status, extent of disease, and the response criteria used for evaluation. No current data suggest that dose–response relationships exist for single-agent therapy, and doses and schedules are generally adjusted to minimize toxicity for an individual patient (Table 8.8).

Combination Therapy

The results of treatment with combination regimens are presented in Table 8.9. The results of GOG 107 comparing doxorubicin (60 mg/m^2 every 3 weeks) with the same doxorubicin dose and cisplatin (50 mg/m^2 every 3 weeks) in 223 patients with advanced or recurrent endometrial cancer

Table 8.8 Single-Agent Trials

Agent	N	Prior Treatment	No. of CR + PR	(%)	95% CI
Alkylating agents					
Cyclophosphamide	37	Some	4	11	3–25
Chlorambucil	11	NS	0	0	0–28
Ifosfamide	56	Some	4 + 4	14	6–26
Hexamethylmelamine	54	Few	2 + 7	17	8–29
Cisplatin					
No prior chemotherapy	63	No	3	21	11–33
Prior chemotherapy	64	Yes	3	25	15–37
Carboplatin	82	No	5	28	19–39
Anthracyclines/ anthraquinones					
Doxorubicin	161	No	18 + 24	26	19–34
Epirubicin	27	No	2 + 5	26	11–46
Liposomal doxorubicin	42	Yes	0 + 4	9.5	2.7–22.6
Pirarubicin	28	7	2 + 0	7	1–30
Mitoxantrone	46	32	0 + 2	4	1–15
Antimetabolites					
Fluorouracil	34	NS	7	21	9–38
Methotrexate	33	No	1 + 1	6	2–20
6-Mercaptopurine	10	NS	0	0	0–31
Vincas/ epipodophyllotoxins					
Vincristine	38	5	1 + 5	16	6–31
Vinblastine	48	Most	1 + 3	8	2–20
Etoposide (VP-16)	29	Yes	0 + 1	3	1–29
Teniposide (VM-26)	22	17	0 + 2	9	1–26
Topoisomerase I inhibitor					
Topotecan	42	No	3 + 5	20	Nr
Microtubule stabilizers					
Paclitaxel	44	Yes	3 + 9	27.3	15–42.8
Docetaxel	35	No	3 + 4	21	Nr
Ixabepilone	50	Yes	1 + 5	12	Nr

95% CI, the 95% confidence interval for complete and partial response; CR, complete response; NS, not stated; Nr, not reported; PR, partial response.

Table 8.9 | Randomized Trials of Combination Chemotherapy[a]

GOG trial #	Drug	Dose (mg/m²)	N	CR/PR	DFS	P	OS	P
48	DOX	60	132	5%/17%	3.2	Nr	6.7	Nr
	vs.							
	CYC	500	144	13%/17%	3.9		7.3	
	DOX	60						
107	DOX	60	150	8%/17%	3.8	0.01	9.2	NS
	vs.							
	DOX	60	131	19%/23%	5.7		9	
	CIS	50						
163	DOX	60	157	15%/25%	7.2	NS	12.6	NS
	CIS	50						
	vs.							
	DOX	50	160	17%/26%	6		13.6	
	PAC	150						
177	DOX	60	129	7%/27%	5.3	<0.01	12.3	0.03
	CIS	50						
	vs.							
	DOX	45	134	22%/35%	8.3		15.3	
	CIS	50						
	PAC	160						
209	DOX							
	CIS							
	PAC							
	vs.							
	CARB							
	PAC							

[a]All trials were conducted in chemonaïve patients, and each regimen is given on a q3 wk schedule.
CYS, cyclophosphamide; DOX, doxorubicin; CIS, cisplatin; PAC, paclitaxel, CR, complete response; PR, partial response.

have shown a significantly higher response rate for the combination (42% vs. 25%, $p = 0.004$) but a PFS and OS of 5.7 versus 3.8 months and 9.2 versus 9.0 months, respectively. This study confirms a higher response rate with combination therapy, but the difference in PFS is modest and likely not clinically meaningful; the OS is identical in the two groups.

The GOG conducted a randomized trial (GOG 163) for patients with primary stage III and IV or recurrent endometrial cancer with measurable disease comparing doxorubicin and cisplatin to doxorubicin with 24-hour paclitaxel and granulocyte colony–stimulating factor (G-CSF). There were no significant differences in response rate (40% vs. 43%), PFS (median, 7.2 vs. 6.0 months), or OS (median, 12.6 vs. 13.6 months) for arms 1 and 2, respectively. The disadvantage of GOG 163 was the lack of platinum in the taxane-containing arm, however. The addition of a taxane was subsequently studied in GOG 177 evaluating doxorubicin (60 or 45 mg/m² in patients with prior radiotherapy) with cisplatin (50 mg/m²) as the standard arm versus paclitaxel (160 mg/m²) with doxorubicin (45 mg/m²) and cisplatin (50 mg/m²) (TAP regimen) and G-CSF as the investigational regimen. Overall, TAP chemotherapy increased 12-month survival to 59% compared to 50% with doxorubicin and cisplatin with a HR of 0.75 (0.56 to 0.998). Although the TAP regimen produced an improvement in response rate and PFS, survival was minimally increased, and it is associated with greater toxicity.

The combination of paclitaxel and carboplatin as a doublet has also been evaluated and is active in the first-line setting. These results were discussed above. In addition, the angiogenesis inhibitor bevacizumab was shown to have activity in this disease. In GOG 229E, 52 patients with recurrent disease were treated with single-agent bevacizumab; the overall response rate was 13.5%, and the 6-month PFS rate was 40.4%. A similar 6-month PFS was reported with another VEGF inhibitor, aflibercept, which was tested in GOG 229F. However, in that trial, the overall response rate was only 13.5%.

SEROUS AND CLEAR CELL HISTOLOGIES—CHEMOTHERAPY

Serous cancer and to a lesser extent clear cell cancer tend to spread in a fashion similar to ovarian cancer, with a high propensity for upper abdominal relapse. With whole-abdomen radiotherapy, the rate of relapse is still substantial, indicating the need for effective systemic therapy. Based on the response rates of paclitaxel and carboplatin in other tumors of serous histology, trials investigating paclitaxel and carboplatin in uterine serous carcinomas have reported response rates of 60% to 70%. Recognizing the limits of retrospective studies, data support the potential benefit of a regimen of platinum-based chemotherapy with cuff irradiation in patients with uterine serous carcinomas. Randomized prospective data are needed to accurately define the best approach in these patients.

Molecular Targeted Therapy

Targeted therapy, which specifically inhibits molecular abnormalities or pathways, has emerged as a novel approach for the innovative and effective medical treatment of malignancies. Multiple molecular pathways of cellular proliferation have been identified, and several targets within these pathways have been explored. A growing understanding of the underlying molecular biology of endometrial cancer has established the mammalian target of rapamycin (mTOR), angiogenesis, and the epidermal growth factor receptor family as relevant therapeutic targets. The limited efficacy of systemic therapy for patients with advanced or recurrent disease has led to the initiation of several clinical trials that have tested targeted approaches against the key drivers of these pathways. Unfortunately, even though there is an initial response with these therapies, some epithelial tumors have intrinsic mutations that make them primarily resistant or eventually resistant during the course of the treatment. The mutations give the tumor the ability to bypass the blockage of one pathway, and, since most pathways are redundant, tumors are still able to grow. Another pathway that may be of relevance involves the fibroblast growth factor receptor. Two agents have been evaluated (brivanib and nintedanib); the overall response rates were 30% and 9%, respectively, with a 6-month PFS of 30% and 22% reported.

FUTURE DIRECTIONS

In 2001, the National Cancer Institute convened an expert panel to develop a national 5-year plan for research priorities in gynecologic cancers. The resulting report, Priorities of the Gynecologic Cancer Progress Review Group (PRG), specified that understanding tumor biology was the central key toward controlling gynecologic cancers. Now, nearly a decade later, some hope for a better understanding of endometrial cancer at a genetic and molecular level is being realized. The GOG 210 study, a prospective surgical–pathologic study that created an annotated tissue repository from over 6,000 patients with more than 36,000 specimens, serves as a resource for discovery and validation of predictive and prognostic biomarkers. In addition, the Genome Atlas Project has completed an analysis of 500 endometrial cancer cases (endometrioid and serous types). It is expected that the knowledge from these data sets will drive clinical research and patient care for the next decade. Increasingly, we can expect that therapies offered to our patients will be based on a more complete understanding of pathways and that therapies may be matched to address specific genetic changes.

SUMMARY

Endometrial cancer is the most common gynecologic malignancy and an understanding of presentation, surgical management, and treatment options is required for gynecologic oncologists. Surgical therapy is the mainstay of endometrial cancer, with lymphadenectomy and laparoscopy increasingly integrated. A thorough knowledge of the relationships between uterine factors and extrauterine disease spread is essential. Surgical staging defines extent of disease and largely defines risk of recurrence. Radiation is associated with better local control but with no improvement in survival for patients with stage I and II endometrial cancers in randomized trials. Chemotherapy is increasingly integrated into upfront management of advanced-stage endometrial cancer and may have a role in early-stage disease. Combination therapy with radiation and chemotherapy is under evaluation. Targeted agents hold promise; however, a better understanding of molecular and genetic changes is required to improve efficacy.

SUGGESTED READINGS

Alektiar KM, McKee A, Venkatraman E, et al. Intravaginal high-dose-rate brachytherapy for Stage IB (FIGO Grade 1, 2) endometrial cancer. *Int J Radiat Oncol Biol Phys.* 2002;53:707–713.

ASTEC Study Group; Kitchener H, Swart AM, Qian Q, et al. Efficacy of systematic pelvic lymphadenectomy in endometrial cancer (MRC ASTEC trial): A randomised study. *Lancet.* 2009;373(9658):125–136.

Connor JP, Andrews JI, Anderson B, et al. Computed tomography in endometrial cancer. *Obstet Gynecol.* 2000;95:692–696.

Creasman WT, Morrow CP, Bundy BN, et al. Surgical pathologic spread patterns of endometrial cancer: A Gynecologic Oncology Group study. *Cancer.* 1987;60:2035.

Creutzberg CL, van Putten WL, Koper PC, et al. Surgery and postoperative radiotherapy versus surgery alone for patients with stage-1 endometrial carcinoma: Multicentre randomised trial. PORTEC Study Group. Post Operative Radiation Therapy in Endometrial Carcinoma. *Lancet.* 2000;355:1404–1411.

Creutzberg CL, van Putten WL, Koper PC, et al. PORTEC Study Group. Survival after relapse in patients with endometrial cancer: Results from a randomized trial. *Gynecol Oncol.* 2003;89:201–209.

Dizon DS. Treatment options of advanced endometrial carcinoma. *Gynecol Oncol.* 2010;117: 373–381.

Fisher B, Costantino JP, Redmond CK, et al. Endometrial cancer in tamoxifen-treated breast cancer patients: Findings from the National Surgical Adjuvant Breast and Bowel Project (NSABP) B-14. *J Natl Cancer Inst.* 1994;86:527.

Fleming GF, Brunetto VL, Cella D, et al. Phase III trial of doxorubicin plus cisplatin with or without paclitaxel plus filgrastim in advanced endometrial carcinoma: A Gynecologic Oncology Group Study. *J Clin Oncol.* 2004;22:2159–2166.

Horowitz NS, Peters WA III, Smith MR, et al. Postoperative high dose-rate intravaginal brachytherapy combined with external beam irradiation for early-stage endometrial cancer: a long-term follow-up. *Int J Radiat Oncol Biol Phys.* 1994;30:831–837.

Kadar N, Homesley H, Malfetano J. Positive peritoneal cytology is an adverse risk factor in endometrial carcinoma only if there is other evidence of extrauterine disease. *Gynecol Oncol.* 1992;46:145–149.

Kelly MG, O'Malley DM, Hui P, et al. Improved survival in surgical stage I patients with uterine papillary serous carcinoma (UPSC) treated with adjuvant platinum-based chemotherapy. *Gynecol Oncol.* 2005;98(3):353–359.

Killackey MA, Hakes TB, Pierce VK. Endometrial adenocarcinoma in breast cancer patients: Findings from the National Surgical Adjuvant Breast and Bowel Project (NSABP) B-14. *J Natl Cancer Inst.* 1994;86:527–537.

Kurman R, Kaminski P, Norris H. The behavior of endometrial hyperplasia. A long-term study of "untreated" hyperplasia in 170 patients. *Cancer.* 1985;56:403–411.

Latif NA, Haggerty A, Jean S, et al. Adjuvant therapy in early-stage endometrial cancer: a systematic review of the evidence, guidelines, and clinical practice in the U.S. *Oncologist.* 2014;19(6):645–653.

Lu K, Dinh M, Kohlman W, et al. Gynecologic cancer as a "sentinel cancer" for women with hereditary nonpolyposis colorectal cancer syndrome. *Obstet Gynecol.* 2005;105:569–574.

Mariani A, Dowdy SC, Cliby WA, et al. Prospective assessment of lymphatic dissemination in endometrial cancer: A paradigm shift in surgical staging. *Gynecol Oncol.* 2008;109:11–28.

Norris HJ, Tavassoli FA, Kurman RJ. Endometrial hyperplasia and carcinoma, diagnostic consideration. *Am J Surg Pathol.* 1988;7:839.

Nout RA, Smit VT, Putter H, et al. Vaginal brachytherapy versus pelvic external beam radio-therapy for patients with endometrial cancer of high-intermediate risk (PORTEC-2): An open-label, non-inferiority, randomised trial. *Lancet*. 2010;375:816–823.

Picchio M, Mangili G, Samanes Gajate AM, et al. High-grade endometrial cancer: Value of [(18) F]FDG PET/CT in preoperative staging. *Nucl Med Commun*. 2010;31(6):506–512.

Rockall AG, Sohaib SA, Harisinghani MG, et al. Diagnostic performance of nanoparticle-enhanced magnetic resonance imaging in the diagnosis of lymph node metastases in patients with endometrial and cervical cancer. *J Clin Oncol*. 2005;23:2813–2821.

Thigpen JT, Blessing JA, DiSaia PJ, et al. A randomized comparison of doxorubicin alone versus doxorubicin plus cyclophosphamide in the management of advanced or recurrent endometrial carcinoma: A Gynecologic Oncology Group study. *J Clin Oncol*. 1994;12:1408.

Trimble CL, Kauderer J, Zaino R, et al. Concurrent endometrial carcinoma in women with a biopsy diagnosis of atypical endometrial hyperplasia: A Gynecologic Oncology Group study. *Cancer*. 2006;106:812–819.

Wheeler D, Bell K, Kurman R, et al. Minimal uterine serous carcinoma: Diagnostic and clinico-pathologic correlation. *Am J Surg Pathol*. 2000;24:797–806.

Zaino RJ, Kurman RJ, Diana KL, et al. Pathologic models to predict outcome for women with endometrial adenocarcinoma. *Cancer*. 1996;77:1115–1121.

The Corpus: Mesenchymal Tumors

Mesenchymal tumors are rare malignancies that account for approximately 7% to 8% of all uterine cancers. Unlike most endometrial adenocarcinomas, uterine sarcomas are generally aggressive, and overall mortality rates approached 90% in early reports. Though recent literature suggests that uterine carcinosarcoma is better classified as a metaplastic carcinoma of the uterus rather than a sarcoma, uterine carcinosarcoma will be described in this chapter for historical reasons.

The World Health Organization classification of mesenchymal uterine corpus tumors is summarized in Table 9.1. Uterine sarcomas are a heterogeneous group with regard to clinical presentation, response to therapy, and outcomes.

EPIDEMIOLOGY AND RISK FACTORS

KEY POINTS
- Leiomyosarcomas are the most common uterine mesenchymal tumor when excluding carcinosarcomas.
- Uterine sarcomas are more common in African American women.
- Prior radiotherapy is a risk factor for carcinosarcoma and undifferentiated sarcoma.

The most common uterine sarcomas are carcinosarcomas and leiomyosarcomas. When carcinosarcomas are excluded, leiomyosarcomas represent more than two thirds of uterine mesenchymal tumors (Fig. 9.1). Endometrial stromal sarcomas (ESS) account for 25% of true uterine sarcomas and are presently by definition "low grade." The preferred current terminology for previously "high-grade" ESS is undifferentiated uterine sarcoma. Patients with carcinosarcomas and adenosarcomas tend to be older at the time of diagnosis compared to those with leiomyosarcomas and ESS.

Women with carcinosarcomas are more likely to be of African American descent than those with endometrial adenocarcinomas. The age-adjusted incidence of uterine sarcomas in African American women is approximately twice that of Caucasian women. Carcinosarcomas and leiomyosarcomas constitute about 4% and 1.5% of all uterine malignancies, respectively. The risk profile of carcinosarcomas closely parallels that of endometrial adenocarcinomas with regard to obesity, diabetes, anovulation, and low

Table 9.1	WHO Classification of Mesenchymal Tumors of the Uterine Corpus

Leiomyoma
 Cellular Leiomyoma
 Leiomyoma with bizarre nuclei
 Mitotically active leiomyoma
 Hydropic leiomyoma
 Apoplectic leiomyoma
 Lipomatous leiomyoma (lipoleiomyoma)
 Epithelioid leiomyoma
 Myxoid leiomyoma
 Dissecting (cotyledonoid) leiomyoma
 Diffuse leiomyomatosis
 Intravenous leiomyomatosis
 Metastasizing leiomyoma

Smooth muscle tissue of uncertain malignant potential

Leiomyosarcoma
 Epithelioid leiomyosarcoma
 Myxoid leiomyosarcoma

Endometrial stroma and related tumors
 Endometrial stromal nodule
 Low-grade endometrial stromal sarcoma
 High-grade endometrial stromal sarcoma
 Undifferentiated uterine sarcoma
 Uterine tumor resembling ovarian sex cord tumor

Miscellaneous mesenchymal tumors
 Rhabdomyosarcoma
 Perivascular epithelioid cell tumor
  Benign
  Malignant

Others

Source: WHO classification of tumours of the uterine corpus. In: Kurman RJ, Carcangiu ML, Herrington CS, et al., eds. *WHO Classification of Tumours of Female Reproductive Organs,* 4th ed. Lyons, France: IARC Press; 2014:122, with permission.

parity, providing additional support that they be regarded as "metaplastic" endometrial carcinomas instead of true sarcomas.

Possible risk factors for uterine sarcoma are prior radiation exposure, hormone exposure, tamoxifen use, and hereditary predisposition. Prior exposure to pelvic radiotherapy is thought to increase the risk of developing subsequent carcinosarcoma and undifferentiated sarcoma. Carcinosarcomas in previously irradiated patients also tend to present in advanced stage, perhaps because radiotherapy is often associated with cervical stenosis and, thus, no telltale uterine bleeding. The association with hormone exposure is strongest for leiomyosarcoma. There may be a small risk of uterine sarcomas associated with hereditary non-polyposis colorectal cancer and hereditary retinoblastoma.

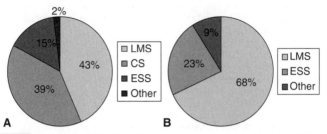

A   **B**

FIGURE 9.1 Histologic distribution of uterine sarcomas in series with at least 100 cases including carcinosarcomas (**A**) and excluding carcinosarcomas (**B**). (ESS, endometrial stromal sarcoma; CS, carcinosarcoma; LMS, leiomyosarcoma; AS, adenosarcoma.) *Source*: From Park J, Kim D, Suh D, et al. Prognostic factors and treatment outcomes of patients with uterine sarcoma: Analysis of 127 patients at a single institution, 1989–2007. *J Cancer Res Clin Oncol.* 2008;134:1277–1287; Koivisto-Korander R, Butzow R, Koivisto A, et al. Clinical outcome and prognostic factors in 100 cases of uterine sarcoma: Experience in Helsinki University Central Hospital 1990–2001. *Gynecol Oncol.* 2008;111:74–81; Kahanpaa K, Wahlstrom T, Grohn P, et al. Sarcomas of the uterus: A clinicopathologic study of 119 patients. *Obstet Gynecol.* 1986;67:417–424; George M, Pejovic MH, Kramar A. Uterine sarcomas: Prognostic factors and treatment modalities—Study on 209 patients. *Gynecol Oncol.* 1986;24:58–67; Olah KS, Gee H, Blunt S, et al. Retrospective analysis of 318 cases of uterine sarcoma. *Eur J Cancer.* 1991;27:1095–1099; Pautier P, Genestie C, Rey A, et al. Analysis of clinicopathologic prognostic factors for 157 uterine sarcomas and evaluation of grading score validated for soft tissue sarcoma. *Cancer.* 2000;88:1425–1431; Abeler VM, Royne O, Thorensen S, et al. Uterine sarcomas in Norway. A histopathological and prognostic survey of a total population from 1970 to 2000 including 419 patients. *Histopathology.* 2009;54:355–364, with permission.

CLINICAL PRESENTATION

Vaginal bleeding is the most common presenting symptom in women with uterine sarcomas in general and is nearly universal in those with carcinosarcomas. Vaginal bleeding occurs in as few as 40% of women with leiomyosarcomas, however. A typical presentation of carcinosarcoma is vaginal bleeding associated with a protuberant, fleshy mass from the cervix. These neoplasms arise in the endometrial lining but often grow in an exophytic pattern within the endometrial cavity (Fig. 9.2).

Uterine enlargement and a presumptive diagnosis of uterine leiomyomata are nearly universal findings in patients with leiomyosarcoma. The incidence of leiomyosarcoma in all patients with the clinical picture of myomas is less than 1% but increases with age to slightly over 1% in the sixth decade of life.

DIAGNOSIS AND EVALUATION

Vaginal bleeding in a postmenopausal female should be evaluated with endometrial sampling and possibly transvaginal ultrasound. Whereas the diagnosis of carcinosarcoma is confirmed, or at least suggested, at the time

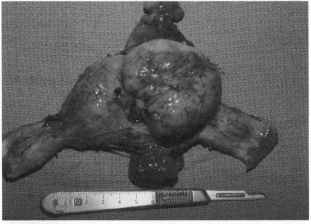

FIGURE 9.2 Exophytic pattern of growth in carcinosarcoma.

of endometrial biopsy or curettage, leiomyosarcomas are rarely diagnosed before hysterectomy.

Laparoscopy has become a standard and preferred approach in the management of benign and malignant gynecologic conditions. Morcellation is often not done in women with carcinosarcoma because they are often older with a preoperative diagnosis. Morcellation of uterine leiomyosarcoma is associated with a worsened outcome. The 5-year overall survival (OS) was 46% after morcellation compared to 73% in those not morcellated ($p = 0.04$). There is literature to support that the combination of serum lactate dehydrogenase and dynamic MRI may help to evaluate uterine lesions for leiomyosarcoma. Recent controversy regarding the use of morcellation has heightened the awareness of these issues and led to cautionary statements from the government and professional societies.

STAGING AND PROGNOSIS

The International Federation of Gynecology and Obstetrics (FIGO) devised a sarcoma-specific staging system in 2009 for leiomyosarcoma, ESS, and adenosarcoma (Tables 9.2 and 9.3). Carcinosarcomas are staged using the system for endometrial carcinoma. A nomogram is also available online at http://www.mskcc.org/cancer-care/adult/endometrial-other-uterine/leiomyosarcoma/prediction-tools (Fig. 9.3).

Staging systems and nomograms have limited prognostic capabilities because they rely on anatomic, clinical, and pathologic criteria that have not been consistently associated with outcome. A better molecular understanding is urgently needed and may provide greater prognostication. Expression patterns of estrogen receptor (ER), progesterone receptor (PR), β-catenin, cyclooxygenase-2, and bcl-2 have all been reported to be associated with survival in leiomyosarcoma.

Table 9.2	The 2009 FIGO Staging System for Uterine Leiomyosarcomas and ESS
I	Tumor limited to the uterus
IA	Less than or equal to 5 cm
IB	More than 5 cm
II	Tumor extends beyond the uterus, within the pelvis
IIA	Adnexal involvement
IIB	Involvement of other pelvic tissues
III	Tumor invades abdominal tissues (not just protruding into the abdomen)
IIIA	One site
IIIB	More than one site
IIIC	Metastasis to pelvic and/or para-aortic lymph nodes
IV	
IVA	Tumor invades the bladder and/or rectum
IVB	Distant metastasis

Source: From D'Angelo E, Prat J. Uterine sarcomas: A review. *Gynecol Oncol.* 2010;116:131–139, with permission.

Table 9.3	The 2009 FIGO Staging System for Uterine Adenosarcomas
Stage	**Definition**
I	Tumor limited to the uterus
IA	Tumor limited to the endometrium/endocervix with no myometrial invasion
IB	Less than or equal to half myometrial invasion
IC	More than half myometrial invasion
II	Tumor extends beyond the uterus, within the pelvis
IIA	Adnexal involvement
IIB	Involvement of other pelvic tissues
III	Tumor invades abdominal tissues (not just protruding into the abdomen)
IIIA	One site
IIIB	More than one site
IIIC	Metastasis to pelvic and/or para-aortic lymph nodes
IV	
IVA	Tumor invades the bladder and/or rectum
IVB	Distant metastasis

Source: From D'Angelo E, Prat J. Uterine sarcomas: A review. *Gynecol Oncol.* 2010;116:131–139, with permission.

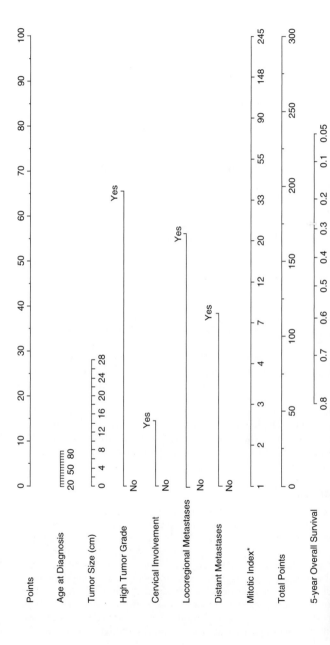

FIGURE 9.3 Nomogram for 5-year OS for uterine leiomyosarcoma. This is the uterine leiomyosarcoma nomogram for 5-year OS. The mitotic index (*asterisk*) was modeled using log transformation; for display purposes, values were converted back to original scale (exponential; concordance probability [CP]$_j$, 0.671; bootstrap-validated CP, 0.651). **Source:** Zivanovic O, Jacks LM, Iasonos A, et al. A nomogram to predict postresection 5-year overall survival for patients with uterine leiomyosarcoma. *Cancer.* 2012;118:660–669.

PATHOLOGY

Malignant mesenchymal tumors can be classified into pure mesenchymal tumors and tumors with a mixed epithelial and mesenchymal component. In the first group, the most common is leiomyosarcoma, followed by endometrial stromal sarcoma, and, rarely, others including rhabdomyosarcoma, liposarcoma, angiosarcoma, chondrosarcoma, osteosarcoma, and alveolar soft part sarcoma. Mixed epithelial and mesenchymal tumors include carcinosarcoma and adenosarcoma. In addition, there are three rare mesenchymal tumors occurring in the uterus: uterine tumors resembling ovarian sex cord tumors, perivascular epithelioid cell tumors, and inflammatory myofibroblastic tumor.

Leiomyosarcoma and Other Smooth Muscle Tumors

Leiomyosarcomas are malignant smooth muscle tumors that usually arise *de novo*. Recent studies have shown that some tumors display areas with benign morphology, suggesting some progression from leiomyoma to leiomyosarcoma; however, clonality studies only support this progression in a small percentage of cases. Microscopically, most leiomyosarcomas are overtly malignant and have hypercellularity, coagulative tumor cell necrosis, abundant mitoses (more than 10/10 hpf), atypical mitoses, marked cytologic atypia, and infiltrative borders. The three most important criteria are coagulative tumor cell necrosis, high mitotic rate, and significant cytologic atypia.

Some smooth muscle tumors have histologic features that are not worrisome enough to render an unequivocal diagnosis of sarcoma. These tumors can be classified as atypical leiomyomas, smooth muscle tumors with low malignant potential (low probability of an unfavorable outcome), or smooth muscle tumors of uncertain malignant potential (STUMP) (insufficient numbers have been studied to predict their behavior). Figure 9.4 summarizes the classification of uterine smooth muscle tumors based on their histologic characteristics. It is recommended that unusual cases be reviewed by a gynecologic pathologist. Histologic parameters of leiomyosarcomas that have been shown to be prognostic indicators include grade, mitotic rate, extensive tumor cell necrosis, lymphovascular invasion, and ER/PR status.

Carcinosarcoma

Uterine carcinosarcomas, also called malignant mixed müllerian tumors, are lesions containing carcinomatous and sarcomatous elements. Numerous studies have shown that these tumors are clonal malignancies derived from a single stem cell and should be considered "metaplastic carcinomas." Microscopically, these tumors have a typical biphasic pattern with carcinomatous and sarcomatous elements. The carcinoma is usually high grade; the sarcomatous component is always high grade and may be homologous or heterologous. Homologous elements are those components that are native to the uterine body and most commonly are high-grade fibrosarcoma, although other varieties such as undifferentiated sarcoma may be found as

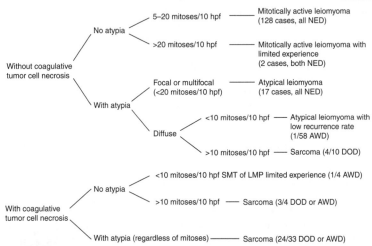

FIGURE 9.4 Uterine smooth muscle tumors (excluding epithelioid and myxoid types and cervical tumors). (AWD, alive with disease; DOD, dead of disease; hpf, high-power fields; LMP, low malignant potential; NED, no evidence of disease; SMT, smooth muscle tumor.)

well. Heterologous elements are those components that are not normally found within the uterus. Heterologous elements are seen in half of the cases. The most common heterologous sarcoma is rhabdomyosarcoma, followed by chondrosarcoma, and, less often, osteosarcoma and liposarcoma.

Most studies suggest that the behavior of carcinosarcomas is predicted by the carcinomatous component. Tumors typically metastasize through lymphatic channels similar to endometrial carcinomas. Most metastases and recurrences are composed of pure carcinoma. In two recent studies, adverse prognostic factors included the following: heterologous elements (in stage I tumors) and high percentage of sarcomatous component in the main tumor and in the recurrences. Data from The Cancer Genome Atlas indicate that approximately 90% of carcinosarcomas harbor TP53 mutations.

Endometrial Stromal Neoplasms

In the current World Health Organization classification, endometrial stromal tumors are classified into endometrial stromal nodules, ESS (by definition low grade), and undifferentiated endometrial sarcoma. Both endometrial stromal nodules and ESS are composed of cells identical to those found in the stroma of proliferative endometrium. Undifferentiated endometrial sarcomas, on the other hand, are high-grade sarcomas that do not resemble endometrial stroma, and a diagnosis is made by excluding other uterine sarcomas.

The differential diagnosis between an endometrial stromal nodule and an endometrial stromal sarcoma is important since the nodules are always benign lesions. Differential diagnosis is based upon the presence of infiltrating margins with or without angioinvasion in endometrial stromal sarcoma. These two features are not seen in stromal nodules, which are always well circumscribed and have pushing margins. It is impossible to render a definitive diagnosis based upon curettage material alone; final diagnosis requires a hysterectomy specimen.

Most ESS have fewer than 10 mitoses/10 hpf, but even mitotically active variants behave in a similar indolent manner. Sixty percent of low-grade endometrial stromal tumors (including ESS and stromal nodule) have cytogenetic abnormalities involving rearrangements of chromosomes 6, 7, and 17. The most characteristic translocation of these tumors, t(T7;17) (Tp15;q21), generates a fusion of the JAZF1 and JJAZ1 genes, both of which encode zinc finger proteins.

Undifferentiated endometrial sarcomas have cytologic atypia to the extent that they cannot be recognized as arising from endometrial stroma. Morphologically, these high-grade lesions resemble undifferentiated mesenchymal tumors and behave as high-grade sarcomas. It is advisable to use a term such as "high-grade sarcoma," "undifferentiated sarcoma," or "poorly differentiated uterine sarcoma" rather than "endometrial stromal sarcoma." This last term may inaccurately suggest an indolent tumor. Undifferentiated uterine sarcomas are usually seen in patients older than 50 years, have a recurrence rate of over 85%, and are usually fatal.

Müllerian Adenosarcoma

Müllerian adenosarcomas are mixed müllerian tumors composed of malignant stromal and benign epithelial components. Microscopically, the tumors have a benign epithelial component usually covering the surface of the polyps and in the form of benign glands uniformly distributed throughout the tumor. The mesenchymal component is usually a low-grade sarcoma that resembles endometrial stroma. Minimal criteria include at least one of the following: two or more stromal mitoses/10 hpf, marked stromal hypercellularity, and significant stromal cell atypia. A minority of cases have "sarcomatous overgrowth," when more than 25% of the tumor is composed of pure sarcoma. In these cases, the sarcoma is typically high grade, and the lesions are aggressive. Most adenosarcomas without stromal overgrowth express ERs in the sarcomatous component, and this may be used for therapeutic purposes. Besides stromal overgrowth, the only other histologic feature associated with decreased survival is myometrial invasion.

SURGERY

KEY POINTS

- Surgery, typically hysterectomy, is a cornerstone of treatment for uterine sarcoma.
- Lymphadenectomy is considered standard of care for carcinosarcoma.
- Surgical cytoreduction and surgery for recurrent disease may be considered in highly select cases.

Surgery is a cornerstone in the treatment of uterine sarcomas. A total hysterectomy (never supracervical) must be performed in the majority of malignant mesenchymal tumors of the uterus, including leiomyosarcoma, undifferentiated sarcoma, or carcinosarcoma. Uterine preservation is an option in younger women who wish to preserve fertility and are diagnosed with STUMP or other atypical leiomyomata of the uterus. The risk of ovarian metastasis is very low in leiomyosarcoma, and oophorectomy is not recommended in premenopausal women with leiomyosarcoma. Occult ovarian metastasis in carcinosarcoma is approximately 12%, so bilateral salpingo-oophorectomy should be recommended. Oophorectomy in ESS may be associated with a decrease in recurrence but is not associated with OS since these patients do very well in general.

Lymph node metastasis in adult soft tissue sarcomas is less than 3%, with some variation among histologic types. There is no clear benefit to routine lymphadenectomy in patients with leiomyosarcoma confined to the uterus and clinically normal lymph nodes. Lymphadenectomy is considered standard for carcinosarcoma, in which the overall and occult rates of lymph node metastasis are 27% and 20%, respectively.

Surgical cytoreduction and surgery for recurrent disease may be considered in highly select cases. Complete gross resection in leiomyosarcoma with extrauterine metastasis was found on multivariate analysis to be independently associated with progression-free survival. Cytoreductive surgery for recurrent disease is considered if there has been a relatively long disease-free interval, and sites of recurrence seem amenable to complete surgical resection. The approach to carcinosarcomas is often extrapolated from data for endometrial carcinomas.

RADIATION THERAPY

KEY POINTS

- Radiation therapy for carcinosarcoma can provide good local control but does not impact OS due to distant failure.
- The role of radiation therapy remains undefined for leiomyosarcoma and endometrial stromal sarcoma.

Since the utilization of radiation therapy for patients with uterine sarcomas has been almost exclusively in the postoperative setting, the role of primary or palliative radiotherapy will not be presented. As they are more fully explored in the chapter on epithelial tumors of the corpus, a detailed discussion of the techniques and complications of adjuvant radiation therapy will not be discussed in this section (Fig. 9.5).

Uterine Sarcomas

Because of the rarity of uterine sarcomas, most literature is retrospective and has often had to combine many types of sarcomas to attain numbers sufficient for evaluation. Thus, most of these retrospective studies have not

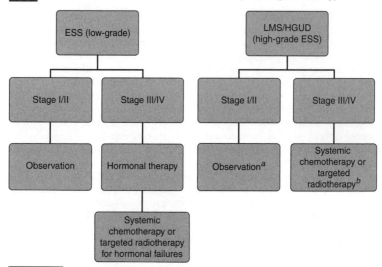

FIGURE 9.5 Adjuvant management algorithm for patients with leiomyosarcoma, endometrial stromal sarcoma, and high-grade undifferentiated sarcoma. [a]Consider adjuvant chemotherapy or pelvic RT for particularly high-risk features. [b]For isolated extrauterine disease, tumor-directed RT may be appropriate, but in general, systemic chemotherapy should be given for advanced-stage disease. *Source:* Adapted from NCCN practice guidelines in oncology v.2.2009; UTSARC-2/3.

achieved statistical power to reach definite conclusions. However, the data from the nonrandomized review of the Surveillance, Epidemiology, and End Results (SEER) analyses of 2,677 cases of all types of uterine sarcomas did demonstrate a statistically significant improvement in survival favoring adjuvant radiotherapy for stage II, III, and IV (but not stage I) uterine sarcomas.

The GOG has previously conducted two prospective clinical trials involving selected patients with uterine sarcomas. The earliest study reported on 156 evaluable patients with surgically staged I or II sarcomas of the uterus (GOG 20). Radiotherapy did not seem to affect recurrence in general. However, there was a notable decrease in vaginal recurrences in patients with carcinosarcomas. Furthermore, there was a significant reduction in pelvic relapses (10%) in treated patients compared with those untreated (23%) (Table 9.4). The second main GOG trial for patients with uterine sarcomas involved a clinicopathologic evaluation of patients with clinical stage I and II diseases (GOG 40). Although adjuvant pelvic external beam therapy was not mandated in this surgical trial, there appeared to be a possibility that adjuvant radiation plays a role in reducing pelvic relapses.

Currently, there is one completed prospective phase III clinical trial that focused on the role of adjuvant radiation therapy for patients with all three main cell types of uterine sarcomas (protocol 55874 of the

Table 9.4	Sites of First Recurrence[a]	
	Pelvic	Extrapelvic
No RT	14/60 (23%)	12/60 (20%)
Pelvic RT	5/49 (10%)	17/49 (35%)

[a]Eighty-five percent of this group (93 patients) with nonleiomyosarcomas of the uterus were stage I/II uterine carcinosarcomas.
RT, radiation therapy.
Source: Modified from Hornback NB, Omura G, Major FJ. Observations on the uterine sarcomas of adjuvant radiation therapy in patients with stage I and II uterine sarcoma. *Int J Radiat Oncol Biol Phys.* 1986;12:2127–2130.

European Organization for Research and Treatment of Cancer [EORTC]). Those subjects in EORTC 55874 with surgical stage I or II disease were randomized to either no further treatment or external beam irradiation of the whole pelvis. For carcinosarcomas, there were 2 of 46 (4.4%) in the adjuvantly irradiated arm and 11 of 45 (24.4%) in the observation subset with isolated local relapses. For leiomyosarcomas, 1 of 50 (2%) in the radiotherapy group and 7 of 49 (14.3%) in the untreated cohort developed isolated local failures. Though local control was improved in both subtypes, patients with isolated local failures evaluated in EORTC 55874 are in the minority for both carcinosarcomas and leiomyosarcomas. The patients treated postoperatively had a nonsignificant median survival advantage of 8.5 years versus 6.7 years for the observational cohort with a hazard ratio of 1.02 (95% confidence interval [CI]: 0.68 to 1.53, $p = 0.92$).

A recently published retrospective review has the largest number to date of patients with uterine sarcomas, with 3,650 evaluable patients. There was no significant impact on OS for patients receiving predominantly postoperative pelvic radiation therapy versus those receiving no adjuvant therapy. However, there was a statistically significant reduction in local recurrence rate in the adjuvantly irradiated cohort, which was preserved on subset analyses of patients with carcinosarcoma ($p < 0.001$), leiomyosarcoma ($p < 0.01$), and ESS ($p < 0.05$). Further studies are needed to evaluate the role of adjuvant "volume-directed" radiation therapy for patients with uterine sarcomas.

Uterine Carcinosarcomas

Other reports have been limited to one histologic type of sarcoma. The most common of these have evaluated uterine carcinosarcomas, which are more appropriately considered metaplastic carcinomas. Results are inconsistent with some studies demonstrating no benefit for radiotherapy, while others have shown a significant impact of adjuvant pelvic radiotherapy on the survival for patients with carcinosarcomas. One of these studies involved a review of the nonrandomized SEER database of 2,461 women with carcinosarcomas from 1973 to 2003. In this data set, 890 patients received adjuvant radiotherapy. The overall 5-year survival rates of those receiving radiotherapy versus no irradiation were 41.5% and 33.2%, respectively ($p < 0.001$). Furthermore, a significant improvement in survival in this study was observed for all stages of disease, including stage IV. Finally, there have been several published retrospective reports suggesting that combined adjuvant radiotherapy and chemotherapy may impart even longer survival, especially for stage I and II diseases.

GOG 150 is the only randomized phase III prospective trial of adjuvant radiotherapy in carcinosarcomas. This study compared whole-abdominal irradiation to three cycles of cisplatin–ifosfamide chemotherapy with respect to recurrence rates, disease free, and OS. Eligible were patients with carcinosarcomas confined to the abdomen who underwent optimal surgical debulking with no postsurgical residual disease greater than 1 cm. After adjusting for stage and age at diagnosis, there was a diminution in death rate reduction of 29% for those receiving chemotherapy compared with radiotherapy (HR = 0.712, 95% CI: 0.484 to 1.048, $p = 0.085$, two-tail test). Of interest is the fact that those patients who received adjuvant radiotherapy had more late complications, mainly gastrointestinal, than those having cytotoxic therapy ($p < 0.001$). In addition, two patients undergoing radiotherapy died as a direct result of radiation-induced hepatitis.

Based on the results of GOG 150, the role of adjuvant radiotherapy for the management of patients with carcinosarcomas continues to remain uncertain. Since there were more vaginal failures in the chemotherapy arm of GOG 150 and other sites of relapse were similar or less common in frequency (abdominal recurrences) than those in the radiotherapy arm, perhaps postoperative vaginal brachytherapy (either high- or low-dose rate) with chemotherapy should be considered for any patient having optimally debulked carcinosarcomas in future trials (Table 9.5).

Table 9.5	Patterns of Failure in GOG 150	
Sites of Recurrence[a]	WAI ($n = 105$), Number of Cases	Chemotherapy ($n = 101$), Number of Cases
Vagina	4	10
Pelvis	14	14
Abdomen	29	19
Distant	27	24

[a]Some patients had multiple sites of relapse.
n, total number of cases in each arm; WAI, whole-abdominal irradiation.
Source: Modified from Wolfson AH, Brady MF, Rocereto T, et al. A Gynecologic Oncology Group randomized phase III trial of whole abdominal irradiation (WAI) vs. cisplatin-ifosfamide and mesna (CIM) as postsurgical therapy in stage I–IV carcinosarcoma (CS) of the uterus. *Gynecol Oncol.* 2007;107:177–185.

Uterine Leiomyosarcomas

The most common uterine sarcoma excluding carcinosarcoma is leiomyosarcoma. There are currently no randomized phase III trials that demonstrate any impact of adjuvant radiation therapy on locoregional relapse or survival. The overall pelvic/extrapelvic relapse rates are approximately 16.6% and 42.0% for patients with uterine leiomyosarcoma. There still remains a paucity of information that specifies between upper abdominal and extra-abdominal distant sites of tumor involvement. The respective pelvic/extrapelvic percentages were 18.5% (22/119)/41.2% (49/119) for nonirradiated and 12.9% (8/62)/43.5% (27/62) for patients treated with postoperative radiotherapy. From this overview, it does not appear that postoperative radiotherapy has any real effect on reducing recurrences for patients with uterine leiomyosarcoma.

However, two of the listed series combined to yield an 11.1% (4/36) pelvic relapse rate with radiation versus 61.1% (22/36) without the implementation of adjuvant radiation therapy. However, the major problem is that the majority of these patients have distant extra-abdominal metastases, such as the lung, despite having local control. This would suggest that adjuvant systemic therapy must be added in order to have an impact on the outcome of these patients. The role of adjuvant radiotherapy in leiomyosarcoma remains undefined.

Endometrial Stromal Sarcomas

The total pelvic and extrapelvic rates of relapse for patients with ESS are 42.2% and 33.3%, respectively. There was a 33.3% (6/18) pelvic recurrence rate of which the majority did not undergo any radiation therapy. This latter finding initially suggested that postoperative external pelvis radiotherapy could be considered for the subset of patients with low-grade ESS.

A more recent report retrospectively reviewed 28 patients with ESS of which 19 were low grade and 9 high grade. Fifty percent of the patients in this series underwent adjuvant pelvic radiotherapy with no difference in the survival of the patients. In addition, almost 30% of those receiving adjuvant radiotherapy relapsed within the treatment field. However, a more recent small series of 13 patients with all stages of ESS showed that the 10 patients undergoing adjuvant radiation therapy had an 89% locoregional control rate versus 50% locoregional control for the 3 not receiving any radiotherapy. Thus, the role of radiotherapy for patients with ESS remains uncertain.

CHEMOTHERAPY

KEY POINTS
- Combined chemotherapy is more effective than single agents.
- Active agents are different for carcinosarcoma and leiomyosarcoma.
- Hormonal therapy is effective for endometrial stromal sarcoma.

Uterine sarcomas, although far less common than endometrial carcinomas, exhibit two features that increase the need for systemic therapy: a recurrence rate of at least 50%, even in early-stage disease, and a high propensity for distant failure. The comparatively low incidence of uterine sarcomas has made randomized controlled trials difficult. Crucial to the understanding of the use of chemotherapy in uterine sarcomas is the observation that these neoplasms are heterogeneous. The first two subtypes, carcinosarcomas and leiomyosarcomas, constitute 90% of cases entered into clinical trials. These two histologic subtypes are usually the only uterine sarcomas with sufficient numbers to permit meaningful phase III studies; however, as these two histologic subtypes appear to respond differently to chemotherapy, they should be studied separately.

Chemotherapy: Limited Disease

Uterine sarcoma has a high rate of distant metastases even in the absence of intraperitoneal or lymph node metastases. It has been concluded that this is due to the high rate of hematogenous and lymphatic dissemination. Even for surgical stage I disease, the recurrence is as high as 53%. The largest randomized trial to date of adjuvant chemotherapy versus no further therapy in patients with uterine sarcoma did not segregate histologic subtypes. Although the recurrence rate and median survival of patients treated with doxorubicin compared to no therapy were 41% versus 53% and 73 months versus 55 months, respectively, this phase III GOG trial of 156 evaluable patients concluded that there was no significant difference. As with advanced disease, more recent trials began to segregate the histologic subtypes.

Uterine Carcinosarcomas

A GOG study reported by Sutton et al. in 2005 of 65 patients with completely resected stage I and II carcinosarcomas of the uterus treated with adjuvant ifosfamide and cisplatin reported 2- and 5-year survival rates of 82% and 62%, respectively. Since more than half of the recurrences involved the pelvis, the study suggested that a combined sequential approach with chemotherapy and radiotherapy might be beneficial for this group of patients, which should be verified in randomized phase III study.

GOG 150, a phase III study of patients with stage I–IV uterine carcinosarcoma who had undergone complete gross resection, compared whole-abdominal radiation with three cycles of cisplatin and ifosfamide as adjuvant therapy. There was a trend toward improved outcome in the chemotherapy group with recurrence and estimated death 21% and 29% lower, respectively, compared to the radiotherapy group.

Leiomyosarcomas

Two factors continue to limit the study of adjuvant therapy in patients with uterine leiomyosarcomas: the relatively low frequency of the disease, which makes it difficult to complete randomized trials in a reasonable period of time, and the lack of highly active agents. The Sarcoma Alliance for Research through Collaboration conducted a phase II adjuvant therapy trial (SARC005) of gemcitabine and docetaxel followed by doxorubicin for women with uterus-limited leiomyosarcoma and reported a progression-free survival at 2 and 3 years of 78% and 50%, respectively. A phase III multicenter randomized trial (GOG 277) will compare gemcitabine and docetaxel followed by doxorubicin to the current standard approach of observation, in order to determine if adjuvant chemotherapy improves outcomes for patients with uterus-limited high-grade leiomyosarcoma.

Chemotherapy: Advanced or Recurrent Disease

Leiomyosarcomas

Numerous single agents have been and continue to be tested in patients with leiomyosarcomas. Doxorubicin and ifosfamide are the most active agents investigated as primary single-agent chemotherapy in advanced and recurrent uterine leiomyosarcomas. Combination chemotherapy yields greater response rates.

In 1996, using a combination of ifosfamide and doxorubicin, the GOG demonstrated an overall response of 30% in patients with advanced leiomyosarcoma with no history of prior treatment. Gemcitabine plus docetaxel was proven highly active and tolerable (40% overall response rate) in treated and untreated patients with leiomyosarcomas. The response rate of this doublet was 36% as initial therapy and 27% in the second-line setting. Given the paucity of survival data available from the randomized trials to compare various chemotherapy regimens, a pooled analysis showed that patients who received first- or second-line chemotherapy for the treatment of metastatic leiomyosarcoma had a higher response rate with combination chemotherapy than with single-agent chemotherapy.

Uterine Carcinosarcomas

Several drugs have been studied in this group of tumors as single agents. However, only three drugs have demonstrated clear-cut activity: ifosfamide, cisplatin, and paclitaxel. Of the three drugs given as a single agent, ifosfamide is the most active single agent studied to date, with a response rate of 36%. In patients with prior chemotherapy, cisplatin produced an 18% response in 28 patients. A repeat trial in patients with no prior chemotherapy documented essentially the same response rate of 19% among a larger group of patients. Paclitaxel, as a single agent, was associated with a response rate of 21% in a group of 33 patients with uterine sarcoma who had prior chemotherapy, with an 8% response rate in patients who failed appropriate local therapy. Doxorubicin, generally regarded as the most active agent in soft tissue sarcomas, unfortunately demonstrated inconsistent activity in three trials of patients with carcinosarcomas.

A phase II study of carboplatin and paclitaxel as first-line chemotherapy for women with advanced uterine carcinosarcoma reported an overall response rate of 54%, with a favorable toxicity profile. The GOG evaluated the addition of cisplatin to ifosfamide in 194 eligible carcinosarcoma patients and found that this improved the overall response rate from 36% to 54% and prolonged the median progression-free interval by an absolute 2 months. However, this advantage was not associated with a significant OS gain. More recently, and based upon the finding of moderate activity (18% response rate) of paclitaxel for this disease, the GOG carried out a phase III trial of ifosfamide with or without paclitaxel in advanced uterine carcinosarcomas. The group found that the addition of paclitaxel produced a 45% response rate compared with 29% in the ifosfamide single agent arm with OS significantly improved. There was a significant decrease in the hazard of death and progression but more sensory neuropathy, as expected. A recent meta-analysis supports the use of combination chemotherapy in advanced or recurrent carcinosarcoma with a reduction in the risk of death and disease progression compared to single-agent therapy. In order to determine the best first-line chemotherapy doublet, the GOG is now conducting a noninferiority phase III trial, GOG 261, comparing carboplatin and paclitaxel with ifosfamide and paclitaxel.

Endometrial Stromal Sarcoma

In recurrent stromal sarcoma, reports support hormone therapy for patients with low-grade subgroup and chemotherapy for high-grade tumors. Current definitions do not include high-grade lesions as a component of endometrial stromal sarcoma. Randomized phase III trials with stromal sarcomas are limited due to the rarity of this disease. The GOG reported a phase II study of ifosfamide treatment in 21 cases with high- or low-grade, recurrent or metastatic ESS, with an overall response of 33%. Another noncontrolled study observed a 50% response rate to doxorubicin therapy in 10 patients with recurrent ESS. Interest in ESS continues owing to the difference in the prognosis of patients with low-grade disease versus those with undifferentiated endometrial sarcomas.

Hormonal Therapy

Although the role of hormonal therapy is clear in breast and endometrial cancers, it has not been extensively evaluated in mesenchymal uterine tumors. Few uterine sarcomas contain sufficient estrogen or progesterone receptor protein to influence therapy, the only exception being low-grade ESS or stromal nodules. Uniquely, low-grade ESS are hormonally responsive in roughly two thirds of cases, and long-term maintenance therapy should be beneficial. Progestins, gonadotropin-releasing hormone analogues, or aromatase inhibitors have been used in the treatment of patients with advanced or recurrent stromal sarcomas. Several papers reported that long-term use of tamoxifen for the treatment of breast cancer was related to the development of uterine sarcomas, likely secondary to the stimulatory estrogenic effects of tamoxifen on the uterus.

Biologic Therapy

Because of the high recurrence rate and poor response to radiotherapy and chemotherapy, biologic therapy may have more promise in uterine sarcoma. The recent advances in the biology of uterine sarcoma related to probable treatments have concentrated on tyrosine kinase receptors, vascular endothelial growth factor, and the phosphatidyl-3-kinase (PI3K)/Akt pathway. The results of a GOG phase II trial of pazopanib in previously treated uterine carcinosarcoma indicate very limited activity. A phase III, placebo-controlled trial of gemcitabine and docetaxel with or without bevacizumab as first-line therapy for advanced or recurrent leiomyosarcoma failed to show benefit. Advances in the understanding of the biology of uterine sarcomas may provide more treatment targets and make long-term control of the disease possible.

Systemic Therapy Summary

The current role of chemotherapy in the management of uterine sarcomas involves the treatment of patients with advanced or recurrent disease, and an emphasis on palliative intent. In leiomyosarcomas, the active drugs are doxorubicin, ifosfamide, gemcitabine, and docetaxel. For carcinosarcomas, the drugs of choice are ifosfamide, cisplatin/carboplatin, and paclitaxel. Hormonal therapy, including progestational agents, gonadotropin-releasing hormone analogues, and aromatase inhibitors, has a role in the treatment of advanced or recurrent ESS. The use of hormonal agents in the treatment of other histologic subtypes has not been well studied.

LONG-TERM RESULTS OF THERAPY

Leiomyosarcoma

The prognosis of patients with uterine leiomyosarcoma is uniformly poor. The reported 5-year survival of uterine leiomyosarcoma varies between 30% and 48%. However, leiomyosarcoma may tender a worse prognosis than carcinosarcoma when adjusting for stage and mitotic count. The mitotic index was the only factor significantly related to progression-free interval.

Carcinosarcomas

Major et al. (1993) reported a recurrence rate of 53% for 301 patients with clinical stage I and II carcinosarcomas. This included 61 patients (20%) who were "upstaged" based upon surgical findings. The prognostic factors based on multivariate analysis were adnexal spread, lymph node metastases, histologic cell type, and grade of sarcoma. Median survival in patients with clinically recurrent or advanced-stage carcinosarcomas ranged from 4 to 13 months despite therapy.

Müllerian Adenosarcomas

Among the 100 adenosarcoma patients, 26.1% developed recurrent disease. Generally, müllerian adenosarcomas are regarded as locally invasive; however, sarcomatous overgrowth has been described in as many as 57% of cases and is associated with a fulminant clinical course and death.

Endometrial Stromal Sarcoma

Virtually, no endometrial stromal nodule will recur after hysterectomy. In comparison with leiomyosarcoma and carcinosarcoma, patients with endometrial stromal sarcoma tend to present with low-grade and early-stage disease with favorable prognosis. In a large series, mitotic count successfully predicted outcome in patients with stage II to IV ESS. Young et al. and Berchuck et al. have suggested that patients with ovarian preservation at the time of hysterectomy for endometrial stromal sarcoma were more likely to develop recurrences. Bilateral salpingo-oophorectomy would seem to be prudent given the potential for low-grade ESS to express ERs and respond to hormonal therapy.

Patterns of Failure
A propensity for carcinosarcoma to relapse in the abdomen or pelvis and leiomyosarcomas to metastasize to the lung has been reported. In the follow-up of the GOG staging study reported by Major et al. (1993), 28 of 301 patients with carcinosarcoma developed lung metastases (9.3%), versus 24 of 59 (40.7%) of those with leiomyosarcomas. Recurrences with a pelvic component were 63 (20.9%) and 8 (13.6%), respectively, for the 2 tumor types. In patients whose tumors were initially confined to the uterus, there were purely distant recurrences in only 4 of 51 (7.8%) patients with carcinosarcoma but 22 of 35 (62.9%) in the patients with leiomyosarcoma.

CONCLUSIONS

There has been a slow evolution in the understanding of the basic science of sarcomas. The majority are felt to be sporadic with no specific etiology and most have complex karyotypes. However, in an increasing number of sarcomas, specific chromosomal translocations resulting in fusion genes that are constitutive and involve the activation of transcription factors have been identified.

Trials of adjuvant chemotherapy are appropriate in early-stage, resected leiomyosarcomas. Recurrence rates after surgery alone are unacceptably high; the risk of mortality associated with recurrent leiomyosarcoma easily offsets any morbidity derived from adjuvant chemotherapy in this population of relatively young patients. Combination or sequential radiation and chemotherapy have a great deal of appeal. A basic understanding of uterine sarcomas and their differences is paramount to the understanding of surgical and adjuvant therapy as well as palliative treatment in patients with these rare neoplasms; this knowledge is critical in the practice of gynecologic oncology.

SUGGESTED READINGS

Berchuk A, Rubin SC, Hoskins WJ, et al. Treatment of endometrial stromal tumors. *Gynecol Oncol.* 1990;36:60–65.

Chi DS, Mychalczak B, Saigo PE, et al. The role of whole-pelvic irradiation in the treatment of early-stage uterine carcinosarcoma. *Gynecol Oncol.* 1997;65:493–498.

Ferguson SE, Tornos C, Hummer A, et al. Prognostic features of surgical stage I uterine carcinosarcoma. *Am J Surg Pathol.* 2007;31(11):1653–1661.

Hensley ML, Blessing JA, Mannel R, et al. Fixed-dose rate gemcitabine plus docetaxel as first-line therapy for metastatic uterine leiomyosarcoma: A Gynecologic Oncology Group phase II trial. *Gynecol Oncol.* 2008;109:329–334.

Hensley ML, Maki R, Venkatraman E, et al. Gemcitabine and docetaxel in patients with unresectable leiomyosarcoma: Results of a phase II trial. *J Clin Oncol.* 2002;20:2824–2831.

Hensley ML, Wathen JK, Maki RG, et al. Adjuvant therapy for high-grade, uterus-limited leiomyosarcoma: Results of a phase 2 trial (SARC 005). *Cancer.* 2013;119:1555–1561.

Homesley HD, Filiaci V, Markman M, et al. Phase III trial of ifosfamide with or without paclitaxel in advanced uterine carcinosarcomas: A Gynecologic Oncology Group study. *J Clin Oncol.* 2007;25:526–531.

Major FJ, Blessing JA, Silverberg SG, et al. Prognostic factors in early-stage uterine sarcoma: A Gynecology Oncology Group study. *Cancer.* 1993;71:1702–1709.

Meredith RJ, Eisert DR, Kaka Z, et al. An excess of uterine sarcomas after pelvic irradiation. *Cancer.* 1986;58:2003–2007.

Norris HJ, Taylor HB. Mesenchymal tumors of the uterus. I. A clinical and pathological study of 53 endometrial stromal tumors. *Cancer.* 1966;19:755–766.

Reed NS, Mangioni C, Malmström H, et al. Phase III randomized study to evaluate the role of adjuvant pelvic radiotherapy in the treatment of uterine sarcoma stages I and II: An EORTC Gynaecological Cancer Group study (protocol 55874). *Eur J Cancer.* 2008;44(6):808–818.

Silverberg SG, Major FJ, Blessing JA, et al. Carcinosarcoma (malignant mixed mesodermal tumor) of the uterus. A Gynecologic Oncology Group pathologic study of 203 cases. *Int J Gynecol Pathol.* 1990;9:1–19.

Sutton G, Brunetto VL, Kilgore L, et al. A phase III trial of ifosfamide with or without cisplatin in carcinosarcomas of the uterus: A Gynecologic Oncology Group study. *Gynecol Oncol.* 2000;79:147–153.

Sutton G, Kauderer J, Carson LF, et al. Adjuvant ifosfamide and cisplatin in patients with completely resected stage I or II carcinosarcomas (mixed mesodermal tumors) of the uterus: A Gynecologic Oncology Group study. *Gynecol Oncol.* 2005;96:630–634.

Wolfson AH, Brady MF, Rocereto TF, et al. A Gynecologic Oncology Group randomized trial of whole abdominal irradiation versus cisplatin-ifosfamide and mesna as post-surgical therapy in stage I–IV carcinosarcomas of the uterus. *Gynecol Oncol.* 2007;107(2):177–185.

Young RH, Prat J, Scully RE. Endometrial stomal sarcomas of the ovary: A clinicopathologic analysis of 23 cases. *Cancer.* 1984;53(5):1143–1155.

Zivanovic O, Jacks LM, Iasonos A, et al. A nomogram to predict postresection 5-year overall survival for patients with uterine leiomyosarcoma. *Cancer.* 2012;118:660–669.

10 Ovarian Cancer (Including the Fallopian Tube)

Ovarian cancer is the fifth most common cause of cancer death in US women. It has been estimated that, in the United States, 1 woman in 70 will develop ovarian cancer and 1 woman in 100 will die of the disease.

Worldwide, ovarian cancer is the eighth most common form of cancer in women. In general, the highest incidence rates are found among European and North American population groups, and the lowest rates in Sub-Sahara African population groups. In the United States, rates for black American women are about two-thirds of those for white women, and rates for women of Asian/Pacific Islander descent are similar to those of black women. Rates of hysterectomy and oophorectomy in a population will affect the rate of ovarian cancer; 40% to 50% of women in the United States have a hysterectomy by 60 to 70 years of age, and about half of them have their ovaries removed at the same time.

Despite some apparent advances in therapy, survival in the United States from ovarian cancer has increased only 22% over the past three decades. Small but significant improvements in survival have been noted for white women but not for black women. Overall 5-year relative survival rates were 44% for white women and 36% for black women during 2003 to 2009. Outcomes in black women are worse even when controlling for age, stage, and histology.

RISK FACTORS

KEY POINTS
- Ovarian cancer is the fifth most common cause of death in US women.
- Risk factors for ovarian cancer include increasing age, nulliparity, and family history.
- Use of oral contraceptives and tubal ligation are protective.
- Carriers of *BRCA1* or *BRCA2* mutations have a 20% to 40% lifetime risk of ovarian cancer and should consider prophylactic salpingo-oophorectomy.

Established risk factors for ovarian cancer include increasing age, family history, nulliparity, early menarche, and late menopause. Breast-feeding is protective. Aside from having a first-degree relative with the disease, age is the most important risk factor for ovarian cancer (Fig. 10.1). Fifty percent of all US cases occur in women over the age of 65. Older women have a worse prognosis overall (Fig. 10.2), which is in part because they have an increased incidence of high-stage and high-grade disease at the time of diagnosis (Table 10.1). However, age remains a poor prognostic factor

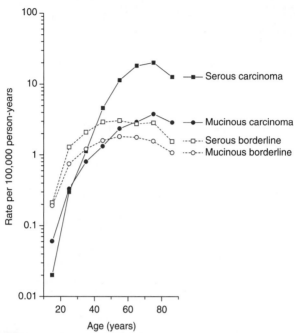

FIGURE 10.1 Incidence of invasive and borderline ovarian tumors in the United States by age. *Source:* Sherman ME, Berman J, Birrer MJ, et al. Current challenges and opportunities for research on borderline ovarian tumors. *Hum Pathol.* 2004;35:961–970.

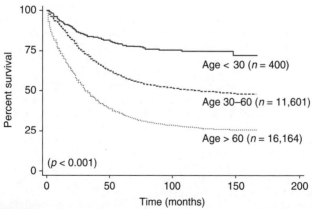

FIGURE 10.2 Disease-specific survival of patients based on age at diagnosis. *Source:* Chan JK, Urban R, Cheung MK, et al. Ovarian cancer in younger vs. older women: A population-based analysis. *Br J Cancer.* 2006;95:1314–1320.

Table 10.1	Incidence of Stage and Grade by Age Grouping in SEER Data 1988 to 2001		
	Total ($n = 28,165$)	Age < 30 ($n = 400$)	Age 30–60 ($n = 11,601$)	Age > 60 ($n = 16,164$)
STAGE				
I	22%	58%	31%	15%
II	8%	8%	9%	8%
III	36%	19%	34%	38%
IV	34%	16%	26%	40%
GRADE				
1	9%	34%	12%	5%
2	18%	24%	21%	16%
3	44%	13%	44%	45%
Unknown	29%	29%	23%	34%

Source: Adapted from Chan JK, Urban R, Cheung MK, et al. Ovarian cancer in younger vs. older women: A population-based analysis. *Br J Cancer*. 2006;95:1314–1320.

even when adjusted for stage, grade, histologic cell type, race, and surgical treatment.

There have been no consistent relationships reported of specific dietary components to ovarian cancer risk. Although some studies had implicated a diet high in meat and animal fat or a diet high in lactose, most large recent studies have failed to demonstrate any relationship between the consumption of animal foods and the development of ovarian cancer. There does appear to be a modest inverse correlation between moderate physical activity and ovarian cancer risk, and obesity has consistently shown a positive association with ovarian cancer risk.

Case–control analyses have consistently documented that users of oral contraceptives (OCP) have a 30% to 60% decreased risk of developing ovarian cancer than do women who have never used OCP. Tubal ligation is also protective. Some reports have suggested an increased risk with use of fertility-inducing drugs such as clomiphene, but most recent studies have found either a weak association or no association between infertility treatment and development of ovarian cancer. There appears to be a modest association between hormone replacement therapy (HRT) and risk of ovarian cancer. Progestins have been proposed to be protective against ovarian cancer, and the risk of ovarian cancer may be greater for estrogen-only HRT than for estrogen–progestin combinations.

Approximately 15% to 20% of cases of invasive epithelial ovarian cancer are the result of autosomal dominant high-penetrant genetic factors, predominantly germline mutations in the *BRCA1* or the *BRCA2* genes. The *BRCA1* and *BRCA2* gene products function in the cellular response to DNA damage. The lifetime risk of ovarian cancer for women with *BRCA1* mutations and *BRCA2* mutations has been estimated to be 40% and 20%, respectively. Risk may be reduced by prophylactic salpingo-oophorectomy. Survival for women with ovarian cancer related to a *BRCA1* or *BRCA2* mutation is longer than for women with a similar stage cancer and no mutation. Issues related to *BRCA* mutations as well as mutations in genes involved in the mismatch repair pathway are discussed in Chapter 3. Epithelial ovarian cancer is also a component of Lynch syndrome (also known as hereditary non-polyposis colorectal cancer syndrome—HNPCC). In addition to a predisposition to develop colorectal and endometrial cancer, women with this syndrome have a 10% to 13% lifetime risk for developing ovarian cancer.

PATHOLOGY

KEY POINTS

- Most fatal ovarian cancers in the United States are high-grade serous neoplasms.
- Most serous ovarian cancers originate in the distal fallopian tube from serous tubal intraepithelial carcinoma (STIC) lesions.
- Borderline tumors are usually confined to the ovary and have a better prognosis.
- Primary mucinous ovarian cancers can be difficult to distinguish from metastases to the ovary from other sites.

Ovarian carcinoma includes many subtypes (Table 10.2). Approximately half of all ovarian tumors are of epithelial origin and account for 90% of malignant tumors. The vast majority of fatal ovarian cancers are high-grade serous carcinomas. Most recently, there have been new insights into the origin of serous "ovarian" cancer. A putative precursor lesion in the fallopian tube, STIC, has been identified, and it is now believed that most serous "ovarian" cancer originates in the distal fallopian tube as STIC lesions. However, it is often not possible to clearly identify where the serous tumor originated. This makes screening and early detection difficult. Most of the remaining cell types of ovarian carcinomas appear to have other precursor lesions. Nearly all clear cell carcinomas and a large proportion of endometrioid carcinomas arise in endometriosis and appear to progress through a hyperplasia–borderline tumor–carcinoma sequence. Similarly, mucinous carcinomas most probably transit through a mucinous cystadenoma–borderline tumor–intraepithelial carcinoma sequence before invasion occurs. Such tumors are much more likely to be diagnosed while still confined to the ovary, and they therefore comprise more curable ovarian carcinomas. Low-grade serous carcinoma is a recently described and relatively small subset of ovarian serous carcinoma that also often appears to follow a stepwise progression from borderline tumor to invasive carcinoma.

Table 10.2	Histologic Classification of Common Epithelial Tumors of the Ovary

SEROUS TUMORS
Benign
Serous cystadenoma
Serous adenofibroma
Serous surface papilloma
Borderline
Serous borderline tumor/atypical proliferative serous tumor
Serous borderline tumor—micropapillary variant/noninvasive low-grade serous carcinoma
Malignant
Low-grade serous carcinoma
High-grade serous carcinoma

MUCINOUS TUMORS
Benign
Mucinous cystadenoma
Mucinous adenofibroma
Borderline
Mucinous borderline tumor/atypical proliferative mucinous tumor
Malignant
Mucinous carcinoma

ENDOMETRIOID TUMORS
Benign
Endometriotic cyst
Endometrioid cystadenoma
Endometrioid adenofibroma
Borderline
Endometrioid borderline tumor/atypical proliferative endometrioid tumor
Malignant
Clear cell carcinoma

CLEAR CELL TUMORS
Benign
Clear cell cystadenoma
Clear cell adenofibroma
Borderline
Clear cell borderline tumor/atypical proliferative clear cell tumor
Malignant
Clear cell carcinoma

BRENNER TUMORS
Benign
Brenner tumor
Borderline
Borderline Brenner tumor/atypical proliferative Brenner tumor
Malignant
Malignant Brenner tumor

Table 10.2	Histologic Classification of Common Epithelial Tumors of the Ovary (*continued*)

SEROMUCINOUS TUMORS
Benign
Seromucinous cystadenoma
Seromucinous adenofibroma
Borderline
Seromucinous borderline tumor/atypical proliferative seromucinous tumor
Malignant
Seromucinous carcinoma

MIXED EPITHELIAL AND MESENCHYMAL TUMOURS
Adenosarcoma
Carcinosarcoma

Source: Modified with permission from Kurman RJ, Carcangiu ML, Herrington CS, et al. *WHO Classification of Tumours of Female Reproductive Organs*, 4th ed. World Health Organization Classification of Tumours. Lyon, France: IARC Press; 2014:12–14.

Serous Tumors

Approximately 20% of serous tumors are malignant, 2% are borderline tumors, and 78% are benign. The mean age for patients with cancer is 56 years. Patients with benign and borderline tumors are generally younger, with mean ages at diagnosis of 45 and 48 years, respectively. Approximately 1 in 6 serous adenomas are bilateral compared to one-third of stage I serous adenocarcinomas. Those of higher stage are bilateral in two-thirds of cases. A recent Stanford series showed a 55% bilateral rate in serous borderline tumors. Borderline tumors that are confined to the ovary are associated with a survival that approaches 100%. The 10-year survival for women with tumors that have associated noninvasive peritoneal lesions still exceeds 95%, while for those with invasive implants it is 67%. Micropapillary serous tumors are a subtype of borderline tumors that are particularly likely to be associated with invasive implants and therefore have a worse prognosis. Microinvasion (defined variously as a maximal invasive focus size of 2, 3, or 5 mm, or an area of 10 mm^2) can be found in up to 10% of borderline tumors. The overall prognosis for the patient with microinvasion in a borderline tumor is currently considered to be no different than that of a borderline tumor without microinvasion. Borderline serous tumors may also spread to lymph nodes, but this does not appear to worsen the overall good prognosis.

Serous adenocarcinomas range in size from small (2 to 3 cm) to quite large. They often present as solid masses bounded by a capsule, often containing areas of necrosis and hemorrhage. The ovary from which the neoplasm has arisen is frequently not apparent grossly or microscopically. The gross appearance of a typical high-grade serous carcinoma is not distinctive, and it may be mimicked by other high-grade epithelial ovarian neoplasms, granulosa cell tumors, and carcinomas metastatic to the ovary. The tumor may appear as large sheets of polygonal cells growing autonomously without stromal support or as broad to fine clusters of cells related to papillae that irregularly dissect through the stroma, accompanied by a host desmoplastic response. The nuclei are typically large and pleomorphic, with variably sized nucleoli and numerous mitotic figures. Two grading systems for serous carcinomas have been proposed and tested in the past decade: a 3-grade system and, more recently, a binary system of high-grade and low-grade serous carcinoma. In contrast to high-grade serous carcinoma, low-grade neoplasms are characterized by cells with only mild-to-moderate nuclear atypia, evenly distributed chromatin, variable nucleoli, and fewer than 10 mitoses/10 hpf. Micropapillary architecture is frequently observed. The binary system separates over 90% of advanced-stage serous carcinomas into the high-grade group. This distribution is reflected in the overall behavior of advanced-stage serous carcinoma, which is associated with a 5-year survival of approximately 25%. In contrast, the 5- and 10-year survivals for women with advanced-stage low-grade serous carcinoma are approximately 85% and 50% to 60%, respectively. Serous carcinomas frequently stain positively with immunohistochemistry for WT1 and cytokeratin (CK) 7, and negative or only focally positive for CK20 and calretinin. A panel that includes these antibodies is frequently employed to evaluate a carcinoma whose primary site is uncertain. Pancreatic and breast carcinomas have the same CK7/20 profile, and thus other markers are needed for these sites. GCDFP-15 (gross cystic disease fluid protein) is often positive in breast carcinoma and only rarely positive in ovarian carcinoma.

Mucinous Tumors

Primary ovarian mucinous tumors include three types: cystadenomas (81%; these are benign), borderline tumors (13%), and primary ovarian mucinous carcinomas (5%). The mean age for patients with mucinous adenocarcinoma is 52 years, which, as with serous adenocarcinoma, is greater than the mean age of patients with benign and borderline tumors (44 and 49 years, respectively).

Mucinous tumors can grow to extremely large sizes, being among the largest of any recorded tumor in the body. Sizes exceeding 40 kg and 30 cm in greatest diameter have been reported. There are two types of borderline mucinous tumors: the gastrointestinal type and the endocervical type. The gastrointestinal type is more common. Both types of borderline mucinous tumors are almost always stage I and have close to 100% survival. As with serous borderline tumors, the presence of microinvasion does not appear to affect the generally benign prognosis of these tumors.

Primary ovarian mucinous carcinomas are typically unilateral multicystic mucinous masses with smooth capsules. They may contain solid areas and regions of necrosis, and rupture with surface involvement can occur. A thick tenacious mucinous material may fill the cysts. Most are stage I cancers. Pseudomyxoma peritonei is a clinicopathologic syndrome in which mucinous ascites is accompanied by low-grade neoplastic mucinous epithelium intimately associated with pools of extracellular mucin and fibrosis. It was thought that this syndrome sometimes resulted from mucinous ovarian tumors, but now it is believed to be derived universally from appendiceal low-grade (adenomatous) mucinous tumors; the ovarian involvement is secondary.

Mucinous carcinomas with secondary spread to the ovary are much more commonly encountered than primary ovarian mucinous carcinomas, and the distinction can be difficult to make. The ovarian metastasis may be the presenting site of disease. Approximately 80% of mucinous carcinomas that involve the ovary are metastatic from other sites. Metastatic mucinous carcinomas are usually readily recognized as such when the ovarian tumors exhibit any or all of the following features: bilateral, smaller size (typically <10 cm), ovarian surface involvement, a nodular pattern of involvement, and an infiltrative pattern of stromal invasion. However, some metastatic mucinous carcinomas, especially those derived from the colorectum, pancreaticobiliary tract, appendix, and endocervix, can exhibit deceptive patterns of invasion. Immunohistochemical analysis with antibodies such as CK7, CK20, CDX-2, and p16 can be useful for identifying some metastatic mucinous carcinomas; however, the utility of currently available markers is limited due to overlapping immunoprofiles of primary ovarian mucinous tumors with other mucinous tumors, particularly those of upper gastrointestinal tract origin.

Endometrioid Tumors

Endometrioid tumors account for a relatively small proportion of the common epithelial tumors, but most endometrioid tumors are malignant. When controlled for stage, the survival rate for endometrioid tumors is similar to that of serous adenocarcinoma in some studies but better in others. About 10% to 40% of cases are associated with endometriosis. Approximately 14% of women with endometrioid ovarian carcinoma also have endometrial cancer of the uterine corpus. Endometrial hyperplasia is also commonly present. The similar histology and subtype and high survival rate of these patients (80% at 10 years) suggest that the majority are synchronous primaries rather than metastases. Many of these patients also have coexisting endometriosis.

Clear Cell Tumors

Clear cell tumors are uncommon in the United States; they are more common in Japan. About half of cases are associated with endometriosis. Clear and "hobnail" cells are the microscopic hallmark, but the diagnosis rests upon architecture as well as optically clear cytoplasm. When present, the clear appearance of the cytoplasm results from glycogen that has leached as the tissue specimen is prepared for microscopic examination. The hobnail cells contain bulbous nuclei that protrude into the lumen at the apparent cytoplasmic limits of the cell.

Mixed Carcinoma

Perhaps, as many as 10% of all ovarian tumors of common epithelial origin are mixed, when defined as a carcinoma in which more than 10% of the neoplasm exhibits a second histologic cell type. One common specific malignant combination is mixed clear cell and endometrioid carcinoma, both being related to endometriosis.

Primary Peritoneal Serous Carcinomatosis

Primary peritoneal carcinoma has been defined by the Gynecologic Oncology Group (GOG) as follows: (i) ovaries are of normal size or enlarged by a benign process; (ii) ovarian involvement is absent or limited to the surface and/or superficial cortex with no tumor nodule within the ovarian cortex exceeding 5 × 5 mm; (iii) serous histology; and (iv) volume of extraovarian disease significantly exceeds that of ovarian disease. The pathology and response to treatment of peritoneal serous carcinomas are essentially identical to that of ovarian serous carcinomas. It has recently become apparent that the tubal fimbriae may be an important source of carcinomatosis in the absence of the typical features of primary tubal carcinomas (i.e., a dilated fallopian tube with a large mucosal lesion). Because the gross and microscopic characteristics, as well as spread, of carcinoma of the fallopian tube are identical to those of the ovary, the determination of the site of origin of a tumor that forms a solid or cystic tuboovarian mass is arbitrary. The fallopian tube may actually be the source of many high-grade serous carcinomas that are considered primary to the ovary.

Fallopian Tube Carcinoma

The gross appearance of the fallopian tube affected by papillary carcinoma is typically described as enlarged, deformed, or fusiform, with agglutination of the fimbriae and, frequently, distal obstruction. When the tumor is confined to the mucosa, the tube is generally soft to palpation, and the initial impression of the surgeon is often hematosalpinx, pyosalpinx, or hydrosalpinx. The most frequent site of origin is the ampulla, followed by the infundibulum. Microscopically, most fallopian tube neoplasms display papillary serous histology. With the recent knowledge that most high-grade serous carcinomas develop in the distal fallopian tube from precursor STIC lesions, the incidence of fallopian tube carcinoma has increased dramatically.

DIAGNOSIS AND CLINICAL EVALUATION

Ovarian carcinomas are distinctive by virtue of their propensity to exfoliate malignant cells into the peritoneal cavity. There the cells follow the normal circulation of peritoneal fluid up the right paracolic gutter and to the undersurface of the right hemidiaphragm, where they may implant and grow as surface nodules. The omentum is also a frequent site of involvement, and, indeed, all intraperitoneal (IP) surfaces are at risk. Ovarian cancer may also spread via the retroperitoneal lymphatics that drain the ovary. These follow the ovarian blood supply in the infundibulopelvic ligament to terminate in lymph nodes lying along the aorta and vena cava up to the level of the renal vessels. Lymph channels also pass laterally through the broad ligament and parametrial channels to terminate in the pelvic sidewall lymphatics, including the external iliac, obturator, and hypogastric chains. Spread may also occur along the course of the round ligament, resulting in involvement of the inguinal lymphatics.

Approximately 75% to 85% of patients with epithelial ovarian cancer are diagnosed at the time when their disease has spread throughout the peritoneal cavity. Several organizations, including the Gynecologic Cancer Foundation, the Society of Gynecologic Oncologists, and the American Cancer Society, released a consensus statement on the symptoms of ovarian cancer in June 2007. It urges women to seek medical attention if they have new and persistent symptoms of bloating, pelvic or abdominal pain, difficulty eating, early satiety, or urinary urgency or frequency. These symptoms were found to be much more likely to occur in women with ovarian cancer than in the general population. There is, however, no evidence that detection based on these factors will shift diagnosis early enough to affect mortality.

The diagnosis of early-stage ovarian cancer (when the tumor is still confined to the pelvis) usually occurs by palpation of an asymptomatic adnexal mass during a routine pelvic examination. However, the vast majority of palpable adnexal masses are not malignant and, in premenopausal women, ovarian cancer represents less than 5% of adnexal neoplasms. In these women, the ovarian enlargement is usually due to either follicular or corpus luteum cysts. The vast majority of these functional cysts will regress in one to three menstrual cycles and, consequently, the initial approach to management for a palpable adnexal mass less than 8 cm in size in a premenopausal woman is to repeat the pelvic examination and imaging studies in 1 to 2 months. In contrast, an adnexal mass in a premenarchal or postmenopausal woman, particularly when complex as seen on ultrasound, has a higher likelihood of being a malignant tumor, and surgical exploration is usually indicated.

Preoperative evaluation of the ovarian cancer patient is shown in Figure 10.3. CT scans of the chest, abdomen, and pelvis are usual. Brain scans and bone scans are unnecessary unless suggested by the patient's symptoms; metastases to these sites are extremely uncommon, particularly at the time of diagnosis. If there is concern for a gastrointestinal primary based on bowel symptoms or heme-positive stools, barium enema or colonoscopy

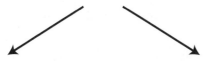

Family history evaluation
Abdominal/pelvic exam
GI evaluation if clinically indicated
Ultrasound and/or abdominal/pelvic CT
Chest imaging
CA-125 or other tumor markers as clinically indicated
Complete blood count
Chemistry profile with liver function tests

Surgery, staging/cytoreduction

- Neoadjuvant chemotherapy for patients not surgical candidates (requires diagnosis by fine needle aspiration, biopsy, or paracentesis)
- Consider surgery after 3–6 cycles

FIGURE 10.3 Suspicious symptoms/palpable mass or ascites.

can be useful. Because of the association of ovarian cancer with breast cancer and because metastatic breast cancer can produce intra-abdominal carcinomatosis as well, mammography is often performed. Serum CA-125 level should be measured. It has been demonstrated that less than 1% of normal nonpregnant women have serum CA-125 levels greater than 35 U/mL. In contrast, 80% to 85% of patients with epithelial ovarian cancer have elevated serum levels. Unfortunately, the percentage of women with an elevated CA-125 level is lower in stage I disease, limiting the usefulness of the marker as a screening test. The serous histologic subset of ovarian cancer has the highest incidence of elevated CA-125 levels (>85%), whereas mucinous tumors are associated with a low incidence of abnormally elevated serum CA-125 levels. In postmenopausal women with asymptomatic pelvic masses, an elevated serum CA-125 (>65 U/mL) had a sensitivity of 97% and a specificity of 78% for ovarian cancer. In contrast, in premenopausal women, there is a higher prevalence of nonmalignant conditions that can produce elevated serum CA-125 levels (e.g., pregnancy, endometriosis, uterine fibroids, and pelvic inflammatory disease).

SCREENING

KEY POINTS

- Ovarian cancer has a low prevalence: 1 case/2,500 women per year.
- Screening with pelvic exam, transvaginal ultrasound, and CA-125 has not been shown to be effective in any group of women, including *BRCA* mutation carriers.
- Premenopausal women frequently have palpable adnexal masses. Most are benign and are due to follicular or corpus luteum cysts.
- Surgical exploration is generally indicated for complex adnexal masses in postmenopausal women.

Despite decades of large trials, no reliable procedures are currently available for the early detection of ovarian cancer. Available potential screening techniques have included pelvic examination (ovarian palpation), ultrasound examinations, CA-125 and other tumor markers, and combined modality approaches. Difficulties include the need for surgery, with its attendant risks, to evaluate a positive test, and the fact that slow-growing tumors detected on screening are often borderline (which are not likely to be lethal) or already in an advanced stage (which are difficult to cure). A representative large multimodal screening trial, the NCI-sponsored Prostate, Lung, Colorectal, and Ovarian (PLCO) Cancer Screening Trial, enrolled over 74,000 women aged 55 to 74 years from 1993 through 2000. Women were randomly assigned to either observation or baseline measurements of CA-125 levels and transvaginal ultrasonography followed by annual CA-125 readings for 6 years and transvaginal ultrasound for 4 years. Baseline screening in the 28,816 women randomized to screening who received at least one test detected 29 neoplasms (26 ovarian, 2 fallopian, and 1 primary peritoneal). Nine were of low malignant potential. Only 2 of the invasive cancers were stage I; 1 of these was a granulosa cell tumor.

Five hundred seventy surgical procedures, including 325 laparotomies, were performed. The authors calculated the positive predictive value for invasive cancer of an abnormal CA-125 as 3.7%, of an abnormal transvaginal ultrasound as 1.0%, and of having both tests abnormal as 23.5%. However, if only subjects in whom both tests were abnormal had been evaluated, 12 of the 20 invasive cancers would have been missed.

Clearly, it is possible that screening may do more harm (complications from needless procedures) than good. At this time, routine screening of the general population should not be performed. Even in women with a positive family history of ovarian cancer or known *BRCA* mutations, there is no evidence that screening can affect mortality from this disease. However, despite the lack of evidence for benefit of screening such high-risk women, it seems prudent to follow them with pelvic and ultrasound examinations with serum CA-125 determinations on a regular basis until/unless they elect a prophylactic bilateral salpingo-oophorectomy. A large ongoing trial in the UK, the UK Collaborative Trial of Ovarian Cancer Screening (UKCTOCS), is expected to be reported in 2015. In this trial, more than 200,000 postmenopausal women were enrolled and randomly assigned to usual care or screening.

SURGICAL STAGING

KEY POINTS

- Surgical stage is the most important prognostic factor for women with ovarian carcinoma.
- Volume of residual disease after surgery is an important prognostic factor in women with advanced disease.
- Grade is a particularly important prognostic factor in women with early-stage disease.

The International Federation of Gynecology and Obstetrics (FIGO) staging system for ovarian carcinomas is presented in Table 10.3. The stage usually can be determined only following exploratory laparotomy and thorough evaluation of all areas at risk. Operations on women with a pelvic or adnexal mass that may represent ovarian cancer should generally be carried out through a vertical abdominal incision to allow access to the upper abdomen, which is difficult to visualize through a low transverse incision. However, advanced minimally invasive techniques are appropriate to evaluate and stage carefully selected patients. On entering the abdomen, aspiration of ascites or peritoneal lavage should be performed to obtain specimens for cytologic examination. Separate specimens should be obtained from the pelvis, right and left paracolic gutters, and the undersurfaces of the right and left hemidiaphragms. An encapsulated adnexal mass should be removed intact, if possible, since rupture and spillage of malignant cells within the peritoneal cavity will increase the patient's stage and may adversely affect her prognosis. Adhesions should be noted and biopsied since they may represent occult areas of microscopic disease. If frozen section indicates the presence of ovarian cancer, a complete abdominal

Table 10.3	Carcinoma of the Ovary: 2014 FIGO Nomenclature
I	Tumor confined to ovaries or fallopian tube(s)
IA	Tumor limited to 1 ovary (capsule intact) or the fallopian tube. No tumor on ovarian or fallopian tube surface. No malignant cells in the ascites or peritoneal washings
IB	Tumor limited to both ovaries (capsule intact) or fallopian tubes No tumor on ovarian or fallopian tube surface No malignant cells in the ascites or peritoneal washings
IC	Tumor limited to 1 or both ovaries or fallopian tubes, with any of the following: IC1 surgical spill intraoperatively IC2 capsule ruptured before surgery or tumor on ovarian surface IC3 malignant cells present in the ascites or peritoneal washings
II	Tumor involves 1 or both ovaries or fallopian tubes with pelvic extension (below pelvic brim) or peritoneal cancer (Tp)
IIA	Extension and/or implants on the uterus and/or fallopian tubes
IIB	Extension to other pelvic intraperitoneal tissues
III	Tumor involves 1 or both ovaries, or fallopian tubes, or primary peritoneal cancer, with cytologically or histologically confirmed spread to the peritoneum outside the pelvis and/or metastasis to the retroperitoneal lymph nodes
IIIA	Metastasis to the retroperitoneal lymph nodes with or without microscopic peritoneal involvement beyond the pelvis
IIIA1	Positive retroperitoneal lymph nodes only (cytologically or histologically proven) IIIA1(i) Metastasis $\leq$10 mm in greatest dimension (note this is tumor dimension and not lymph node dimension) IIIA1(ii) Metastasis >10 mm in greatest dimension
IIIA2	Microscopic extrapelvic (above the pelvic brim) peritoneal involvement with or without positive retroperitoneal lymph nodes
IIIB	Macroscopic peritoneal metastases beyond the pelvic brim $\leq$2 cm in greatest dimension, with or without metastasis to the retroperitoneal lymph nodes
IIIC	Macroscopic peritoneal metastases beyond the pelvic brim >2 cm in greatest dimension, with or without metastases to the retroperitoneal nodes[a]
IV	Distant metastasis excluding peritoneal metastases Stage IV A: Pleural effusion with positive cytology Stage IVB: Metastases to extra-abdominal organs (including inguinal lymph nodes and lymph nodes outside the abdominal cavity)[b]

[a]Includes extension of tumor to capsule of the liver and spleen without parenchymal involvement of either organ.
[b]Parenchymal metastases are stage IVB.
Source: Mutch DG, Prat J. 2014 FIGO staging for ovarian, fallopian tube and peritoneal cancer. *Gynecol Oncol*. 2014;133:401–404, with permission.

exploration should be carried out, including the evaluation of all intestinal surfaces. Any suspicious areas should be biopsied. Omentectomy and random peritoneal biopsies should be performed. Pelvic and aortic lymph node sampling should be performed. Several reports have demonstrated that the pelvic lymph nodes are involved by ovarian cancer at the same frequency as are paraaortic nodes and suggest the need for comprehensive nodal sampling in presumed early-stage disease.

Prognostic Factors

The 5-year survival of patients with epithelial ovarian cancer is directly correlated with the tumor stage (Fig. 10.4). Prognosis for stage I disease has been reported to be from 60% to over 80% and is strongly dependent on tumor grade and whether the patient was fully staged (as patients with apparent stage I disease may have stage III disease found with careful surgical exploration and node biopsy). Similarly, initial studies of patients with stage II disease reported the range of 5-year survivals from 0% to 40%. However, stage II disease frequently is upstaged to stage III disease, particularly when patients present with large-volume disease in the pelvis. The small numbers of patients who are found to have stage II disease following completion of a comprehensive laparotomy have a 5-year survival rate of approximately 80%. Patients with stage III disease have a 5-year survival rate of approximately 15% to 30%, whereas patients with stage IV disease have a 5% 5-year survival rate.

In women with advanced-stage disease, the volume of residual disease following cytoreductive surgery is directly correlated with survival. Patients who have been optimally cytoreduced have a 22-month improvement in median survival compared to those patients undergoing less than optimal resection.

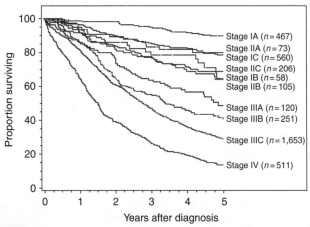

FIGURE 10.4 Carcinoma of the ovary; patients treated from 1996 to 1998. Survival of FIGO stage. *Source:* Heintz AP, Odicino F, Maisonneve P, et al. Carcinoma of the ovary. *Int J Gynecol Obstet.* 2003;83:135–166, with permission.

In general, the histologic type has less prognostic significance than the other clinical factors, such as stage, volume of disease, and histologic grade. However, there is a high correlation between histologic type, stage, and grade. The histologic grade of the tumor is a particularly important prognostic and decision-making factor in patients with early-stage ovarian cancer. In surgically staged patients from the FIGO database, the overall 5-year survivals are 87%, 82%, and 69% for stage I grade 1, 2, and 3 tumors, respectively.

TREATMENT

A general algorithm for the management of ovarian cancer is shown in Figure 10.5.

Early-Stage Ovarian Cancer

Although the benefits of chemotherapy in advanced-stage ovarian cancer have been well demonstrated, they have been much harder to show in early-stage disease. The number of patients available is smaller and the prognosis better than with more advanced-stage disease, making adequately powered randomized trials difficult to complete. Some patients treated postsurgically with observation alone may be salvaged with chemotherapy after recurrence. In addition, early-stage epithelial ovarian cancer is composed of a rather different mix of grades and histologies than does advanced-stage disease, in particular a much larger percentage of low-grade, mucinous, and clear cell carcinomas and a smaller percentage of serous carcinomas (Table 10.4). The current standard of care for most early-stage ovarian cancer patients is chemotherapy. This is based on the positive results of the combined ACTION and ICON-1 trials, which randomized women with early-stage disease to chemotherapy versus no postoperative treatment (Fig. 10.6).

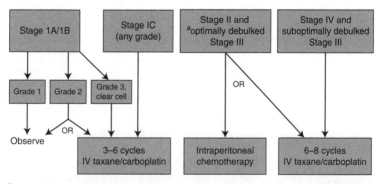

^{a}Less than 1-cm maximal size residual lesion

FIGURE 10.5 Postoperative chemotherapy.

Table 10.4	Histology and Stage in Ovarian Cancer	
	IA ($n = 550$)	IIIC ($n = 1,793$)
Serous	23%	67%
Mucinous	38%	7%
Endometrioid	19%	14%
Clear cell	10%	4%
Undifferentiated	3%	7%
Mixed	6%	2%

Source: Adapted from Heintz AP, Odicino F, Maisonneuve P, et al. *Int J Gynecol Obstet.* 2003;83(suppl 1):135–166, with permission.

The benefit of adjuvant chemotherapy was found to be restricted to patients with incomplete surgical staging, and incompletely staged patients with a poorly differentiated grade III tumor were found to derive the greatest benefit from adjuvant chemotherapy. Duration of therapy for early-stage disease remains controversial. The GOG randomized 427 eligible patients with early-stage disease to receive either three or six cycles of

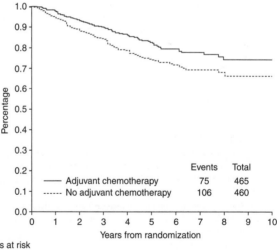

		Events	Total
—— Adjuvant chemotherapy		75	465
------ No adjuvant chemotherapy		106	460

Patients at risk

	0	1	2	3	4	5	6	7	8	9	10
Adjuvant chemotherapy	465	432	362	301	244	187	145	101	52	16	7
No adjuvant chemotherapy	460	407	347	290	230	175	128	83	41	12	3

FIGURE 10.6 Kaplan-Meier curves for overall survival in early-stage ovarian cancer patients treated with adjuvant chemotherapy (*solid line*) and no adjuvant chemotherapy (*dotted line*). *Source*: Trimbos JB, Parmar M, Vergote I, et al. International Collaborative Ovarian Neoplasm Trial 1 and Adjuvant Chemotherapy in Ovarian Neoplasm Trial: Two parallel randomized phase III trials of adjuvant chemotherapy in patients with early-stage ovarian carcinoma. *J Natl Cancer Inst.* 2003;95:105–112.

carboplatin/paclitaxel chemotherapy. Overall 5-year survival was 84% for stage I disease and 73% for stage II disease and did not differ by treatment regimen (HR 1.02). However, after adjusting for initial FIGO stage and tumor grade, the recurrence rate was 25% lower for patients receiving six cycles (HR 0.76), and many physicians therefore prefer to use six cycles of chemotherapy.

At this time, it is recommended that patients with comprehensively staged stage IA or IB grade 1 epithelial ovarian cancer receive no post-operative chemotherapy. Patients with grade 3 or stage IC disease have a relapse risk of at least 20%, and this can be reduced with platinum-based chemotherapy. Paclitaxel/carboplatin for three to six cycles is the usual treatment in the United States. Based on the frequency of early-stage disease, future data to better address which women with early-stage ovarian cancers actually derive benefit from therapy will be difficult to generate.

Early-Stage Fallopian Tube Carcinomas

Unlike ovarian carcinoma, in which two thirds of patients present with advanced-stage disease, about half of patients diagnosed with fallopian tube carcinoma using traditional criteria have been diagnosed in stage I or II. Prognosis of early-stage disease has been reported to be dependent on depth of invasion of the tumor into the fallopian tube. Most recent data have suggested that the survival for women with fallopian tube cancer is similar or superior to that of women with ovarian cancer when standardized for stage. No meaningfully sized series to inform about benefits of treatment exist. As advanced-stage fallopian tube carcinomas appear to respond to platinum-based therapies in a manner similar to that of ovarian carcinomas, adjuvant chemotherapy is currently used for early-stage fallopian tumor in most situations.

Management of Borderline Tumors

KEY POINTS
- Surgery is the primary management for borderline tumors.
- There is no evidence that postoperative chemotherapy improves outcomes for women with borderline ovarian cancer even with advanced-stage disease.
- Borderline tumors may recur after 10 to 15 years.
- Twenty to thirty percent of ovarian tumors diagnosed as borderline at the time of frozen section examination may return as invasive carcinomas on final pathology.

Borderline tumors comprise 10% to 20% of ovarian malignancies. Most are of serous or mucinous histology, and most are diagnosed at an early stage. Even when they present with more advanced-stage disease, they progress very slowly. A review of borderline tumors entered into the NCI SEER database between 1988 and 1997 showed 10-year relative survivals of 99% for stage I, 98% for stage II, 96% for stage III, and 77% for stage IV disease. Borderline tumors are particularly likely to affect young women (Fig. 10.1), in whom therapeutic decisions regarding fertility-sparing, premature hormonal deprivation, and adjuvant chemotherapeutic treatments are particularly pertinent.

Surgery is the cornerstone of treatment for early-stage as well as advanced-stage ovarian borderline tumors. There is no evidence that a conservative surgical approach has an adverse effect on survival in patients with stage I borderline tumors. Even though patients treated with a unilateral oophorectomy have a higher recurrence rate than patients treated with a total hysterectomy and bilateral oophorectomy, effective surgery for recurrent disease leads to equivalent survival. Chemotherapy is not indicated for stage I or II borderline tumors.

Approximately 5% to 10% of early-stage serous borderline tumors will ultimately recur, either as borderline tumors or low-grade carcinomas. Recurrences can present 10 to 15 years after the initial diagnosis, making long-term follow-up necessary. Although their very slow growth would seem to predispose them to resistance to traditional cytotoxic agents, serous borderline tumors are not completely chemotherapy resistant, and response rates of 15% to 57% to frontline therapy have been reported. Surgery is often used as sole primary treatment for women with serous borderline tumor of the ovary with noninvasive implants, for whom 5-year survivals are 94% to 95%, and chemotherapy is often used in women with invasive implants. However, there is no clear evidence that chemotherapy can decrease relapse rates or improve survival in any subset of patients. Over 90% of serous borderline ovarian tumors are estrogen receptor positive, and there are case reports of major responses to tamoxifen, leuprolide, and anastrozole.

Most mucinous borderline ovarian tumors are stage I and present as large unilateral ovarian masses; bilaterality suggests the possibility of metastatic tumor from another site. Appendectomy and evaluation of the GI tract should be performed to rule out a primary gastrointestinal tumor. Advanced-stage pure borderline mucinous tumors are exceedingly uncommon. Twenty to thirty percent of ovarian tumors diagnosed as borderline of any histologic subtype at the time of frozen section examination proved to be invasive carcinomas on final pathology.

Advanced Epithelial Ovarian Cancer

KEY POINTS

- Cytoreductive surgery is standard in the management of ovarian cancer, with the goal being complete resection of all visible tumor.
- Six cycles of carboplatin/paclitaxel represents standard therapy for most women with advanced-stage ovarian cancer in the United States.
- There is no confirmed survival benefit for platinum dose escalation. Recent trials (GOG 218 and ICON-7) have shown statistically significant but modest benefit with the addition of bevacizumab to frontline therapy.
- IP therapy may benefit women with small-volume residual disease.
- Advanced-stage clear cell and mucinous tumors appear to be relatively chemotherapy resistant.

Cytoreductive Surgery

The majority of cases of ovarian cancer are not diagnosed until the disease has spread beyond the ovary. Often, patients with advanced disease will present with an abdomen distended with ascites and obviously bulky tumor masses in the pelvis and upper abdomen. The goal of surgical cytoreduction in patients with advanced stage III/IV ovarian cancer should be a complete resection of all visible tumors. Removal of bulky tumor masses in a patient with advanced ovarian cancer may improve the patient's comfort, reduce the adverse metabolic consequences of the tumor, and enhance the patient's ability to maintain her nutritional status. Removal of large tumor masses may also enhance the response of the remaining tumor to chemotherapy. Large tumor masses with a relatively poor blood supply may provide a pharmacologic sanctuary where viable tumor cells can escape exposure to adequate concentrations of cytotoxic drugs. Additionally, such poorly vascularized masses may have a low growth fraction (i.e., a larger proportion of cells in the nonproliferating [G_0] phase of the cell cycle) when they are relatively insensitive to the effects of cytotoxic drugs. In clinical trials in which the percentage of patients who were optimally cytoreduced was reported, the median survival for optimally cytoreduced patients (i.e., those with a maximum remaining lesion size of less than a centimeter) was 39 months as compared to 17 months for those not optimally cytoreduced. However, randomized clinical trial data supporting aggressive debulking surgery do not exist. It is possible that patients who present with small volume disease have disease that is biologically less aggressive than do patients who are anatomically cytoreduced to the same amount of residual disease after surgical removal of bulky tumor.

Surgery prior to chemotherapy, for diagnosis and tumor debulking, has been the standard in the United States. However, since some patients cannot be successfully cytoreduced at initial surgery, the benefit of a brief induction course of chemotherapy prior to debulking surgery has been explored. Two to three cycles of chemotherapy substantially increase the percentage of patients who will be successfully cytoreduced and decrease operative morbidity. This approach clearly seems appropriate in patients who are poor surgical candidates at presentation. Whether it should be more universally applied remains controversial due to the overall poor survival reported in randomized trials of neoadjuvant chemotherapy.

Interval debulking is a term traditionally used to describe surgery performed in the middle of a chemotherapy course for patients in whom initial debulking surgery was attempted but was unsuccessful and whose disease appears to be responding to therapy. There is conflicting evidence from two large prospective randomized trials (EORTC and GOG) as to whether interval debulking can improve survival in certain patients with advanced ovarian cancer, with an EORTC trial showing substantial benefit and a GOG trial showing no benefit in either progression-free or overall survival. It has been hypothesized that the differences in outcome result from a more aggressive initial surgical attempt in the United States. Select patients may benefit from interval debulking depending on the aggressiveness of the initial cytoreductive surgery, the geographic distribution and size of the remaining disease, and the response to the initial several cycles of chemotherapy.

Interval debulking is appropriate for patients who have received initial neoadjuvant chemotherapy without attempted primary cytoreductive surgery.

Chemotherapy

Surgery is rarely curative for women with advanced-stage ovarian carcinoma, even when there is no residual disease. The most standard regimen in the United States is currently six cycles of postoperative intravenous paclitaxel/carboplatin; areas of uncertainty exist not only regarding the use of neoadjuvant therapy and interval debulking but the role of single-agent carboplatin, use of IP chemotherapy, and use of maintenance therapy.

Platinum Use

Platinum agents represent the most active group of chemotherapy drugs in the treatment of ovarian cancer. Multiple randomized trials comparing carboplatin to cisplatin in ovarian carcinoma have been performed, and both individual studies and meta-analyses have confirmed that there is no difference in efficacy between the two agents. No evidence supports the use of doses of cisplatin above 50 to 100 mg/m^2 every 3 weeks or carboplatin AUC 5 to 7.5 every 3 weeks. Weekly carboplatin is thought to increase the rate of serious allergic reactions in addition to potentially less efficacy. Oxaliplatin also has activity against ovarian cancer but has not been shown to be superior to, non–cross-resistant with, or less toxic than carboplatin. Therefore, in general, carboplatin, which is less emetogenic and produces less neurotoxicity and nephrotoxicity than cisplatin, is the first-line platinum agent in the treatment of ovarian cancer in the United States. However, as discussed below, there are no randomized data showing that IP carboplatin produces benefits similar to those seen with IP cisplatin, and cisplatin remains the standard platinum drug for IP administration.

Addition of a Taxane to Platinum Chemotherapy

In the 1980s, a great deal of excitement was generated by the demonstration that single-agent paclitaxel had substantial activity against platinum-resistant ovarian cancer.

A number of randomized trials were rapidly launched comparing platinum-based regimens with and without taxane in the first-line treatment of ovarian cancer. The four largest studies are summarized in Table 10.5. The results of the first two of these trials completed (GOG 111 and OV-10) clearly demonstrated that combination chemotherapy with paclitaxel and cisplatin prolongs both progression-free and overall survival as compared with cyclophosphamide/cisplatin. However, the other two trials did not clearly support the addition of paclitaxel to frontline therapy. GOG-132 compared single-agent paclitaxel to single-agent cisplatin to the combination of cisplatin and paclitaxel. The response rate to single-agent paclitaxel in patients with measurable disease was significantly lower than to either of the platinum-containing regimens (42% vs. 67%, $p < 0.01$). However, there was no difference in overall survival (30.2, 25.9, and 26.3 months) between the regimens. It is possible that sequential therapy with platinum and taxane would produce the same results as combined therapy, but this has not been prospectively demonstrated, and combination platinum/taxane therapy remains the standard in the United States.

Table 10.5 Randomized Trials ± Taxane in First-Line Chemotherapy for Ovarian Cancer

Author (Year)	n	Eligibility	Regimens	Median PFS	Median OS
McGuire (1996) GOG-111	386	Suboptimal III any IV	Cisplatin 75 mg/m² + paclitaxel 13.5 mg/m²/24 h vs. Cisplatin 75 mg/m² + cyclophosphamide 750 mg/m²	18 mo vs. 13 mo $p < 0.001$	38 mo vs. 24 mo $p < 0.001$
Piccart (2000) OV-10	680	IIb–IV	Cisplatin 75 mg/m² + paclitaxel 175 mg/m²/3 h vs. Cisplatin 75 mg/m² + cyclophosphamide 750 mg/m²	15.5 mo vs. 11.5 mo $p = 0.0005$	35.6 mo vs. 25.8 mo $p = 0.0016$
Muggia (2000) GOG-132	614	Suboptimal III any IV	Cisplatin 75 mg/m² + paclitaxel 135 g/m²/24 h vs. Paclitaxel 200 mg/m²/24 h vs. Cisplatin 100 mg/m²	14 mo vs. 11 mo vs. 16 mo Paclitaxel worse $p < 0.001$	26 mo vs. 26 mo vs. 30 mo $p = NS$
ICON-3 (2002)	2,075	I–IV	Carboplatin AUC 6 + paclitaxel 175 mg/m² vs. Carboplatin AUC 6 or CAP ($n = 421$) Cyclophosphamide 500 mg/m² + Cisplatin 50 mg/m² + doxorubicin 50 mg/m²	17 mo vs. 16 mo $p = NS$	39 mo vs. 36 mo $p = NS$

Alternate Taxanes/Taxane Schedules

Docetaxel plus carboplatin has been prospectively compared to paclitaxel plus carboplatin. There were no apparent differences in progression-free or overall survival between the two drugs. Docetaxel was associated with less neurotoxicity but more myelotoxicity. It represents an attractive option for patients with or at risk for neurotoxicity. Higher doses or more prolonged infusions of paclitaxel have not been shown to be of benefit. However, phase II trials of weekly paclitaxel have reported response rates of 32% to 47% in platinum-refractory patients, and there is substantial interest in the incorporation of weekly paclitaxel into frontline therapy of ovarian cancer. Results from a trial conducted in Japan comparing weekly paclitaxel plus every-3-week carboplatin to every-3-week paclitaxel plus every-3-week carboplatin have suggested superior outcomes but increased toxicity with the weekly paclitaxel schedule.

Addition of a Third Agent to Frontline Chemotherapy

There are no data to prove that the addition of any third cytotoxic agent to frontline chemotherapy of ovarian cancer improves outcomes. An international multi-arm randomized study was led by the GOG (GOG-182—ICON5) to definitively answer whether triplet cytotoxic chemotherapy improves survival. A total of 4,312 advanced-staged ovarian cancer patients were randomized to carboplatin/paclitaxel or carboplatin/paclitaxel combined with gemcitabine, liposomal doxorubicin, or topotecan. Progression-free survival (PFS) was not statistically different among any of the combination regimens studied.

Recent interest has focused on the role of combining some of the newer molecular targeted agents with chemotherapy. The most promising agent to date has been bevacizumab, a monoclonal antibody targeting vascular endothelial growth factor (VEGF). It has produced single-agent response rates in the range of 20% in the setting of recurrent ovarian cancer and has improved survival when combined with chemotherapy in the treatment of metastatic colon cancer and lung cancer. Two large randomized trials testing the addition of bevacizumab to frontline therapy (GOG-218 and ICON-7) have recently been completed. Results from GOG-218 showed a significant improvement in PFS (3.8 months) with the addition of bevacizumab to upfront intravenous chemotherapy when the bevacizumab was continued as a maintenance regimen after chemotherapy. In the ICON-7 trial, PFS at 42 months was 22.4 months without bevacizumab versus 24.1 months with bevacizumab ($p = 0.04$). Additionally, the benefits were greater among patients at high risk for disease progression. The clinical results are modest, and these trials have been interpreted with global controversy. Unanswered questions include whether bevacizumab given as part of initial treatment is more favorable than bevacizumab given in the recurrent disease setting. Furthermore, neither study demonstrated an overall survival benefit.

Intraperitoneal Chemotherapy

IP chemotherapy provides a means by which high concentrations of drugs and long durations of tissue exposure can be attained at the peritoneal surface. As IP progression of disease remains the major source of morbidity and mortality in ovarian cancer, it is a theoretically attractive approach in the treatment of this disease. It should be noted that (i) the theoretical benefit is only for very small tumor volumes and (ii) agents that do not reach therapeutic systemic levels when given by the IP route need to be administered intravenously as well. For a given dose of cisplatin, peak concentrations are higher with intravenous cisplatin, and this has resulted in somewhat decreased toxicity in a randomized comparison of the same doses of cisplatin given intraperitoneally versus intravenously, including less hearing loss and neuromuscular toxicity. However, the amount of cisplatin recovered in the urine, reflecting total systemic exposure, is similar regardless of whether the administration is intravenous or IP. Similarly, carboplatin administered IP at an AUC of 6 has been shown to give an AUC in the peritoneal cavity of about 17 times higher than that of carboplatin given intravenously, while producing a very similar serum AUC. For paclitaxel, on the other hand, serum concentrations in patients treated with IP paclitaxel at feasible doses are low. However, significant levels persist in the peritoneal cavity 1 week after drug administration.

Clinical Use of IP Therapy for Ovarian Cancer

Numerous prospective randomized clinical trials have tested the benefit of IP cisplatin in the treatment of ovarian cancer; the three largest are summarized in Table 10.6. In January 2006, the NCI issued a clinical alert suggesting the use of IP cisplatin chemotherapy in women with optimally debulked ovarian cancer. A meta-analysis of eight trials comparing IP to intravenous platinum-based chemotherapy (all but one used cisplatin) showed an average 21.6% decrease in the risk of death (HR = 0.79). As the expected median duration of survival for women with optimally debulked ovarian cancer receiving standard treatment is approximately 4 years, this size reduction in death rate was estimated to translate into about a 12-month increase in overall median survival. Despite these results, IP therapy has not yet been consistently adopted for the treatment of women with optimally debulked ovarian cancer in the United States and has not been widely adopted internationally. There are several reasons for this. First, IP therapy, as used in the reported trials, is technically demanding. Administration of paclitaxel over 24 hours, which has been used to reduce the neurotoxicity when paclitaxel is combined with cisplatin, is inconvenient and, if it requires hospitalization, expensive. Use of IP catheters is not routine in many oncology practices and is associated with a number of complications including intestinal injury, catheter blockage, and infections. Second, all of the large randomized studies used cisplatin in both the IP and intravenous arms, whereas carboplatin, which is less toxic and easier to administer, has become the standard intravenous platinum agent in the treatment of ovarian cancer. While IP carboplatin can be safely used and appears to have favorable pharmacokinetics (pharmacologic advantage combined with good systemic drug exposure), there is no clinical trial evidence that it will provide the same survival benefits as IP cisplatin. Finally, the heterogeneity and toxicity of the IP regimens used have left some confusion as to what the most important elements of the ideal IP therapy regimen are and which could be modified to improve safety and tolerability while maintaining efficacy. Despite these uncertainties, a potential 1-year survival advantage is

Table 10.6 Selected Randomized Trials of Intraperitoneal versus Intravenous Chemotherapy in Optimally Debulked Ovarian Cancers

Author (Year)	N	Regimens	Median PFS	Median OS	Comments
Alberts (1996)	546	IV cyclophosphamide 600 mg/m² + IP cisplatin 100 mg/m² × 6 vs. IV cyclophosphamide 600 mg/m² + IV cisplatin 100 mg/m² × 6	N/A	49 mo vs. 41 mo $p = 0.02$	<2 cm residual disease permitted; 58% of patients in both groups completed six cycles of cisplatin
Markman (2001)	462	IV carboplatin AUC 9 × 2 followed by IV paclitaxel 135 mg/m²/24 h + IP cisplatin 100 mg/m² × 6 vs. IV paclitaxel 135 mg/m²/24 h + IV cisplatin 75 mg/m² × 6	28 mo vs. 22 mo $p = 0.01$	63 mo vs. 52 mo $p = 0.05$	18% of patients on IP arm got ≤ 2 cycles of IP therapy
Armstrong (2006)	416	D1 IV paclitaxel 135 mg/m²/24 h + D2 IP cisplatin 100 mg/m² + D8 IP paclitaxel 60 mg/m² vs. D1 IV paclitaxel 135 mg/m²/24 h + D2 IV cisplatin 75 mg/m²	24 mo vs. 19 mo $p = 0.027$	67 mo vs. 50 mo $p = 0.0076$	49% of patients received ≤ 3 cycles of IP therapy

certainly meaningful, and the option of IP therapy should be discussed with healthy patients who have optimally debulked ovarian cancer. Ongoing trials may clarify the benefit of simplified, less toxic regimens.

Prolongation of Primary Therapy/Consolidation/Maintenance

Many women with ovarian cancer have an excellent response to first-line chemotherapy, but most will nonetheless relapse and die of their disease. Further therapy after a clinical complete remission would clearly be warranted if an effective treatment could be found. Strategies tested in randomized trials include whole-abdominal radiotherapy, IP P32, IP cisplatin, greater than six cycles of primary therapy, consolidation with a different agent such as topotecan or epirubicin, and high-dose chemotherapy with stem cell support. However, none of these approaches have produced any convincing survival benefit to date.

The most promising trial of maintenance therapy to date has been an SWOG/GOG trial, which randomized women in clinical complete remission to either 3 or 12 cycles of intravenous paclitaxel 175 mg/m^2 every 4 weeks. The trial was halted by its data and safety monitoring board after a planned interim efficacy analysis at a point when there was a statistically significant improvement in time to progression (PFS 28 months vs. 21 months) but no difference in overall survival between the treatment arms. A preliminary report on results of an Italian trial randomizing women in complete remission after frontline therapy to observation or 6 cycles of paclitaxel 175 mg/m^2 every 3 weeks showed no benefit in either progression-free or overall survival. The GOG is attempting to confirm the beneficial results it observed with a larger study randomizing women after clinical complete remission to 1 of 3 arms: no further therapy, paclitaxel 135 mg/m^2 every 4 weeks for 12 cycles, or Xyotax (a microparticle-bound paclitaxel) 135 mg/m^2 every 4 weeks for 12 cycles. This trial currently has overall survival as the end point and has completed accrual. Current treatment recommendations for women with advanced-stage fallopian tube carcinoma or primary peritoneal serous carcinomas are the same as for women with advanced-stage ovarian carcinomas.

Implications of Clear Cell and Mucinous Histology

Advanced clear cell carcinomas are unusual in the United States. Clear cell carcinoma is more common in Japan, where it accounts for about 20% of ovarian carcinomas. Even in Japan, early-stage clear cell carcinoma is more common than advanced-stage disease; in one review, stage I made up 51% of clear cell disease, stage II 13%, stage III 30%, and stage IV 6%. The implications of clear cell histology in early disease are not clear; in some reports, it seems to portend a high risk of recurrence, and in others, it appears to have little prognostic significance. However, it has become increasingly clear that advanced-stage clear cell tumors may not respond well to platinum chemotherapy. For example, the Hellenic Cooperative Oncology Group reviewed outcomes for women with an advanced clear cell carcinoma of the ovary treated on protocols from 1987 to 2003 ($n = 35$) and compared them to outcomes for women with serous tumors treated on the same trials. Response rates were 45% versus

81% ($p = 0.008$), and median survival was 25.1 months versus 49.1 months ($p = 0.141$). Clinical data regarding differential chemotherapy sensitivity to various agents of clear cell carcinomas are sparse and inconsistent. A multinational phase III study for stage I to IV clear cell carcinomas of the ovary has been launched by the Japanese Gynecologic Oncology Group. Women are randomized to therapy with either carboplatin/paclitaxel or cisplatin/irinotecan. It has also been hypothesized that antiangiogenic agents will benefit women with clear cell carcinomas, but this remains unproven. Interestingly, multiple reports suggest that women with clear cell carcinomas are more likely to have a thromboembolic event. Clear cell carcinomas may also be associated with hypercalcemia.

Early-stage mucinous tumors tend to be low grade and have a good prognosis. Advanced-stage mucinous tumors are uncommon in the United States and are difficult to distinguish from mucinous tumors metastatic from other sites. They respond poorly to chemotherapy and are associated with a short survival. Investigators from the Royal Marsden Hospital reviewed all patients with stage III or IV mucinous epithelial ovarian cancer ($n = 27$, 19 with measurable disease) treated with first-line platinum-based therapy at their unit between 1992 and 2001 and compared them to controls with nonmucinous epithelial ovarian cancer. The response rate for patients with measurable mucinous cancer was only 26%; 63% of patients experienced disease progression while on platinum-based chemotherapy. The response rate for the controls with measurable disease was 65%. Median overall survival was 12 months versus 37 months ($p < 0.001$). Specific trials are being developed for patients with advanced-stage mucinous tumors.

Second-Look Surgery

The term *second-look laparotomy/laparoscopy* refers to an abdominal procedure after chemotherapy to assess whether or not residual disease remains. At least half of patients in clinical complete remission with a normal CA-125 level will have residual disease at laparotomy. Second-look procedures used to be routine and provided important information about the natural history of ovarian cancer. However, although surgery is the most accurate way to assess the response to therapy, there is no evidence that any type of routine surgical procedure after initial chemotherapy prolongs overall survival or that any further therapy administered to patients with clinically inapparent residual disease will prolong survival. Moreover, even patients with negative second-look laparotomy have a 50% recurrence risk. This type of procedure is therefore no longer current standard of practice.

Follow-Up of Patients in Remission

Because of the high relapse risk, most patients with ovarian cancer who enter a clinical complete remission have been followed with a combination of pelvic examinations, computerized tomography (CT) scans, and monitoring of serum CA-125 levels. However, none of these have been shown to decrease symptoms or improve survival. Unlike the situation in general screening, rise in CA-125 after primary treatment for ovarian cancer is fairly specific, particularly if a confirmatory test is obtained. However, a randomized trial testing initiation of chemotherapy at the time of CA-125 rise versus at the time of clinical recurrence did not show any benefit in terms of survival or quality of life.

TREATMENT OF PERSISTENT/RECURRENT DISEASE

KEY POINTS

- Recurrent ovarian cancer is generally incurable, but patients who recur more than 6 months after completion of primary therapy may have significant benefit from further chemotherapy.
- Combination therapy produces higher response rates than single-agent chemotherapy in women with platinum-sensitive disease, but data regarding overall survival benefit are conflicting.
- The value of secondary debulking surgery is being tested in the clinical trial setting.

Second-Line Chemotherapy

Ovarian cancer that is resistant to primary chemotherapy or recurs at some point after primary chemotherapy is generally not curable. However, some patients benefit from further treatment, in particular those who relapse after a substantial disease-free interval. The GOG defines ovarian cancers with progression on platinum-based therapy as "platinum refractory," those that recur in less than 6 months after completion of platinum-based therapy as "platinum resistant," and those that recur in more than 6 months after completing treatment with a platinum-based regimen as "platinum sensitive" (short for "potentially platinum sensitive"). Women with primary platinum-refractory therapy have a very poor prognosis, and response to any subsequent treatment is unlikely. General principles of treating recurrent disease include the following:

1. Although platinum-sensitive tumors are more sensitive than platinum-resistant tumors to any cytotoxic agent tested to date, most data suggest that platinum compounds are the most active single agents in women with platinum-sensitive recurrent disease.
2. Platinum-based combinations of cytotoxic agents produce superior response rates and PFS compared with single-agent platinum therapy in women with platinum-sensitive disease; the effect on overall survival is less certain, and toxicity may be increased. In women with platinum-resistant disease, combination therapy is not of proven benefit.
3. No agents except possibly taxanes have consistently produced response rates over 20% in women with platinum-resistant disease.
4. Treatment must be recognized as primarily palliative, and decisions about treatment regimens should include patient convenience and toxicity as well as efficacy.

Platinum-Sensitive Disease

Several randomized trials comparing platinum-containing combinations including paclitaxel, gemcitabine, and liposomal doxorubicin to single-agent platinum therapy produce superior PFS to single-agent platinum therapy in the setting of platinum-sensitive disease. As a group, they show a superior response rate and superior PFS with combination therapy. Results regarding any benefit to overall survival are conflicting, and any such benefit is probably small. The addition of bevacizumab to a platinum doublet has demonstrated a 4-month benefit in PFS. Secondary debulking surgery has been hypothesized to be of benefit in this group, and a randomized trial testing this approach is underway.

Repeated courses of carboplatin-based therapy place patients at risk for hypersensitivity reactions. The incidence in patients treated with seven or more cycles of platinum-based therapy (typically the second dose of the second regimen) has been reported to be 27%. The reactions that occur during drug infusion are associated with flushing, nausea, and hypertension. A number of desensitization protocols have been published and appear to be generally effective; moreover, not all patients allergic to carboplatin will be allergic to cisplatin. However, the reactions are frightening and may be fatal, and desensitization protocols are time consuming for the patient and decrease the convenience of carboplatin therapy. Routine use of diphenhydramine premedication has been reported to produce a nonsignificant decrease in reaction rate.

Treatment of Platinum-Resistant Disease

Response rates to any conventional single-agent therapy in this group of women are 10% to 20%; median PFS is 3 to 4 months, and median overall survival is 9 to 12 months. A list of agents with some activity in the treatment of platinum-resistant recurrent ovarian cancer is shown in Table 10.7. At this time, pegylated liposomal doxorubicin is one of the agents commonly used in this setting, based on the ease of administration and tolerable toxicity. The addition of bevacizumab to single-agent salvage

Table 10.7	Agents in Treatment of Platinum-Resistant Ovarian Cancer
Bevacizumab	
Docetaxel	
Epirubicin	
p.o. Etoposide	
Gemcitabine	
Ifosfamide	
Tamoxifen	
Weekly paclitaxel	
Topotecan	
Vinorelbine	
Pegylated liposomal doxorubicin	
Irinotecan	

chemotherapy has demonstrated approximately a 3-month benefit in PFS with a 2% rate of bowel perforation.

Hormonal therapies, such as tamoxifen, have also been tested. Response rates to hormonal treatment by modern standards are hard to gauge, as most of the trials are quite old; however, it does appear that selected patients, perhaps those with borderline tumors, may respond, and toxicities are minimal. Antiangiogenic agents appear promising in the treatment of ovarian cancer. None, including bevacizumab, an anti-VEGF monoclonal antibody that has produced single-agent response rates in the range 15% to 20% in the treatment of ovarian cancer, are currently FDA approved for the treatment of ovarian cancer. All are exceedingly expensive, and bevacizumab has been associated with a number of toxicities, including an increased number of bowel perforations.

SUGGESTED READINGS

Alberts DS, Liu PY, Hannigan EV, et al. Intraperitoneal cisplatin plus intravenous cyclophosphamide versus intravenous cisplatin plus intravenous cyclophosphamide for stage III ovarian cancer. *N Engl J Med.* 1996;335:1950–1955.

Bell J, Brady MF, Young RC, et al. Randomized phase III trial of three versus six cycles of adjuvant carboplatin and paclitaxel in early stage epithelial ovarian carcinoma: A Gynecologic Oncology Group study. *Gynecol Oncol.* 2006;102:432–439.

Buys SS, Partridge E, Greene MH, et al. Ovarian cancer screening in the Prostate, Lung, Colorectal and Ovarian (PLCO) cancer screening trial: Findings from the initial screen of a randomized trial. *Am J Obstet Gynecol.* 2005;193:1630–1639.

Eisenhauer EA, Vermorken JB, van Glabbeke M. Predictors of response to subsequent chemotherapy in platinum pretreated ovarian cancer: A multivariate analysis of 704 patients. *Ann Oncol.* 1997;8:963–968.

Markman M, Liu PY, Wilczynski S, et al. Phase III randomized trial of 12 versus 3 months of maintenance paclitaxel in patients with advanced ovarian cancer after complete response to platinum and paclitaxel-based chemotherapy: A Southwest Oncology Group and Gynecologic Oncology Group trial. *J Clin Oncol.* 2003;21:2460–2465.

Markman M, Rothman R, Hakes T, et al. Second-line platinum therapy in patients with ovarian cancer previously treated with cisplatin. *J Clin Oncol.* 1991;9:389–393.

McGuire WP, Hoskins WJ, Brady MF, et al. Cyclophosphamide and cisplatin compared with paclitaxel and cisplatin in patients with stage III and stage IV ovarian cancer. *N Engl J Med.* 1996;334:1–6.

Medeiros F, Muto MG, Lee Y, et al. The tubal fimbria is a preferred site for early adenocarcinoma in women with familial ovarian cancer syndrome. *Am J Surg Pathol.* 2006;30:230–236.

Rubin SC, Benjamin I, Behbakht K, et al. Clinical and pathological features of ovarian cancer in women with germ-line mutations of BRCA1. *N Engl J Med.* 1996;335:1413–1416.

Seidman JD, Kurman RJ. Ovarian serous borderline tumors: A critical review of the literature with emphasis on prognostic indicators. *Hum Pathol.* 2000;31:539–557.

Trimble CL, Kosary C, Trimble EL. Long-term survival and patterns of care in women with ovarian tumors of low malignant potential. *Gynecol Oncol.* 2002;86:34–37.

Trimble EL. NCI Clinical Announcement on Intraperitoneal Chemotherapy in Ovarian Cancer (January 5, 2006); 2006. http://ctep.cancer.gov/highlights/ovarian.html. Accessed March 1, 2009.

van der Burg ME, van Lent M, Buyse M, et al. The effect of debulking surgery after induction chemotherapy on the prognosis in advanced epithelial ovarian cancer. Gynecological Cancer Cooperative Group of the European Organization for Research and Treatment of Cancer. *N Engl J Med.* 1995;332:629–634.

van Nagell JR Jr, DePriest PD, Puls LE, et al. Ovarian cancer screening in asymptomatic postmenopausal women by transvaginal sonography. *Cancer.* 1991;68:458–462.

Whittemore AS, Harris R, Itnyre J. Characteristics relating to ovarian cancer risk: Collaborative analysis of 12 US case–control studies. II. Invasive epithelial ovarian cancers in white women. Collaborative Ovarian Cancer Group. *Am J Epidemiol.* 1992;136:1184–1203.

Nonepithelial Ovarian Cancer

PATHOLOGY

KEY POINTS

- Nonepithelial ovarian cancers predominantly consist of germ cell tumors and sex cord–stromal tumors.
- The most common malignant germ cell tumors in females are (i) dysgerminomas, (ii) endodermal sinus tumors, and (iii) immature teratomas (ITs).
- Ovarian sex cord–stromal tumors are associated with endocrinologic abnormalities with granulosa cell, theca cell, and Sertoli cell tumors predominantly estrogenic, and Sertoli–Leydig cell tumors androgenic.

Germ Cell Tumors

The current World Health Organization classification of ovarian germ cell tumors includes dysgerminoma, yolk sac tumor (endodermal sinus tumors), embryonal carcinoma, polyembryoma, nongestational choriocarcinoma, mixed germ cell tumors, and teratomas (immature, mature, and monodermal types).

Dysgerminoma

Dysgerminoma represents the most common ovarian malignant germ cell tumor. Most dysgerminomas are seen in patients with a normal karyotype, but it is the most frequent neoplasm in patients with gonadal dysgenesis. Clinically, they tend to present as abdominal enlargement, a mass, or pain due to torsion. About 10% of dysgerminomas are bilateral on gross examination and another 10% have microscopic involvement of the contralateral ovary.

On gross examination, dysgerminomas are usually large, white to gray, fleshy lobulated masses. At surgery, abundant hemorrhage, necrosis, or cystic areas in a well-fixed tumor should raise the question of a mixed germ cell tumor. Microscopically, dysgerminomas display nests and cords of primitive-appearing germ cells with clear to eosinophilic cytoplasm and prominent cytoplasmic borders. The number of mitotic figures does not have any therapeutic or prognostic significance.

Dysgerminomas contain cytoplasmic glycogen that can be demonstrated with a periodic acid–Schiff stain. In addition, they stain diffusely for placenta-like alkaline phosphatase (PLAP). Because dysgerminoma is the only ovarian germ cell tumor that displays c-kit staining, positive stains for this marker (and nuclear transcription factor OCT3/4) can also help to confirm the diagnosis. Tumors may also stain positively for human chorionic gonadotropin (hCG) due to the presence of syncytiotrophoblast cells within these tumors. Poor fixation can result in artifacts that mimic embryonal carcinoma and yolk sac tumor histology.

Yolk Sac Tumor

Yolk sac tumor (endodermal sinus tumor) is the second most common ovarian germ cell tumor. These tumors grow very rapidly, often becoming clinically evident acutely. Yolk sac tumors are typically large and unilateral, with a smooth external surface. On cut section, these neoplasms are tan to gray, with abundant hemorrhage and necrosis. They may be partially solid, but they usually contain cysts that vary in size from a few millimeters to several centimeters in diameter. The cut surface appears mucoid, slimy, or gelatinous. Yolk sac tumors display many different histologic patterns. The most common is the reticular or microcystic pattern. The tumor has a meshlike pattern, and it displays a network of flattened or cuboidal epithelial cells with varying degrees of atypia. The endodermal sinus (festoon) pattern contains Schiller-Duvall bodies (Fig. 11.1), which have a central capillary surrounded by connective tissue and a peripheral layer of columnar cells. When present, Schiller-Duvall bodies are diagnostic of yolk sac tumor. Yolk sac tumors generally, though not always, display cytoplasmic staining for cytokeratin and α-fetoprotein (AFP).

Embryonal Carcinoma

Embryonal carcinoma is rarely seen in the ovary. On gross examination, embryonal carcinoma characteristically displays areas of hemorrhage and necrosis. Microscopically, this tumor is composed of very crowded cells that display overlapping nuclei in paraffin sections. The nuclei are very pleomorphic, and they contain large, prominent nucleoli. The mitotic rate

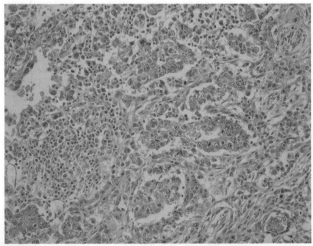

FIGURE 11.1 Schiller-Duvall bodies, papillary structures with central blood vessels, are seen in the endodermal sinus pattern of yolk sac tumor.

is high in these tumors. Glandular, solid, and papillary patterns may be seen. Vascular invasion is common. Embryonal carcinoma stains positively for PLAP, pancytokeratin (AE1/AE3 and CAM 5.2), CD30, and OCT3/4. Some embryonal carcinomas display focal AFP positivity that may represent partial transformation to yolk sac tumor. Syncytiotrophoblast cells may be present, resulting in positive stains for hCG.

Polyembryoma

Polyembryoma is a very rare malignant ovarian tumor. In the few cases reported, the embryoid bodies characteristic of this germ cell tumor have coexisted with other germ cell tumor types. The microscopic appearance of embryoid bodies with an embryonic disc separating a yolk sac and an amniotic cavity may actually be due to an admixture of yolk sac tumor and embryonal carcinoma.

Choriocarcinoma

Primary nongestational ovarian choriocarcinoma is rare. It is most often seen as a component of mixed germ cell tumors of the ovary. Choriocarcinomas display abundant hemorrhage and necrosis on gross examination. Microscopically, these neoplasms show a plexiform pattern composed of an admixture of syncytiotrophoblast and cytotrophoblast cells. Numerous mitoses are usually easily identified in the histologic specimen. These tumors produce hCG due to the presence of syncytiotrophoblast cells. Choriocarcinoma may also stain for cytokeratins, epithelial membrane antigen, and carcinoembryonic antigen. Nongestational choriocarcinoma must be distinguished from gestational choriocarcinoma because the former has a worse prognosis and requires more aggressive therapy. The identification of paternal genetic material indicates that the tumor is of gestational origin.

Mixed Germ Cell Tumors

Mixed germ cell tumors of the ovary contain two or more different types of germ cell neoplasm, either intimately admixed or as separate foci within the tumor. They are much less common in the ovary than in the testis, accounting for only about 8% of malignant ovarian germ cell tumors.

The diagnosis and prognosis of malignant mixed germ cell tumors depend on adequate tumor sampling in order to detect small areas of different types of germ cell tumor because the types of tumor identified may affect therapy and prognosis.

Teratomas

Teratomas are germ cell tumors that contain tissue derived from two or three embryonic layers. Teratomas are subclassified according to whether the tumor elements represent mature or immature tissue types. In addition, some teratomas are composed of a predominance of one tissue type such as thyroid tissue (struma ovarii).

Most teratomas are mature cystic teratomas that contain differentiated tissue components such as skin, cartilage, glia, glandular elements, and bone. Any tissue type present in adults may be represented in teratomas. Mature cystic teratomas represent benign neoplasms unless they contain a somatic malignancy such as squamous carcinoma, papillary thyroid carcinoma, or other non–germ cell tumors arising in differentiated elements of the teratoma.

ITs in adult women, in contrast to mature cystic teratomas, are uncommon tumors. They represent only about 3% of all ovarian teratomas, but ITs are the third most common form of malignant ovarian germ cell tumors.

Most immature ovarian teratomas are unilateral, although they can metastasize to the opposite ovary and can also be associated with mature teratoma in the opposite ovary. They are predominantly solid tumors, but they may contain some cystic areas. The cut surface of an IT is soft and fleshy in appearance. Areas of hemorrhage and necrosis are common. Microscopically, these tumors contain a variety of mature and immature tissue components. The immature elements almost always consist of immature neural tissue in the form of small round blue cells focally organized into rosettes and tubules (Fig. 11.2). There is a correlation between the disease prognosis and the degree of immaturity in the teratoma.

A three-tiered grading system is still the one most often used:

- Grade 1 neoplasms display some immaturity, but the immature neural tissue does not exceed in aggregate the area of one low-power field (40×) in any slide.
- Grade 2 teratomas contain more immaturity, but immature neural tissue occupies no more than an area equal to three low-power fields in any slide.
- Grade 3 neoplasms contain immature neural tissue that occupies an area greater than three low-power fields in at least one slide.

The amount of mitotic activity and immature neural tissue (characterized as rosettes and tubules) increases with increasing tumor grade. In patients whose neoplasm has disseminated beyond the ovary, the grade of the tumor metastasis is important in predicting survival and determining treatment. Occasionally, patients may have peritoneal implants that contain only mature tissue, but these mature glial implants may represent host tissue and not actual tumor

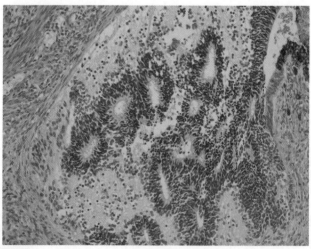

FIGURE 11.2 Ovarian IT. Immature neural tissue forms tubules.

implants. It is extremely important to sample peritoneal disease thoroughly in order that foci of IT (that may coexist with mature glia) are identified.

Sex Cord–Stromal Tumors

The current World Health Organization classification of ovarian sex cord–stromal tumors includes granulosa cell tumors, thecomas, fibromas, sclerosing stromal cell tumors, Sertoli cell tumors, Sertoli–Leydig cell tumors, sex cord tumors with annular tubules, gynandroblastomas, and steroid cell tumors.

Granulosa Cell Tumors

Granulosa cell tumors comprise 5% of all ovarian malignancies, but account for approximately 70% of malignant sex cord–stromal tumors. The peak incidence for these tumors occurs during the perimenopausal decade. They are subdivided into adult type and juvenile type.

The majority of patients with adult-type granulosa cell tumors present with one or a combination of the following clinical findings: abnormal vaginal bleeding, abdominal distention, and abdominal pain. The endocrine function of adult-type granulosa cell tumors, specifically the production of estrogens, has been demonstrated by assessments of the end organ, the endometrium, and measurements of peripheral levels of estrogen. Adult-type granulosa cell tumors have an average diameter of 12 cm. They are predominately cystic, with numerous loculi filled with fluid or blood and separated by solid tissue. The solid tissue may be gray-white or yellow and soft or firm. Microscopic examination reveals a population of granulosa cells often with an additional component of theca cells, fibroblasts, or both. In well-differentiated tumors, the granulosa cells have a microfollicular pattern characterized by numerous small cavities (Call-Exner bodies).

Approximately 90% of the granulosa cell tumors diagnosed in prepubertal girls and women less than 30 years of age will be of the juvenile type. The majority of prepubertal patients present with clinical evidence of isosexual precocious pseudopuberty. Serum estradiol levels are reported as increased in these cases with pseudopuberty. The appearance of juvenile-type granulosa cell tumors is similar to the adult form: a solid and cystic neoplasm in which cysts contain hemorrhagic fluid. Microscopic examination typically reveals a predominately solid cellular tumor with focal follicle formation. Call-Exner bodies are rarely encountered.

Thecoma

Theca cell tumors, or thecomas, are composed of lipid-laden stromal cells, occasionally demonstrating luteinization, and are almost invariably clinically benign. Thecomas account for approximately 1% of ovarian neoplasms. The primary presenting signs and symptoms are abnormal vaginal bleeding and/or pelvic mass. Thecomas are considered to be among the most hormonally active of the sex cord–stromal tumors.

Fibroma–Fibrosarcoma

Fibromas are the most commonly encountered sex cord–stromal tumor, accounting for approximately 4% of all ovarian neoplasms. These endocrine-inert tumors are seldom bilateral and vary in size. As their size increases, fibromas tend to become more edematous, leading to the escape of increasing quantities of fluid from the tumor surfaces. Ascites is detected with 10% to 15% of ovarian fibromas exceeding 10 cm. Furthermore, 1% of patients develop a hydrothorax in addition to hydroperitoneum (Meigs syndrome).

Ovarian fibromas are generally benign, but 10% will demonstrate increased cellularity and varying degrees of pleomorphism and mitotic activity. Fibromatous tumors characterized histologically by an increased cellular density and brisk mitotic activity are considered to be of low malignant potential. In contrast, fibrosarcomas are highly malignant neoplasms distinguished by their greater cellular density and marked pleomorphism.

Sclerosing Stromal Tumors

Accounting for less than 5% of sex cord–stromal tumors, sclerosing stromal cell tumors are a rare tumor characteristically different from both thecomas and fibromas. Histologically, the presence of pseudolobulation of cellular areas separated by edematous connective tissue, increased vascularity, and prominent areas of sclerosis are distinguishing features. The signs and symptoms that most commonly necessitate medical evaluation include menstrual irregularities and/or pelvic pain.

Sertoli Cell Tumors

Sertoli cell tumors are rare. Evidence of estrogen production is observed in approximately two thirds of cases. Consistent with estrogen excess, isosexual precocious puberty has been witnessed during the first decade of life, menstrual disorders during the reproductive decades, and postmenopausal bleeding in the decades after the climacteric. These rare tumors are typically solid, lobulated, and yellow.

Sertoli–Leydig Tumors

Sertoli–Leydig tumors are extremely uncommon, accounting for less than 0.2% of all ovarian tumors. As implied by their designation, the tumors contain both Sertoli and Leydig cell elements. The average patient age at diagnosis is approximately 25 years old. The most frequent complaints at the time of presentation are menstrual disorders, virilization, and nonspecific symptoms resulting from abdominal mass. Frank virilization occurs in 35% of the patients with Sertoli–Leydig cell tumors, and another 10% to 15% have some clinical manifestations consistent with androgen excess. The majority of these tumors are solid, often yellow, and lobulated. Well-differentiated Sertoli–Leydig cell tumors are characterized by a predominately tubular pattern. A nodular architecture is often conspicuous, with fibrous bands intersecting lobules composed of small, round, hollow, or—less often—solid tubules, separated by Leydig cells.

Sex Cord Tumor with Annular Tubules

These unique ovarian tumors are characterized by either simple or complex ring-shaped tubules, giving them the morphologic designation ovarian sex cord tumor with annular tubules. The distinctive cellular elements of these neoplasms are judged to be histologically representative of an intermediate between Sertoli cell tumors and granulosa cell tumors. Approximately one in three sex cord tumors with annular tubules occurs in association with Peutz-Jeghers syndrome. Abnormal vaginal bleeding is the most common presenting complaint, including menstrual irregularities during the reproductive era and postmenopausal bleeding during the mature years.

Gynandroblastoma

Gynandroblastoma is an extremely rare sex cord–stromal tumor. Microscopically these tumors must demonstrate readily identifiable granulosa cells and tubules of Sertoli cells. Patients present at an average age of 29.5 years with primary symptoms of menstrual disturbances consistent with the predominant functional status of the tumor.

Steroid Cell Tumors

Steroid cell tumors constitute only 0.1% of all ovarian neoplasms. The predominant components of these tumors are steroid hormone–secreting cells including lutein cells, Leydig cells, and adrenocortical cells. Steroid cell tumors are stratified into subclasses based on their hormone secretion.

Stromal luteomas are relatively small (<3 cm) tumors localized within the parenchyma of the ovary, accounting for approximately 25% of steroid cell tumors. Eighty percent occur after the climacterium. The predominant functional profile is estrogenic, with abnormal vaginal bleeding being the primary complaint.

Leydig cell tumors account for 15% to 20% of steroid cell tumors. Histologically, the cellular elements are indistinguishable from lutein cells or adrenocortical cells except for the presence of crystals of Reinke. The initial clinical manifestations are usually consistent with a hyperandrogenic state. Overt signs of virilization are observed in over 80% of the patients.

Neoplasms identified as steroid cell tumors but lacking the specific characteristics of stromal luteomas or Leydig cell tumors are collectively classified as *steroid cell tumors not otherwise specified*. These generally solid yellow tumors are larger than other steroid cell tumors, with a higher frequency of bilaterality. Clinical signs and/or symptoms of androgen excess ranging from heterosexual precocity in prepubertal girls to amenorrhea, hirsutism, and virilization during the reproductive and postmenopausal ages prompt the majority of patients to seek medical advice.

CLINICAL FEATURES OF GERM CELL TUMORS

KEY POINTS

- Germ cell tumors account for 2% to 3% of all ovarian cancers and usually occur in girls or young women.
- Most patients present with stage I disease.
- hCG and AFP are useful tumor markers for some subsets of germ cell tumors.

Abdominal pain associated with a palpable pelvic–abdominal mass is present in approximately 85% of patients with germ cell tumors. Approximately 10% of patients present with acute abdominal pain, usually caused by rupture, hemorrhage, or ovarian torsion. This finding is somewhat more common in patients with endodermal sinus tumor or mixed germ cell tumors. Less common signs and symptoms include abdominal distention (35%), fever (10%), and vaginal bleeding (10%). A few patients exhibit isosexual precocity, presumably due to hCG production by tumor cells.

Many germ cell tumors possess the unique property of producing biologic markers that are detectable in serum. The development of specific

Table 11.1	Serum Tumor Markers in Malignant Germ Cell Tumors of the Ovary	
Histology	AFP	hCG
Dysgerminoma	−	±
Endodermal sinus tumor	+	−
IT	±	−
Mixed germ cell tumor	±	±
Choriocarcinoma	−	+
Embryonal carcinoma	±	+
Polyembryoma	±	+

and sensitive radioimmunoassay techniques to measure hCG and AFP led to dramatic improvement in patient monitoring. Serial measurements of serum markers aid the diagnosis and, more importantly, are useful for monitoring response to treatment and detection of subclinical recurrences. Table 11.1 illustrates typical findings in the sera of patients with various tumor histologic types. Endodermal sinus tumor and choriocarcinoma are prototypes for AFP and hCG production, respectively. Embryonal carcinoma can secrete both hCG and AFP, but most commonly produces hCG. Mixed tumors may produce either, both, or none of the markers, depending on the type and quantity of elements present. Dysgerminoma is commonly devoid of hormonal production, although a small percentage of tumors produce low levels of hCG. The presence of an elevated level of AFP or high level of hCG (>100 U/mL) denotes the presence of tumor elements other than dysgerminoma. Therapy should be adjusted accordingly. Although ITs are associated with negative markers, a few tumors can produce AFP. A third tumor marker is lactic dehydrogenase, which is frequently elevated in patients with dysgerminoma or other germ cell tumors. Unfortunately, it is less specific than hCG or AFP, which limits its usefulness. CA-125 can also be nonspecifically elevated in patients with ovarian germ cell tumors.

CLINICAL FEATURES OF SEX CORD–STROMAL TUMORS

KEY POINTS

- The sex cord–stromal tumors account for approximately 7% of all ovarian neoplasms.
- The majority of these tumors are benign or of low malignant potential and are associated with a favorable long-term prognosis.
- With the exception of fibromas, the clinical presentation of patients with sex cord–stromal tumors is frequently governed by their clinical manifestation resulting from endocrinologic abnormalities.

Adult granulosa cell tumors are low-grade malignancies with propensity to remain localized and demonstrate indolent growth. Ninety percent are diagnosed at stage I. For patients who recur, the median time to recurrence is 6 years, and the median survival after recurrence is 5.6 years. Serum estrogens are generally produced by granulosa cell tumors and have been utilized as an indicator of disease status. Although the adult form frequently includes a latency period, the juvenile counterpart is characteristically aggressive in advanced stages, and the time to relapse is generally within 3 years of initial diagnosis.

Ovarian thecomas, fibromas, and sclerosing stromal cells tumors are considered to be benign neoplasms, and any associated morbidity or mortality is attributable to the treatment modalities or the sequelae of concurrent disease. The prognosis for patients with cellular fibromas is generally quite favorable. Fibrosarcomas are associated with an extremely poor prognosis.

The great majority of Sertoli cell tumors are well differentiated, and only rare tumors are malignant. Excision of the tumor results in prompt resolution of the hyperestrogenic state.

Only 2% to 3% of Sertoli–Leydig cell tumors have demonstrable extra-ovarian spread at the time of detection. The more favorable prognosis reflects the abrupt onset of androgenic manifestations that promote prompt medical assessment. Nevertheless, the natural history of the malignant variant includes early recurrences, with approximately two thirds becoming evident within 1 year of treatment and only 6% to 7% recurring after 5 years.

The difference in the natural history and, hence, long-term prognosis of sex cord tumor with annular tubules associated with Peutz-Jeghers syndrome and those independent of Peutz-Jeghers syndrome are readily apparent. Those detected in women with Peutz-Jeghers syndrome are benign. Patients with sex cord tumor with annular feature without Peutz-Jeghers syndrome have a clinical malignancy rate of approximately 20%. The tumor characteristically has a relatively long doubling time, a propensity for lymphatic dissemination, and an aptness to remain lateralized.

SURGERY

KEY POINTS

- A substantial majority of patients with ovarian germ cell tumors and sex cord–stromal tumors are long-term survivors and suffer minimal morbidity from treatment.
- Surgery remains the cornerstone of treatment.
- Fertility-sparing surgery procedures enable a large proportion of young women with early-stage disease to preserve their reproductive potential.
- Secondary cytoreduction may be important for women whose tumors contain IT.

Operative Findings

Malignant germ cell tumors of the ovary tend to be quite large at the time these patients go to surgery. Bilaterality of tumor involvement is exceedingly rare except for dysgerminoma. Ascites may be noted in approximately 20% of cases. Rupture of tumors, either preoperatively or intraoperatively, can occur in approximately 20% of cases.

Benign cystic teratoma is associated with malignant germ cell tumors in 5% to 10% of cases. These coexistent teratomas may occur in the ipsilateral ovary, in the contralateral ovary, or bilaterally. Likewise, a preexisting gonadoblastoma may be noted in association with dysgerminoma and dysgenetic gonads related to a 46,XY karyotype.

Malignant germ cell tumors generally spread in one of two ways: along the peritoneal surface or through lymphatic dissemination. They more commonly metastasize to lymph nodes than epithelial tumors. The stage distribution is also very different from that of epithelial tumors. In most large series, approximately 60% to 70% of tumors will be stage I, with stage III accounting for 25% to 30% of tumors. Stages II and IV are relatively uncommon.

Extent of Primary Surgery

The initial treatment approach for a patient suspected of having a nonepithelial ovarian tumor is surgery, both for diagnosis and for therapy. A thorough determination of disease extent by inspection and palpation should be made. If the disease is confined to one or both ovaries, it is imperative that proper staging biopsies be performed (see Surgical Staging section, below).

The type of primary operative procedure depends upon the surgical findings. Because many of these patients are young women, for whom the preservation of fertility is a priority, minimizing the surgical resection while ensuring the removal of tumor bulk must be thoughtfully balanced. As noted previously, bilateral ovarian involvement is rare, except for the case of pure dysgerminoma. Bilateral involvement may be found in cases of advanced disease (stages II to IV), in which there is metastasis from one ovary to the opposite gonad. Therefore, fertility-sparing unilateral salpingo-oophorectomy with preservation of the contralateral ovary and of the uterus can be performed in most patients. If the contralateral ovary appears grossly normal on careful inspection, it should be left undisturbed. However, in the case of pure dysgerminoma, biopsy may be considered because occult or microscopic tumor involvement occurs in a small percentage of patients. Unnecessary biopsy may result in future infertility due to peritoneal adhesions or ovarian failure. If the contralateral ovary appears abnormally enlarged, a biopsy or ovarian cystectomy should be performed. If frozen examination reveals a dysgenetic gonad, or if there are clinical indications suggesting a hermaphrodite phenotype, then bilateral salpingo-oophorectomy is indicated. It is difficult to establish this diagnosis on frozen section; therefore, this determination should be made by determining a normal female karyotype preoperatively. If benign cystic teratoma is found in the contralateral ovary, an event that can occur in 5% to 10% of patients, then ovarian cystectomy with the preservation of remaining normal ovarian tissue is recommended.

The advent of *in vitro* fertilization technology has had an impact on operative management. Convention has dictated that if a bilateral salpingo-oophorectomy is necessary, a hysterectomy should also be performed. However, with current assisted reproduction technologies (ART) involving donor oocyte and hormonal support, a woman without ovaries could potentially sustain a normal intrauterine pregnancy. Similarly, if the uterus and one ovary are resected because of tumor involvement, current techniques provide the opportunity for oocyte retrieval from the remaining ovary, *in vitro* fertilization with sperm from her male partner, and embryo implantation into a surrogate's uterus. As the field of ART is evolving, traditional guidelines concerning surgical treatment in young patients with gynecologic tumors have to be thoughtfully adapted to individual circumstances.

Surgical Staging

Surgical staging information is essential for determining the extent of disease, providing prognostic information, and guiding postoperative management. It is of critical importance for those patients with early clinical disease in order to detect the presence of occult or microscopic metastases. Staging of nonepithelial ovarian tumors follows the same principles applicable to epithelial ovarian tumors, as described by the International Federation of Gynecologists and Obstetricians (FIGO, see Table 11.2). Proper staging procedures consist of the following:

1. Although a transverse incision is cosmetically superior, a vertical midline incision is usually necessary for adequate exposure, appropriate staging biopsies, and resection of large pelvic tumors or metastatic disease in the upper abdomen.
2. Ascites, if present, should be evacuated and submitted for cytologic analysis. If no peritoneal fluid is noted, cytologic washings of the pelvis and bilateral paracolic gutters should be performed prior to manipulation of the intraperitoneal contents.
3. The entire peritoneal cavity and its structures should be carefully inspected and palpated in a methodical manner. The subdiaphragmatic areas, omentum, colon, all peritoneal surfaces, the entire retroperitoneum, and small intestinal serosa and mesentery should be checked. If any suspicious areas are noted, they should be submitted for biopsy or excised.
4. Next, the primary ovarian tumor and pelvis should be examined. Both ovaries should be assessed for size, presence of obvious tumor involvement, capsular rupture, external excrescences, or adherence to surrounding structures.
5. If disease seems to be limited, that is, confined to the ovary or localized to the pelvis, then random staging biopsies of structures at risk should be performed. These sites should include the omentum (with generous biopsies from multiple areas) and the peritoneal surfaces of the following sites: bilateral paracolic gutters, cul-de-sac, lateral pelvic walls, vesicouterine reflection, and subdiaphragmatic areas. Any adhesions should also be generously sampled.
6. The para-aortic and bilateral pelvic lymph node–bearing areas should be carefully palpated. Any suspicious nodes should be excised or sampled. If no suspicious areas are detected, these areas should be sampled. There is no evidence that a complete para-aortic or pelvic lymphadenectomy is advantageous.
7. If obvious gross metastatic disease is present, it should be excised if feasible, or at least sampled to document disease extent. The concept of cytoreductive surgery is discussed below.

Table 11.2	FIGO Staging of Ovarian Germ Cell Tumors

Stage	Description

I	Tumor limited to ovaries
	IA: Tumor limited to one ovary, intact capsule, no tumor on surface, negative washings
	IB: Tumor involves both ovaries, otherwise like IA
	IC: Tumor limited to 1 or both ovary with one of the following
	  IC1: Surgical spill
	  IC2: Capsule rupture before surgery or tumor on ovarian surface
	  IC3: Malignant cells in the ascites or peritoneal washings

II	Tumor involving one or both ovaries with extension to the pelvis IIA: Extension and/or implant on the uterus and/or fallopian tubes IIB: Extension to other pelvic intraperitoneal tissues

III	Tumor involving one or both ovaries with tumor implants outside the pelvis or with positive retroperitoneal or inguinal lymph nodes. Superficial liver metastases qualify as stage III
	IIIA: Positive retroperitoneal lymph nodes and/or microscopic metastasis beyond the pelvis
	  IIIA1(i) Metastasis ≤ 10 mm
	  IIIA1(ii) Metastasis > 10 mm
	  IIIA2 Microscopic, extrapelvic (above the brim) peritoneal involvement ± positive retroperitoneal lymph nodes
	IIIB: Macroscopic, extrapelvic, peritoneal metastasis ≤ 2 cm ± positive retroperitoneal lymph nodes. Includes extension to capsule of the liver/spleen
	IIIC: Macroscopic, extrapelvic, peritoneal metastasis > 2 cm ± positive retroperitoneal lymph nodes. Includes extension to capsule of the liver/spleen

IV	Distant metastasis IVA: Pleural effusion with positive cytology IVB: Hepatic and/or splenic parenchymal metastasis, metastasis to extra-abdominal organs (including inguinal lymph nodes and lymph nodes outside of the abdominal cavity)

Source: Adapted from FIGO Committee on Gynecologic Oncology. Current FIGO staging for cancer of the vagina, fallopian tube, ovary, and gestational trophoblastic neoplasia. *Int J Gynaecol Obstet* 2009;105:3–4, with permission.

Most patients still undergo initial surgery in community hospitals and are inadequately staged. Upon referral of such a patient to a university or tertiary care center, the oncologist is faced with the dilemma of inadequate staging information. In such cases, postoperative studies including computed tomography of the abdomen are recommended. If histopathologic and limited anatomic information from the first surgery clearly indicates the use of systemic chemotherapy, it is generally inadvisable to consider reexploration solely for the purpose of precise staging information. Reoperation to complete comprehensive staging may be appropriate under clinical circumstances where careful surveillance observation after complete staging may be a sensible alternative to chemotherapy.

Cytoreductive Surgery

If widely spread tumor is encountered at initial surgery, it is recommended that the same principles concerning primary cytoreductive surgery applied in the surgical management of advanced epithelial ovarian cancer be followed. As much tumor should be resected as is technically feasible and safe. It is clear that patients with completely resected disease do better than those with bulky postoperative residual disease. However, as with epithelial tumors, the relative influence of tumor biology, surgical skill, and aggressiveness remain uncertain. Germ cell tumors, especially dysgerminomas, are generally much more chemosensitive than epithelial ovarian tumors. Therefore, aggressive resection of metastatic disease in these cases is questionable. Even in the face of extensive metastatic disease, it is generally possible to perform a fertility-sparing procedure with preservation of a normal contralateral ovary.

The value of secondary cytoreductive surgery in the management of non-epithelial ovarian tumors is even less clear than that of primary cytoreductive surgery. The finding of a residual mass after completion of chemotherapy is less common in patients with ovarian germ cell tumors than in men with testis cancer, because the women are likely to have considerable tumor debulking at the time of the diagnostic surgical procedure and thus enter chemotherapy with significantly less tumor burden. In patients with bulky dysgerminoma, residual masses after chemotherapy are very likely to represent desmoplastic fibrosis. Although a number of patients with pure ovarian ITs or mixed germ cell tumors have persistent mature teratoma at the completion of chemotherapy, the majority are left with multiple small peritoneal implants rather than with a dominant mass. However, occasional patients who have received chemotherapy for IT or mixed germ cell tumor containing teratoma will have bulky residual teratoma after chemotherapy. The natural history or biologic implications of this finding are not clear. Mature teratoma is not chemotherapy sensitive. Considering this information, it seems appropriate to resect persistent masses in patients with negative markers after chemotherapy for germ cell tumors containing IT. If viable malignant neoplasm is found, additional chemotherapy should be considered. However, if only mature teratoma is resected, observation is generally recommended. Repeat cytoreduction for patients with sex cord–stromal tumors frequently affords these patients extended palliation.

CHEMOTHERAPY FOR OVARIAN GERM CELL TUMORS

KEY POINTS

- The risk of relapse with surgery alone is unacceptably high for most women with germ cell tumors. Therefore, chemotherapy using a platinum-based regimen is recommended for most patients. Exceptions to this include stage IA grade I IT and stage IA and IB dysgerminomas.
- The current standard of care is to administer three to four cycles of bleomycin, etoposide, and cisplatin.
- Dysgerminomas are particularly chemotherapy sensitive.

Chemotherapy

Presently, the overwhelming majority of patients with ovarian germ cell tumors survive their disease with the judicious use of surgery and cisplatin-based combination chemotherapy. Based on promising results obtained in men with testicular cancer, a prospective Gynecologic Oncology Group (GOG) study that evaluated bleomycin, etoposide, and cisplatin (BEP) was performed in patients with ovarian germ cell tumors. The regimen was highly effective, with 91 of 93 enrolled patients free of disease at follow-up. Although randomized trials have not been feasible, these data (and others from single-institution and retrospective studies) have led to the widespread adoption of BEP for these patients.

Management of Residual or Recurrent Disease

The large majority of patients with ovarian germ cell tumors are cured with surgery and platinum-based chemotherapy. However, a small percentage of patients have persistent or progressive disease during treatment or recur after the completion of treatment. As in testicular cancer, these treatment failures are categorized as platinum resistant (progression during or within 4 to 6 weeks of completing treatment) or platinum sensitive (recurrence beyond 6 weeks from platinum-based therapy).

The management of recurrent disease is complex and is preferably performed in a specialized center. Data to guide the management of patients with recurrent ovarian germ cell tumors are scant and largely extrapolated from the clinical experience with testicular cancer. In general, options include an alternative platinum-based regimen (such as vinblastine, ifosfamide, and plus cisplatin) or consideration of a high-dose chemotherapy regimen with stem cell rescue.

Immature Teratoma

The management of patients with IT is complex. ITs are categorized as grades 1, 2, or 3 depending on the amount of immature neuroepithelium in the tumor. Our current appreciation of recurrence risk in these patients is based on an early study by Norris. Only 1 of 14 patients with grade 1 IT recurred, while 13 of 26 patients with grade 2 and 3 tumors recurred. This study set the current standard of care for women with stage I teratoma, which is surveillance for grade 1 IT and adjuvant chemotherapy with three courses of BEP for patients with grade 2 and 3 tumors. A significant limitation of the Norris report is the probable underestimation of tumor stage. In the modern era of complete surgical staging of ovarian neoplasms, it might be appropriate to reconsider the role of routine adjuvant therapy in these patients. However, in the absence of prospectively obtained data that reevaluate this paradigm, caution should be applied.

Dysgerminoma

Dysgerminoma is the female equivalent of seminoma. This disease differs from its nondysgerminomatous counterparts in several respects. First, it is more likely to be localized to the ovary at the time of diagnosis (stage I). Bilateral involvement is more common, as is spread to retroperitoneal lymph nodes. While it is less relevant now than before the era of modern chemotherapy, dysgerminoma is very sensitive to radiation.

As many as 75% to 80% of dysgerminoma patients used to be considered stage I at diagnosis. With more precise surgical staging, the true figure is probably somewhat lower. Currently, patients with well-staged IA dysgerminoma can be observed after unilateral salpingo-oophorectomy, regardless of the size of the primary tumor. Careful follow-up is required, because as many as 15% to 25% of patients will experience a recurrence. With the tumor's chemosensitivity, virtually all dysgerminoma patients can be salvaged successfully at the time of recurrence, if detected early.

Dysgerminoma is very responsive to cisplatin-based chemotherapy, even more so than other germ cell tumors. Therefore, less toxic chemotherapy has been considered. An alternative regimen tested by the GOG consists of a 3-day regimen with carboplatin and etoposide. On this protocol, all 39 patients with pure dysgerminoma remained free of disease at a median follow-up of 7.8 years. Although highly active, this regimen is not recommended for routine use, because significantly less experience has accumulated with its use, and there is concern that it is not as effective in tumors containing nondysgerminomatous elements.

The implications of elevated hCG or AFP levels in patients with dysgerminoma should be emphasized. These tumor markers are usually increased in patients with nondysgerminomatous tumors. Therefore, AFP elevation denotes the presence of elements other than dysgerminoma, and treatment should be tailored accordingly. An elevated hCG level can be seen occasionally in pure dysgerminoma. This finding should not alter therapy, but prompt reexamination of the tumor specimen to determine whether syncytiotrophoblastic cells are present or if the tumor contains nondysgerminomatous elements.

CHEMOTHERAPY FOR SEX CORD–STROMAL TUMORS

KEY POINTS

- Most sex cord–stromal tumors present with endocrinologic abnormalities, allowing diagnosis at an early stage.
- Surgical resection alone is sufficient for sex cord–stromal tumors lacking malignant potential.
- Postoperative adjunctive therapy should be considered for patients with advanced disease and Sertoli–Leydig cell tumor with poor differentiation.
- Standard postoperative treatment consists of platinum-based chemotherapy, with three to four cycles of bleomycin, etoposide, and cisplatin being the most popular combination.
- The sex cord–stromal tumors infrequently develop recurrences, many of which will be delayed.

The vast majority of women with sex cord–stromal tumors present with unilateral, localized neoplasms that retain hormone-secreting functions. They are characteristically of low malignant potential, carrying with them an excellent prognosis after surgery alone. For those with IC disease, consideration can be given to adjuvant therapy on an individual basis. Most women presenting with stages II to IV disease would be advised to have postoperative therapy depending on their individual characteristics.

The Gynecologic Oncology Group has reported the largest series of women with ovarian sex cord–stromal tumors treated with chemotherapy in GOG 115. They used four cycles of BEP. This chemotherapy combination is considered to be active, but recognizing the prolonged natural history of these tumors' longer follow-up is important. Brown et al. have reported taxane activity in sex cord–stromal tumors, including a retrospective comparison of the efficacy and side effects of the taxanes with or without platinum, to the combination of BEP. The outcomes in the two groups were similar, but the side effects associated with the BEP regimen appeared to be greater. A GOG randomized phase II study of paclitaxel and carboplatin versus BEP in patients with sex cord–stromal tumors is ongoing (GOG 264). Additionally, antiangiogenesis drugs have also been reported to have activity in the treatment of recurrent sex cord–stromal tumors of the ovary. Specifically, in GOG 251, Brown et al. reported bevacizumab as an active agent with acceptable toxicity.

Granulosa Cell Tumors

Given the characteristic indolent growth pattern of patients with granulosa cell tumors, with long disease-free intervals, surgical resection of disease recurrence is often the initial step in the management of appropriate patients. Considerable rationale exists for the utilization of hormone-based approaches to advanced or recurrent granulosa cell tumors. A proportion of these tumors express steroid hormone receptors. Responses to medroxyprogesterone acetate and GnRH antagonists have been reported. Aromatase inhibitors have also been used in granulosa cell tumors.

Sertoli–Leydig Cell Tumors

Therapy for those few individuals presenting with high-stage Sertoli–Leydig cell tumors, as well as or individuals with recurrent disease, must be individualized. The effectiveness of radiation therapy is unknown. Reports exist of responses to vincristine, actinomycin D, and cyclophosphamide or cisplatin, doxorubicin, and cyclophosphamide. Given the functional hormonal nature of many of these neoplasms, consideration can be given to some form of hormonal manipulation, such as luteinizing hormone–releasing agonists or antagonists.

Immediate Toxicity of BEP Chemotherapy

KEY POINTS
Acute toxicities of BEP chemotherapy include the following:
- Neutropenic fever
- Nausea/vomiting
- Pulmonary fibrosis (bleomycin)
- Renal toxicity (cisplatin)
- Ototoxicity (cisplatin)
- Peripheral neuropathy (cisplatin)

Acute adverse effects of chemotherapy can be substantial, and these patients should be treated by physicians experienced in their management. About 25% of patients develop febrile neutropenic episodes during chemotherapy and require hospitalization and broad-spectrum antibiotics. Cisplatin is associated with nephrotoxicity, which can be minimized by ensuring adequate hydration during and immediately after chemotherapy and by avoidance of aminoglycoside antibiotics. Bleomycin can cause pulmonary fibrosis. The most effective method for monitoring patients is careful physical examination of the chest. Findings of early bleomycin lung disease are a lag or diminished expansion of one hemithorax or fine basilar rales that do not clear with cough. These findings can be very subtle but if present mandate immediate discontinuation of bleomycin.

Patients with advanced nonepithelial tumors should receive three to four courses of treatment given in full dose and on schedule. As most patients are young and will not develop neutropenic fever or infection, hematopoietic growth factors are not routinely necessary. However, it is reasonable to use them to avoid dose reductions for patients with previous episodes of neutropenic fever or in unusually ill patients who are at a higher risk of myelosuppressive complications, or those who received prior radiotherapy. Modern antiemetic therapy has greatly lessened chemotherapy-induced emesis. Chemotherapy-related mortality should be less than 1%.

LATE EFFECTS OF TREATMENT

KEY POINTS

Late toxicities of BEP chemotherapy:
- Secondary leukemia and other malignancies (etoposide).
- Most young women maintain fertility after BEP.

Sequelae of Surgery

Although there is little available information on the long-term effects of surgery in patients with nonepithelial ovarian tumors, future infertility related to pelvic surgery with subsequent peritoneal and tubal adhesions is well described. Therefore, meticulous surgical technique and avoidance of unnecessary operative maneuvers (e.g., biopsy of a normal contralateral ovary) are required for preventing future complications.

GOG 9901 reported that among 132 survivors of ovarian germ cell tumors treated with surgery and platinum-based chemotherapy, 71 patients had fertility-sparing procedures. Of those potentially fertile survivors, 62 (87.3%) maintained menstrual periods and 24 reported 37 successful pregnancies. Although the survivors reported an increased incidence of gynecologic problems and diminished sexual pleasure, they also tended to have stronger, more positive relationships with their significant others.

As with any group of patients with the history of pelvic surgery, patients with malignant nonepithelial ovarian tumors may develop functional cysts in the residual ovary. A trial of oral contraceptives and serial ovarian surveillance with sonography is helpful in distinguishing functional cysts from tumor recurrence.

Sequelae of Chemotherapy

A recognized effect of chemotherapy used for the treatment of nonepithelial tumors is the risk of secondary malignancies. The epipodophyllotoxins, including etoposide, are associated with the development of acute myelogenous leukemia (AML). Morphologically, these leukemias are monocytic or myelomonocytic (M4 or M5). Characteristic chromosomal translocations (mostly involving the 11q23 region) are frequently, but not always, present. Leukemia after etoposide treatment occurs within 2 to 3 years, compared to alkylating agent–induced AML, which has a longer latency period. This treatment complication appears to be dose and schedule dependent. In the GOG protocol testing the efficacy of BEP in women with ovarian germ cell tumors, one case of AML was recorded among 91 patients treated.

There continues to be considerable focus on the long-term effects of chemotherapy on gonadal function. Studies of patients with a variety of cancers suggest that although ovarian dysfunction or failure is a risk of chemotherapy, the majority of survivors can anticipate normal menstrual and reproductive function. Factors such as older age at initiation of therapy, greater cumulative drug dose, and longer duration of therapy have adverse effects on future gonadal function.

The GOG has completed an analysis evaluating the quality of life and psychosocial characteristics of survivors of ovarian germ cell tumors compared to matched controls. In this analysis, the survivors appeared to be well adjusted, were able to develop strong relationships, and were free of significant depression. The impact on fertility was modest or none in patients undergoing fertility-sparing surgeries. Overall, these women appeared to be free of any major physical illnesses at a median follow-up of 10 years.

SUGGESTED READINGS

Brown J, Brady WE, Schink J, et al. Bevacizumab shows activity in treating recurrent sex cord stromal ovarian tumors: Results of a phase II trial of the Gynecologic Oncology Group. *Cancer.* 2014;120(3):344–351.

de Wit R, Stoter G, Kaye SB, et al. Importance of bleomycin in combination chemotherapy for good-prognosis testicular nonseminoma: A randomized study of the European Organization for Research and Treatment of Cancer Genitourinary Tract Cancer Cooperative Group. *J Clin Oncol.* 1997;15:1837–1843.

Einhorn LH, Brames MJ, Juliar B, et al. Phase II study of paclitaxel plus gemcitabine salvage chemotherapy for germ cell tumors after progression following high-dose chemotherapy with tandem transplant. *J Clin Oncol.* 2007;25:513–516.

Einhorn L, Williams SD, Chamness A, et al. High-dose chemotherapy and stem-cell rescue for metastatic germ-cell tumors. *N Engl J Med.* 2007;357:340–348.

Homesely HD, Bundy BN, Hurteau JA, et al. Bleomycin, etoposide, and cisplatin combination therapy of ovarian granulosa cell tumors and other stromal malignancies: A Gynecologic Oncology Group Study. *Gynecol Oncol.* 1999;72:131–137.

Gershenson DM, Miller AM, Champion VL, et al. Reproductive and sexual function after platinum-based chemotherapy in long-term ovarian germ cell tumor survivors: A Gynecologic Oncology Group Study. *J Clin Oncol.* 2007;25(19):2792–2797.

Gershenson DM, Morris M, Cangir A, et al. Treatment of malignant germ cell tumors of the ovary with bleomycin, etoposide, and cisplatin. *J Clin Oncol.* 1990;8:715–720.

Horwich A, Sleijfer DT, Fossa SD, et al. Randomized trial of bleomycin, etoposide, and cisplatin compared with bleomycin, etoposide, and carboplatin in good-prognosis metastatic nonseminomatous germ cell cancer: A Multiinstitutional Medical Research Council/European Organization for Research and Treatment of Cancer Trial. *J Clin Oncol*. 1997;15:1844–1852.

Marina NM, Cushing B, Giller R, et al. Complete surgical excision is effective treatment for children with immature teratomas with or without malignant elements: A Pediatric Oncology Group/Children's Cancer Group Intergroup Study. *J Clin Oncol*. 1999;17:2137–2143.

Murugaesu N, Schmid P, Dancey G, et al. Malignant ovarian germ cell tumors: Identification of novel prognostic markers and long-term outcome after multimodality treatment. *J Clin Oncol*. 2006;24:4862–4866.

Williams SD, Blessing JA, DiSaia PJ, et al. Second-look laparotomy in ovarian germ cell tumors: The Gynecologic Oncology Group experience. *Gynecol Oncol*. 1994;52:287–291.

Williams S, Blessing JA, Liao SY, et al. Adjuvant therapy of ovarian germ cell tumors with cisplatin, etoposide, and bleomycin: A trial of the Gynecologic Oncology Group. *J Clin Oncol*. 1994;12:701–706.

KEY POINTS
- The frequency of molar pregnancy in Asia is seven to ten times greater than in the United States or Europe.
- One in three pregnancies in women over the age of 50 is molar.
- Gestational trophoblastic neoplasms most commonly follow a molar pregnancy but may develop after any gestation.

Gestational trophoblastic disease (GTD) comprises a diverse range of both benign and malignant pathologic processes including the following:

- Complete hydatidiform mole (CHM) and partial hydatidiform mole (PHM)
- Invasive mole
- Choriocarcinoma
- Placental site trophoblastic tumor (PSTT)
- Epithelioid trophoblastic tumor

Whereas both complete and partial hydatidiform moles are benign processes that generally resolve after uterine evacuation, they have the potential to persist despite attempts at evacuation and become invasive. Collectively, invasive mole, choriocarcinoma, and PSTT are malignant processes and referred to as gestational trophoblastic neoplasia (GTN); these disease processes have varying propensities for both local invasion and metastasis.

GTN are among the rare human malignancies that are highly curable with chemotherapy in the presence of widespread metastases. It is important to note that although GTN most commonly follow a molar pregnancy, they may develop after any gestation including a normal delivery, ectopic pregnancy, or miscarriage.

The reported incidence of GTN varies dramatically in different regions of the world. The frequency of molar pregnancy in Asian countries is seven to ten times greater than the reported incidence in North America or Europe. Whereas hydatidiform mole occurs in Taiwan in 1 per 125 pregnancies, the incidence of molar gestation in the United States is about 1 per 1,500 live births.

Increased risk for complete mole has been linked to diets deficient in vitamin A and animal fat, as well as extremes of maternal age (teenage women and women over the age of 40). Women over 40 years of age have a 5- to 10-fold greater risk of complete hydatidiform mole. In fact, one out of three pregnancies in women over 50 years of age is molar, and the risk of developing GTN is significantly increased as well. Interestingly, neither age nor diet appears to play a role in the development of partial mole. However, the risk for both complete and partial molar pregnancies is also increased in women with a history of prior spontaneous abortion and infertility.

MOLAR PREGNANCY

KEY POINTS

- Hydatidiform moles may be categorized as either complete or partial based upon gross morphology, histopathology, and karyotype.
- Most complete moles have a 46,XX karyotype with entirely paternal chromosomes.
- Most partial moles have a triploid karyotype.
- Complete moles often present with bleeding and a markedly elevated human chorionic gonadotropin (hCG).
- Partial moles generally present as a missed abortion.

Complete moles have no identifiable embryonic or fetal tissues. The chorionic villi have generalized swelling and diffuse trophoblastic hyperplasia, and the implantation site trophoblast has diffuse, marked atypia. Complete moles usually have a 46,XX karyotype, with a 46,XY karyotype present in approximately 10% of cases. The molar chromosomes are derived entirely from paternal (androgenetic) origin. Most cases of 46,XX complete moles appear to arise from an anuclear ovum that has been fertilized by a haploid (23X) sperm, which then duplicates its own chromosomes. In contrast, complete moles that possess a 46,XY karyotype arise from the fertilization of an anuclear ovum by two sperm. Whereas chromosomes in the complete mole are entirely of paternal origin, the mitochondrial DNA is of maternal origin.

Familial recurrent hydatidiform mole (FRHM) is a rare syndrome characterized by recurrent complete moles of biparental, rather than the more usual androgenetic, origin. This rare syndrome has been linked to a missense mutation in the *NLRP7* locus on chromosome 19; studies have shown this mutation to be present in up to 60% of patients with FRHM (2–4). Subsequent pregnancies in women diagnosed with this condition are markedly more likely to be a complete mole. Molar pregnancies in women with FRHM are associated with consanguinity and have a risk of progressing to GTN similar to that of nonfamilial cases.

Studies have recently shown that immunohistochemistry for p57 (as well as many other nonroutine markers) is useful for confirming the diagnosis of a complete mole. Almost all complete moles have absent or near-absent villous stromal and cytotrophoblastic nuclear activity for p57, while all other types of gestations (including partial moles) show nuclear reactivity in more than 25% of villous stromal and cytotrophoblastic nuclei.

Partial moles are characterized by the following pathologic features: (i) varying-sized chorionic villi with focal swelling and focal trophoblastic hyperplasia; (ii) focal, mild atypia of implantation site trophoblast; (iii) marked villous scalloping and prominent stromal trophoblastic inclusions; and (iv) identifiable fetal or embryonic tissues (Fig. 12.1). Partial moles generally have a triploid karyotype, which results from the

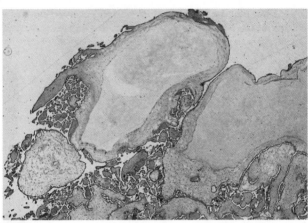

FIGURE 12.1 Photomicrograph of a PHM demonstrating varying-sized chorionic villi with focal swelling and focal trophoblastic hyperplasia.

fertilization of an apparently normal ovum by two sperm. If an identifiable fetus is present in partial mole, they generally have stigmata of triploidy including growth retardation and multiple congenital anomalies.

Complete Hydatidiform Mole

Vaginal bleeding is the most common presenting symptom in patients with a complete mole, with onset between weeks 6 and 16 of the pregnancy. The finding of a markedly elevated hCG value is suggestive of the diagnosis, with serum hCG levels of greater than 100,000 frequently detected. In the presence of significantly elevated hCG levels, symptoms such as excessive uterine enlargement for gestational age, hyperemesis gravidarum, thyrotoxicosis, and preeclampsia may be present, although they are less common now than in previous years due to earlier detection as a result of the advancements in ultrasonography, early prenatal care, and improved sensitivity of hCG testing. On pelvic ultrasound, half of patients are found to have ovarian theca lutein cysts, resulting from hyperstimulation of the ovaries by high circulating levels of hCG.

The diagnosis of complete mole is made via ultrasonography, which is a sensitive and reliable technique for diagnosis. Because of marked swelling of the chorionic villi, a complete mole produces a characteristic vesicular sonographic pattern known as a "snowstorm" appearance.

Complete moles have the potential for uterine invasion or distant spread. Following molar evacuation, uterine invasion and metastasis occur in 15% and 4% of the patients, respectively. Interestingly, the trend to earlier diagnosis of a complete mole does not appear to have affected the incidence of postmolar tumors.

Factors that predispose to postmolar tumors include signs of marked trophoblastic proliferation; these include hCG level of more than 100,000 mIU/mL, uterine size greater than that at gestational age, and theca lutein cysts more than 6 cm in diameter. An increased risk of postmolar GTN has also been observed in women over 40 years of age and in women with multiple molar pregnancies.

Partial Hydatidiform Mole

Patients with a partial mole generally present with the signs and symptoms of a missed or incomplete abortion. Hence, the diagnosis of partial mole is usually made after histologic review of curettage specimens. Sonographic findings significantly associated with the diagnosis of partial mole include focal cystic changes in the placenta and a ratio of the transverse to antero-posterior dimension of the gestational sac greater than 1.5. Patients with partial moles do not present with markedly elevated hCG values as often as patients with complete moles.

Complete and partial moles also differ in their levels of free β- and α-subunits of hCG. Whereas complete moles have higher levels of free β-hCG, partial moles have higher levels of free α-hCG. The mean ratios of percentage free β-hCG to free α-hCG in complete and partial moles are 20.9 and 2.4, respectively. The risk of developing GTN following PHM has been reported from 0% to 11%.

Surgical Evacuation

> ### KEY POINTS
> - Surgical evacuation is the treatment of choice for molar pregnancy.
> - The use of prophylactic chemotherapy at the time of surgery remains controversial.
> - After molar evacuation, women should be followed with hCG levels until the levels have been normal for at least 6 months.
> - Women should avoid pregnancy during the period of hormonal follow-up. Unless contraindicated, oral contraceptive pills should be prescribed.

After diagnosis of a molar pregnancy, the patient should be carefully evaluated to identify the potential presence of medical complications including preeclampsia, electrolyte imbalance, hyperthyroidism, and anemia because any of these may complicate a planned surgical evacuation.

Although hysterectomy is an option for women who no longer desire fertility and are at high a priori risk for development of GTN (age > 40, hCG > 100,000), suction curettage is recommended in most patients because it is a highly effective therapeutic option with minimal perioperative risks.

As the cervix is being dilated, the surgeon may encounter brisk uterine bleeding. Therefore, all patients should be typed and crossed for blood products in advance. Shortly after commencing suction evacuation, uterine bleeding is generally well controlled and in most cases the uterus will rapidly regress in size. When suction evacuation is thought to be complete, a sharp curettage should be gently performed to remove any residual chorionic tissue.

Patients who are Rh negative should receive Rh immune globulin at the time of evacuation because Rh D factor is expressed on trophoblast.

Role of Prophylactic Chemotherapy

The use of prophylactic chemotherapy at the time of molar evacuation remains controversial. In one trial, chemoprophylaxis significantly reduced the incidence of postmolar tumor from 15%–20% to 3%–8%. However, routine administration of chemotherapy exposes all patients to toxicity while benefiting only a relative few. In light of this, most institutions reserve the use of chemoprophylaxis to patients who are at particularly high risk for GTN or are unable or unwilling to comply with serial hCG assays. Massad et al. observed that among 40 indigent women with molar pregnancy, 33 (82%) did not fully comply with hCG follow-up and 5 (13%) were lost to follow-up before remission.

Hormonal Follow-Up

After molar evacuation, patients should be followed with weekly hCG values until they are normal for 3 weeks, and then with monthly values until they are normal for at least 6 months. After achieving nondetectable hCG levels, the risk of relapse appears to be very low.

All patients should be encouraged to use effective contraception during the entire interval of follow-up. Oral contraceptive pills are the contraception of choice because they also have the added benefit of hormonal suppression of the hypothalamic–pituitary–ovarian axis. This mitigates the risk of having an erroneously elevated hCG assay due to cross-reactivity with endogenous LH. Intrauterine devices should not be inserted until the patient achieves normal hCG levels because of the risk of uterine perforation, bleeding, and infection if residual tumor is present. Patients who have an absolute contraindication to oral contraceptives should be educated about the importance of barrier protection.

GESTATIONAL TROPHOBLASTIC NEOPLASMS

KEY POINTS

- The diagnosis of GTN should be considered in any woman in the reproductive age group with unexplained systemic or pulmonary symptoms.
- Metastases are very vascular and bleed easily. Biopsy should be avoided. If deemed necessary, it should be approached with caution.
- Staging differs from that of most common solid tumors and involves a "risk score."

Diagnosis

Postmolar GTN is diagnosed when hCG levels plateau or rise during follow-up after molar evacuation. A plateau is defined as a less than 10% decline in four measurements taken over three weeks; a rise is defined as greater than 20% increase in three measurements taken over two weeks. Therefore, the diagnosis of GTN is based on laboratory data and does not require histologic confirmation.

Pathologic Considerations

GTN may have the histologic pattern of molar tissue, choriocarcinoma, or PSTT. Choriocarcinoma does not contain chorionic villi but is composed of sheets of both anaplastic cytotrophoblast and syncytiotrophoblast. PSTT is uncommon and is composed almost entirely of mononuclear intermediate trophoblast and does not contain chorionic villi. Measurement of serum hCG is not reliable in PSTT because secretion occurs focally. Instead, PSTT secretes human placental lactogen and should be drawn in any patient in whom this diagnosis is suspected.

Natural History of GTN

Nonmetastatic Disease

Locally invasive GTN develop in 15% of patients following evacuation of a complete mole and infrequently after other gestations. An invasive trophoblastic tumor may perforate through the myometrium, producing intraperitoneal bleeding, or erode into uterine vessels, causing vaginal hemorrhage. A bulky necrotic tumor may also serve as a nidus for infection.

Metastatic Disease

Metastatic GTN occurs in 4% of patients after evacuation of a complete mole and infrequently after other pregnancies. The most common metastatic sites are the lung (80%), vagina (30%), brain (10%), and liver (10%). Because fragile vessels perfuse trophoblastic tumors, metastases are often hemorrhagic, making biopsy of any suspected metastases high risk. Patients may present with signs and symptoms of bleeding from metastases such as hemoptysis, intraperitoneal bleeding, or acute neurologic deficits. Cerebral and hepatic metastases are uncommon unless there is concurrent involvement of the lungs and/or vagina.

Patients with pulmonary metastases commonly have asymptomatic lesions on chest radiography, although they may present with dyspnea, chest pain, cough, or hemoptysis. Trophoblastic emboli may cause pulmonary arterial occlusion and lead to right heart strain and pulmonary hypertension.

Gynecologic symptoms may be minimal or absent, and the antecedent pregnancy may be remote in time. The patient may be thought to have a primary pulmonary disease because respiratory symptoms may be dramatic. Vaginal lesions may present with irregular bleeding or purulent discharge and are most commonly located in the fornices or suburethrally. As with other metastatic lesions, these are also notorious for brisk bleeding.

Staging System

The International Federation of Gynecology and Obstetrics (FIGO) reports data on GTN, using an anatomic staging system (Table 12.1). Patients with stage IV tumors generally have a choriocarcinoma, commonly following a nonmolar pregnancy and tend to be diagnosed after protracted delays in diagnosis brought about after the development of a large tumor burden.

The World Health Organization (WHO) has published a prognostic scoring system that reliably predicts the potential for chemotherapy

Table 12.1	FIGO Anatomic Staging for Gestational Trophoblastic Neoplasia
Stage I	Disease confined to the uterus
Stage II	GTN extends outside of the uterus but is limited to the genital structures (adnexa, vagina, and broad ligament)
Stage III	GTN extends to the lungs, with or without known genital tract involvement
Stage IV	All other metastatic sites

Source: Adapted from FIGO Committee on Gynecologic Oncology. Current FIGO staging for cancer of the vagina, fallopian tube, ovary, and gestational trophoblastic neoplasia. *Int J Gynaecol Obstet.* 2009;105:3–4, with permission.

resistance (Table 12.2). A prognostic score of 7 or greater is considered "high risk" and identifies the subset of patients in whom intensive combination chemotherapy is recommended. However, patients with a risk score of 5 to 6 appear to have more treatment failures, and there is discussion that these patients should be separated out into an "intermediate-risk" category. To date, no changes have yet been made to the current staging system.

Table 12.2	Modified WHO Prognostic Scoring System as Adapted by FIGO (2000)			
Scores	0	1	2	4
Age	≤39	>39	—	—
Antecedent pregnancy	Mole	Abortion	Term	—
Interval months from index pregnancy	<4	4–6	7–12	>12
Pretreatment serum hCG (IU/L)	$<10^3$	10^3–10^4	10^4–10^5	$>10^5$
Largest tumor size, cm (including the uterus)	<3	3–4	≥5	—
Site of metastases		Spleen, kidney	GI	Liver, brain
Number of metastases	—	1–4	5–8	>8
Previous failed chemotherapy	—	—	Single drug	Two or more drugs

Note: Format for reporting to FIGO Annual Report: In order to stage and allot a risk factor score, a patient's diagnosis is allocated to a stage as represented by a Roman numerals I, II, III, and IV. This is then separated by a colon from the sum of all the actual risk factor scores expressed in Arabic numerals, for example, stage II:4, stage IV:9. This stage and score will be allotted for each patient. FIGO, International Federation of Gynecology and Obstetrics; WHO, World Health Organization.
Source: From FIGO Oncology Committee. FIGO staging for gestational trophoblastic neoplasia 2000. *Int J Gynaecol Obstet.* 2002;77:285–287, with permission.

In general, patients with stage I disease have a low-risk score, and patients with stage IV disease have a high-risk score. Therefore, the distinction between low risk and high risk primarily applies to stages II and III.

Diagnostic Evaluation

All patients should undergo a complete history and physical examination, baseline hCG level, hepatic, thyroid, and renal function tests, CBC and type and screen, and imaging studies for organ sites at risk for metastasis. The burden of pelvic disease should be assessed by a CT scan of the abdomen and pelvis. For the chest, imaging should start with a PA and lateral chest x-ray. If the chest x-ray has any suspicious findings, a CT scan of the chest should be obtained as well as a brain MRI, as patients with lung metastases have a 20% chance of brain metastases. Asymptomatic patients with a normal pelvic examination and negative chest CT are very unlikely to have liver or brain metastases identified by further radiographic studies.

Management

> ### KEY POINTS
> - Most patients will be cured with chemotherapy, regardless of stage.
> - Low-risk patients (prognostic score ≤6) should be treated with single-agent chemotherapy.
> - High-risk patients (prognostic score ≥7) should receive combination chemotherapy.
> - The use of etoposide appears to improve outcomes in high-risk patients but carries a risk of secondary malignancies, including leukemia.

Stage I, Low-Risk Disease

Table 12.3 reviews the New England Trophoblastic Disease Center (NETDC) protocol for the management of stage I, low-risk disease. The selection of treatment is based mainly on the patient's desire to preserve fertility. If the patient no longer wishes to retain fertility, hysterectomy with adjuvant single-agent chemotherapy is also an option as primary treatment. Chemotherapy may be safely administered postoperatively without increasing the surgical complication rate.

Single-agent chemotherapy is the preferred treatment in patients with stage I disease. Whereas methotrexate (MTX) and actinomycin D (ACT D) are the two most commonly used single agents in the treatment of GTN in the United States and in most parts of the world, 5-fluorouracil has been the preferred single-agent chemotherapy in China. Multiple series have shown impressive efficacy of a single-agent regimen, with survival rates ranging from 77% to 100%. Chemotherapy is continued until hCG levels become normal, and then one additional dose is administered.

Although multiple treatment protocols have been described, the 5-day MTX or ACT D protocols or the 8-day MTX–folinic acid protocol are more effective than weekly MTX or biweekly single-dose ACT D protocols. Side effects include stomatitis, mucositis, pleuritis, conjunctivitis, and rash. However, ACT D is associated with alopecia, whereas MTX is not.

Table 12.3	Treatment Protocols for Stage I GTN

INITIAL
Methotrexate
Actinomycin D
Hysterectomy (with adjunctive single-agent chemotherapy)

SUBSEQUENT LINE[a]
Low risk: alternative single-agent therapy
High risk: MAC or EMA-CO
EMACO, if MAC fails
Hysterectomy (with adjunctive multiagent chemotherapy)
Local uterine resection (for localized lesion, to preserve fertility)

FOLLOW-UP
At least 6 consecutive months of normal hCG levels
Contraception strongly advised

---

[a]Patients should be restaged if they experience progression on their prior line of treatment.
MTX, methotrexate; ACT D, actinomycin D; MAC, methotrexate, actinomycin D, Cytoxan;
EMACO, etoposide, methotrexate, actinomycin D, Cytoxan, Oncovin.

Nonmetastatic PSTT should generally be treated with primary hysterectomy because this tumor responds less well to chemotherapy. A long interval from the antecedent pregnancy to clinical presentation has been reported to be the most important prognostic factor for women with nonmetastatic PSTT. In one series, all 27 patients survived when the interval from the antecedent pregnancy was less than 4 years; all 7 patients died when the time interval exceeded 4 years.

Stages II and III

Low-risk patients (prognostic score <7) can be optimally treated with primary single-agent chemotherapy (Table 12.4). Summarizing the experience from four centers, single-agent chemotherapy induced complete remission in 128 (87%) of 147 patients with low-risk metastatic GTN, and all but two patients who were resistant to single-agent chemotherapy later achieved remission with combination chemotherapy. It is imperative that high-risk patients (prognostic score of 7 or above) receive combination chemotherapy as the primary modality. In high-risk patients who inappropriately received single-agent therapy as their initial treatment, subsequent success rate of multidrug therapy drops to 20% to 50%.

Approximately 50% of patients with high-risk metastatic disease will eventually require some form of surgical intervention. Thoracotomy has a limited role in the management of stage III GTN and should be performed only in the setting of serious diagnostic doubt or a nidus of persistent viable tumor despite administration of chemotherapy. Providers should remember that fibrotic nodules may persist indefinitely on the chest radiograph after complete hCG remission is achieved. If a metastasis is persistent on radiography, but is of questionable viability, either a scan with a radioisotope-labeled antibody to hCG or a PET scan may be useful.

Table 12.4	Treatment Protocol for Stage II or III GTN

LOW RISK

Initial therapy	Single-agent therapy (MTX or ACTD)
Subsequent therapy[a]	Alternative single agent (low-risk disease only)
	MAC or EMACO (if high risk)
	Surgery, as indicated

HIGH RISK

Initial therapy	EMACO
Subsequent therapy	EMAEP[b]; VBP

FOLLOW-UP

Twelve consecutive months of nondetectable hCG levels
Contraception for 12 months

---

[a]Patients should be restaged if they experience progression on their prior line of treatment.
[b]EMA-EP may be the first choice for patients with placental site or epithelioid trophoblastic tumor.
ACT D, actinomycin D; EMACO, etoposide, methotrexate, actinomycin D, cyclophospha-mide (Cytoxan), vincristine (Oncovin); EMAEP, etoposide, methotrexate, actinomycin D, carboplatin; GTN, gestational trophoblastic neoplasia; hCG, human chorionic gonadotropin; MAC, methotrexate, actinomycin D, cyclophosphamide (Cytoxan); MTX, methotrexate; VBP, vinblastine (Velban), bleomycin, carboplatin.

Hysterectomy may be required in patients with metastatic GTN to control uterine hemorrhage, sepsis, or to debulk a large uterine tumor burden, which could contribute to chemoresistance. Angiographic embolization can also be effective in the management of profuse uterine bleeding in lieu of hysterectomy, especially in those patients who are hemodynamically stable and wish to retain their fertility potential.

Stage IV

Table 12.5 outlines the NETDC protocol for the management of stage IV disease. All patients with stage IV disease should be treated with intensive combination chemotherapy and the selective use of radiation therapy and surgery. In patients presenting with brain metastases, radiation or surgical excision with adjuvant radiation is indicated and should be performed prior to chemotherapy to lower the risk of hemorrhage. Alternatively, intrathecal MTX may be used in patients with brain metastases.

An 83% remission rate in patients with metastatic disease and a high-risk score has been achieved using EMACO, a combination regimen that includes etoposide, MTX, ACT D, cyclophosphamide, and vincristine (Oncovin). EMACO is currently the preferred treatment for patients with high-risk metastatic GTN; however, EMA–etoposide cisplatin (EP) may be the first-line choice for women presenting with PSTT or epithelioid tropho-blastic tumor.

In general, combination chemotherapy is administered as frequently as toxicity permits until the patient attains three consecutive normal hCG values. After the patient achieves normal hCG levels, two to three additional courses of chemotherapy are administered to reduce the risk of relapse.

Table 12.5	Treatment Protocol for Stage IV GTN (NETDC, July 1965 to June 2006)

INITIAL
EMACO
With brain metastases—radiation; craniotomy for peripheral lesions OR intrathecal methotrexate
With liver metastases—embolization; resection to manage complications

RESISTANT
Second-line chemotherapy—EMAEP; VBP; experimental protocols
Surgery, as indicated
Hepatic artery infusion or embolization, as indicated

FOLLOW-UP
Weekly hCG levels until undetectable for 3 weeks, and then monthly for 24 months
Contraception for 24 months

EMACO, etoposide, methotrexate, actinomycin D, cyclophosphamide, vincristine; EMAEP, etoposide, methotrexate, actinomycin D, carboplatin; VBP, vinblastine (Velban), bleomycin, carboplatin.

Unfortunately, the use of etoposide has been reported to increase the risk of secondary tumors including myeloid leukemia, melanoma, colon cancer, and breast cancer. The relative risk for leukemia, melanoma, colon cancer, and breast cancer was increased by 16.6, 3.4, 4.6, and 5.8, respectively, in patients who received more than 2 g/m^2. Etoposide should therefore be used only with high-risk metastatic disease. When patients with nonmetastatic and low-risk metastatic GTN experience resistance to MTX and ACT D, it is reasonable to consider administering triple therapy before the treatment with regimens containing etoposide.

Follow-Up

All patients with GTN who enter remission should be followed with weekly hCG tests until normal for 3 consecutive weeks and then monthly for 12 months. Patients should be encouraged to use contraception during the entire interval of follow-up. Patients with stage IV disease are followed with weekly hCG values until normal for 3 weeks and then monthly for 24 months. These patients require prolonged follow-up because they have an increased risk of late recurrence.

False-Positive hCG Tests

hCG molecules in GTN are more degraded or heterogeneous in serum than they are in normal pregnancy. Trophoblastic disease samples contain high proportions of free β-hCG, nicked hCG, hyperglycosylated hCG, and β-core fragment. When monitoring patients with GTN, it is therefore desirable to use an assay that detects not only intact hCG but also all of its metabolites and fragments.

Many hCG assays have a degree of cross-reactivity with luteinizing hormone. Following multiple courses of combination chemotherapy, ovarian steroidal function may be damaged, particularly in patients in their late 30s and 40s, which may cause luteinizing hormone levels to rise, and owing to cross-reactivity, the patient may be falsely thought to have persistent low levels of hCG. Patients who receive combination chemotherapy should therefore be placed on oral contraceptives to suppress luteinizing hormone levels and prevent problems with cross-reactivity, even in the presence of ovarian failure.

Some patients may also have a false-positive elevation in serum hCG measurement owing to the presence of circulating heterophilic antibody, called "phantom hCG." More of a historical problem, modern assays rarely demonstrate cross-reactivity with heterophilic antibody. The possibility of false-positive hCG measurement should be assessed by sending both serum and urine samples to a reference hCG laboratory. Patients with phantom hCG generally have no measurable hCG in a parallel urine sample.

Quiescent GTD

Some women with a history of GTD or GTN may have a consistent, low level of hCG with levels typically less than 200 mIU/mL. This may persist for months despite there being no evidence of active disease. It is believed that this "quiescent GTD" is due to individual, slow growing syncytiotrophoblastic cells with limited invasive potential. For women who present with this clinical scenario, chemotherapy is not indicated. Close follow-up of these patients with administration of combined oral contraceptive pills and routine hCG assays is usually the management of choice. Consistent follow-up is crucial as almost one quarter of these women will go on to develop GTN, diagnosed by a concomitant increase in hCG and hyperglycosylated hCG. Only once GTN is diagnosed should patients undergo active treatment.

Recurrent GTN

In patients who do not achieve remission to initial single-agent therapy, restaging is important, including recalculation of their prognostic score. For those who remain at low-risk, alternative single-agent treatment should be used. Combination chemotherapy should be reserved for those with a high-risk prognostic score after restaging.

Mutch and colleagues reported recurrences after initial remission in 2% of patients with nonmetastatic GTN, 4% of patients with good prognosis metastatic GTN, and 13% of patients with poor prognosis disease. Relapses developed within 3 and 18 months in 50% and 85% of patients, respectively. Most patients with stages I, II, and III GTN who develop recurrence are subsequently cured.

For patients who recur after combination chemotherapy (usually EMA-CO), remission may be possible with EMA-EP. Bower et al. reported that EMAEP induced remission alone or in conjunction with surgery in 16 (76%) of 21 patients who were resistant to EMACO. Beyond EMA-EP, administration of other regimens, such as cisplatin, vinblastine, and bleomycin, or surgical intervention to remove the sites of drug-resistant tumor may be indicated.

Subsequent Pregnancies

Pregnancies after Hydatidiform Mole

In general, patients with a prior history of a complete or partial mole can anticipate normal reproduction in the future. However, they are at increased risk of developing molar disease in later conceptions. After having one molar pregnancy, the risk of subsequent molar pregnancy increases to 1%, or 10- to 20-fold higher risk than the general population. An ultrasound should be performed in the first trimester of any subsequent pregnancy to confirm normal gestational development. An hCG measurement should also be obtained 6 weeks after the completion of any future pregnancy to exclude occult trophoblastic disease.

Pregnancies after GTN

Patients with successfully treated GTN can also generally expect normal reproduction in the future. The frequency of congenital malformations or obstetric complications does not appear to be increased. Patients occasionally become pregnant before the recommended 12-month follow-up period has elapsed. When a patient's hCG level reelevates after completing chemotherapy, the use of ultrasound can help the clinician to distinguish between an intercurrent pregnancy and disease recurrence.

SUGGESTED READINGS

Berkowitz RS, Cramer DW, Bernstein MR, et al. Risk factors for complete molar pregnancy from a case control study. *Am J Obstet Gynecol.* 1985;152(8):1016–1020.

Kou YC, Shao L, Peng HH, et al. A recurrent intragenic genomic duplication, other novel mutations in NLRP7 and imprinting defects in recurrent biparental hydatidiform moles. *Mol Hum Reprod.* 2008;14(1):33–40.

Kashimura Y, Kashimura M, Sugimori H, et al. Prophylactic chemotherapy for hydatidiform mole: Five to 15 years of follow up. *Cancer.* 1986;58(3):624–629.

Messaed C, Chebaro W, Di Roberto RB, et al. NLRP7 in the spectrum of reproductive wastage: Rare non synonymous variants confer genetic susceptibility to recurrent reproductive wastage. *J Med Genet.* 2011;48(8):540–548.

Wang CM, Dixon PH, Decordova S, et al. Identification of 13 novel NLRP7 mutations in 20 families with recurrent hydatidiform mole; missense mutations cluster in the leucine-rich region. *J Med Genet.* 2009;46(8):569–575.

Index

Page numbers in *italics* denote figures; those followed by a "t" denote tables.